Diagnosis and Treatment of Autism

Diagnosis and Treatment of Autism

Edited by

Christopher Gillberg

University of Göteborg
Göteborg, Sweden

Plenum Press • New York and London

Library of Congress Cataloging-in-Publication Data

State-of-the-Art-Conference on Autism: Diagnosis and Treatment (1989 :
Göteborg, Sweden)
    Diagnosis and treatment of autism / edited by Christopher Gillberg.
        p.   cm.
    "Proceedings of the State-of-the-Art-Conference on Autism:
Diagnosis and Treatment, held May 8-10, 1989, in Göteborg,
Sweden"--T.p. verso.
    Includes bibliographical references.
    ISBN 0-306-43481-4
    1. Autism--Congresses.   I. Gillberg, Christopher, 1950-   .
II. Title.
    [DNLM: 1. Autism, Infantile--diagnosis--congresses. 2. Autism,
Infantile--therapy--congresses.   WM 203.5 S797d 1989]
RJ506.A9S74 1989
618.92'8982--dc20
DNLM/DLC
for Library of Congress   89-71050
                                                               CIP

Proceedings of The State-of-the-Art-Conference on Autism:
Diagnosis and Treatment, held May 8-10, 1989, in
Göteborg, Sweden

© 1989 Plenum Press, New York
A Division of Plenum Publishing Corporation
233 Spring Street, New York, N.Y. 10013

Printed in the United States of America

Foreword

In 1987, The Swedish Medical Research Council's Group for Evaluation of Medical Technology approached me on the subject of organizing a conference on Autism - Diagnosis and Treatment. The original idea for this conference had come from a Stockholm politician, Leni Björklund, who had felt that, at least in Sweden, autism appeared to be an area in which conflicting views on etiology and treatment had led to children and parents not always receiving adequate help. Professors Agne Larsson, MD, Tore Scherstén, MD and Björn Smedby, MD in particular showed a keen interest and it was decided to hold a State-of-the-Art-Conference on autism in Gothenburg.

The State-of-the-Art-Conference on Autism - Diagnosis and Treatment was held in Gothenburg May 8 - 10, 1989. A panel of international experts was selected because of outstanding research or clinical activity in the field and in order to represent a wide variety of professional and theoretical approaches ranging from epidemiology, neurobiology and cognitive psychology to psychiatry, neurology, education, behavioural treatment and psychoanalysis. A group of professional observers involved in the field of autism was chosen so as to cover Sweden in a representative fashion. This group consisted of administrators, child psychiatrists, psychologists, social workers, pediatricians, nurses and teachers.

The aim of the conference was for the expert panel to provide a review of the state-of-the-art in their particular field of autism and for the organizer to compile a document of basics in the field of Autism - Diagnosis and Treatment on which all the members of the expert panel could agree. The task for the invited observers was to receive the information from the expert panel and then, hopefully convey this information locally in their professional capacities.

The conference resulted in a State-of-the-Art document on Autism - Diagnosis and Treatment which is published at the end of this book.

This book covers all the presentations from the conference. I thank all the authors for their dedicated efforts to meet the manuscript deadlines and for the high quality of their contributions. I am very grateful to Inger Sahlström and particularly to Carina Löf for typing and word-processing work. I am deeply indebted to Gun Jakobsson for her unselfish secretarial assistance in all matters concerned with producing this book. The people at Plenum have been very helpful at all stages. The conference would not have taken place without the initiative and financial support of the Swedish Medical Research Council, and their help has been gratefully appreciated.

It is hoped that this book will be seen to represent a small but important step forward in the history of autism and that it will receive a wide readership.

Christopher Gillberg

Contents

Introduction

CHRISTOPHER GILLBERG

This book surveys recent important research and clinical developments in the field of autism from infancy to adulthood.

It opens with an expert and broadminded chapter on diagnosis by Lorna Wing and ends with a common-sensical and visionary overview on issues relating to autism in adulthood by the same author. Needless to say, both these chapters are well-rooted in empirical research, but they seem to me to be remarkably useful for the clinician who needs guidelines in everyday practice. Lorna Wing's chapters are far from the narrow, exclusive view of autism as a single disease entity with one etiology, which tended to prevail in the 1950s and 60s. Rather, autism is conceptualized as a behavioural syndrome - diagnosed on the basis of a particular set of social and communication problems and unusual activity patterns - with a wide variety of possible underlying etiologies and the course of a developmental disorder. Psychiatric problems may or may not complicate the clinical picture and might be particularly prevalent among high-functioning persons with autism, who are now often referred to as people with Asperger syndrome. Lorna Wing raises the possibility that high-functioning autism may sometimes be the "precursor" of various adult psychiatric problems such as depression and paranoid symptoms. Indeed, according to limited research, there is reason to believe that a primary history of Asperger syndrome may not be altogether uncommon in an adult psychiatric clientele.

Wing's first chapter is followed by a fascinating account of the "theory of mind theory" by Uta Frith. Frith and her group have led the field in the development and reformulations of an adequate cognitive psychological theory which can account for central autistic symptoms. Their experiments have definitely broken new ground and there is now some hope that, in the future, testing hypotheses which link specific psychological typifying features with variation in function of certain central nervous system circuitries, will be possible.

Lynn Waterhouse and Deborah Fein in their chapter establish that the social and cognitive deficits seen in autism are not clearly distinguishable from each other and should be seen as aspects of the same disorder. Waterhouse and Fein also lucidly identify roadblocks to current research on the social deficits in autism. Indeed, the failure by some researchers to acknowledge the spectrum of social impairments associated with autism has narrowed our vision so much that progress as regards the understanding of the autism spectrum disorders has been slowed down. Maybe it is time to move forward from the position gained by Leo Kanner already in 1943 and accept the plural form of the "autistic disturbances of affective contact". In our stubborn efforts to capture a narrow syndrome of "classic" infantile autism à la Kanner, we may be doing the man behind the syndrome a disservice. If we cling to the idea of classic autism to the exclusion of spectrum viewpoints, Kanner's original writings will in the end be seen as having impeded rather than accelerated development in the field.

In the chapter by Gillberg on early symptoms, two recent studies concerning the first few years in the lives of children with autism are summarized and practical guidelines for clinical diagnostic purposes are suggested. It is obvious that we know very little about the first symptoms of autism and that there is great need for research in this area.

The following section deals more with etiologic and neurobiological pathogenetic mechanisms. First there is a general overview by Suzanne Steffenburg and Christopher Gillberg which provides a state-of-the-art picture of the established facts and some theories with regard to autism etiology. This is then followed by a more detailed account of some of the recent developments in the neurobiology of autism by Luke Tsai. Randi Hagerman's chapter is a succinct account of genetic and chromosomal factors in autism. In particular, it focuses on the fragile X syndrome and its numerous links with the field of autism spectrum disorders. Some interesting findings from new immunologic investigations are reported by Audrius Plioplys. The section ends with an overview of what should be included in the first evaluation of a child with clear or suspected autism by Christopher Gillberg. The recommendations in this respect draw on the empirical data presented in the preceeding chapters. Emphasis is placed on the importance of a thorough neuropsychiatric evaluation in each case as a basis for all future treatment strategies.

The next section provides overviews of various treatment measures and evaluations as to their current status in overall intervention programmes in the field of autism. Margaret Lansing provides us with an up-to-date account of the basis for educational programmes currently used in the North Carolina TEACCH- set-up. Pat Howlin brilliantly summarizes her own and Rutter's data from the London treatment studies with a specific emphasis on providing help for the parents. Magda Campbell then comprehensively covers the whole field of psychopharmacology in autism in a most useful chapter. Mary Coleman presents important examples of "non-psychopharmacological" treatment strategies rationally based on biological/etiological information in each particular case of autism. Her results in some cases appear to be striking indeed, but one should keep in mind that she is reporting on single cases and that larger scale studies are needed before any conclusions can be drawn. Nevertheless, it seems that interventions of the kind she reports may prove very fruitful in the long run. This section ends with a summary of the current status in respect of psychoanalytical thinking in the field of autism by Sheila Spensley.

Much of the remainder of the book is left over to the presentation of different treatment programmes from various parts of the world (England, USA, France, Denmark and Sweden). Pat Howlin gives some excellent examples of how behavioural modes of treatment can make a positive difference both for the child and parents. Again she draws on the empirical data from her own and Rutter's London treatment study. Eric Schopler reviews the educational treatment programme from his own TEACCH-institution at Chapel Hill. The TEACCH-programme now is probably the most widely "copied" model in the world for dealing with diagnostic, treatment and follow-up issues relating to autism spectrum disorders. Gilbert Lelord reports on methods used in Tours, France, where the rationale for treating children with autism is a thorough neurophysiological work-up in each individual case. Ivar Lovaas then reports results from his own treatment study. He describes the intensive behaviour modification programme which he originally reported on in 1987, when he claimed that almost half of a group of 19 young autistic children had been cured. This study is so far the only one of its kind and it is clear that no firm conclusions can yet be drawn as to the clinical applicability and appropriateness of these methods. More research in this area is needed. After Lovaas follows a very instructive chapter on the "Copenhagen model" as applied at the Sofieskolen by Demetrious Haracopos. Two Swedish programmes - one from a rural and one from an urban area - are outlined by Michael Bohman on the one hand and Lena Andersson and Christopher Gillberg on the other. The section closes with a very interesting account of a behavioural treatment service in Chatham, Massachussetts by Stephen Luce.

The next section deals with problems of adolescence and adult life. It opens with a general overview of adolescent problems in autism and is followed by useful reviews of the (admittedly limited) know-how with respect to pharmacological and psychotherapeutical treatment approaches by Magda Campbell and Henrik Pelling respectively. Borgny Rusten, parent and teacher, summarizes her views on educational issues in adolescence. Lorna Wing´s chapter on adulthood then follows (see above).

In an addendum, Annica Dahlström puts forward her case for focusing more research attention to the locus coeruleus in the future study of autism.

The book ends with the state-of-the-art-document on Autism - Diagnosis and Treatment. This document existed in a highly preliminary version already before the conference and had been circulated among all the authors of the book for review. During the three-day conference new drafts were circulated, altered and re-circulated. Just before the closing of the conference a "hearing" was held and the final version - printed here - agreed upon by all the authors. The document is important in that it brings together facts and thinking from various clinical and theoretical "schools" and focuses on those diagnostic and treatment aspects of autism which were considered uncontroversial at the conference.

The Diagnosis of Autism

LORNA WING

The problems of diagnosing autism will be discussed in the light of historical attempts to define specific syndromes and the difficulty of differentiating autism from other similar conditions. The story of the development of the concepts of the triad of social impairments and the autistic continuum will be outlined. An approach to diagnosis based on these concepts and its relevance to clinical practice and research will be described. In this chapter, diagnosis will refer to recognition of patterns of behaviour and psychological impairments, and will not be concerned with any underlying aetiology.

THE NAMING OF SYNDROMES

References to "insanity" in children can be found in the psychiatric literature of the nineteenth century (Connolly, 1862; Haslam, 1809; Maudsley, 1867). In the first half of the present century a number of writers each described and named different clusters of features that they considered were specific syndromes within the general category of childhood "psychosis".

These authors included De Sanctis, (1906, 1908), Earl (1934), Heller (see Hulse, 1954), Kanner, (1943) and Mahler, (1953). Asperger (1944) also wrote about children with related abnormalities, though he conceptualised the problem as an innate disorder of personality.

Kanner's Syndrome

Of all this group, it was Kanner whose syndrome of "early infantile autism" became the most widely known and accepted, followed a long way behind by Asperger, whose original paper is now beginning to arouse interest in many countries (Gillberg, 1985; Van Krevelen, 1971; Wing 1981a). Kanner's influence in the field is probably due to the clarity and vividness of his descriptions, with many illustrations of the behaviour of children known to him personally. From the multiplicity of abnormalities to be found among those with his syndrome, Kanner (1943; 1949) selected the following as characteristic and diagnostic: profound lack of affective contact with other people; an anxiously obsessive desire for the preservation of sameness in the child's repetitive activity pattern; a fascination for objects, which are handled with skill in fine motor movements; mutism, or the kind of language that does not seem to be intended to serve inter-personal communication; good cognitive potential manifested by feats of memory or skill in performance tasks, especially the Seguin form board. Later, Kanner and Eisenberg (1956) emphasized the first two of these points as of primary importance, and pointed out that, for a diagnosis of autism, the repetitive activities must be elaborate and not just simple motor stereotypies.

Kanner excluded children with known organic brain dysfunction. He also stated that the abnormalities invariably were present from birth or began within the first 30 months of life.

Asperger's Syndrome

Asperger's descriptions of children in his group were rather less precise than those of Kanner, but the major features his children had in common were an odd, naive, egocentric style of social interaction; long winded, pedantic, repetitive speech; a limited range of circumscribed interests pursued to the exclusion of other activities; poor coordination of movements; and a conspicuous lack of common sense.

PROBLEMS OF DIAGNOSIS

Diagnosis of Kanner's and Asperger's groups, as of any of the other so-called syndromes within the domain of childhood "psychoses", depends upon recognition of a pattern of behaviour, as there are no psychological or physical tests for positive identification. Young classically autistic children of the kind Kanner described are easy to recognise for anyone with some experience in the field. Diagnosis would present no problems at all if all the children were seen between 2.5 and 5 years of age, had only the one condition as described by Kanner and were all affected at the same level of severity. The trouble is that the majority of autistic children with the autistic behaviour pattern have multiple impairments, the manifestations change with increasing age, they can vary in different environments, they are influenced by each child's own personality and all the features occur at any level on a continuum of severity ranging from profound to minimal. The situation is further complicated by the fact that workers after Kanner have observed that his classic autistic behaviour pattern can occur in children of any level of intelligence as measured on standardised tests, although most are in the moderate to mild range of mental retardation. It is also now clear that autism can be associated with conditions known to cause brain dysfunction, and with any kind of additional handicap, for example hearing or visual impairments or epilepsy (DeMyer 1975; Lotter, 1966; 1967; Rutter, 1970; Wing & Gould, 1979). Kanner's exclusion of those with mental retardation and brain dysfunction reflected the limitations of psychological and neurological techniques of assessment at the time when infantile autism was first described. Difficulties in establishing the exact age of onset retrospectively and accounts of individual children developing the autistic behaviour pattern well after the age of 30 months (Gillberg, 1986; Lotter, 1966; Wing & Gould, 1979) make it inappropriate to include age of onset among the diagnostic criteria, although in most cases abnormalities date from before 3 years of age (Lotter, 1966; Wing & Gould, 1979).

The diagnostic problems are well illustrated by the fact that all the named syndromes, including Kanner's autism, overlap with each other and are difficult to distinguish in clinical practice (Anthony, 1958a;b; Wing, 1988a). There have been changes in the diagnostic criteria in different editions of the International Classification of Diseases (ICD) (World Health Organisation, 1977, 1987) and the Diagnostic and Statistical Manual (DSM) (American Psychiatric Association, 1980; 1987). Autism prevalence rates for autism derived from population-based epidemiological studies have tended to increase over the years (Wing, 1988b) varying from 4.5 per 10.000 children (Lotter, 1966) to 13.9 per 10.000 (Tanoue et al., 1988). Problems in defining the boundaries of a complex behaviour pattern and changes in the two standard systems of classification have influenced the results of such studies, making it difficult to know if there has been any real change in prevalence.

Kolvin and his colleagues (Kolvin, 1971) carried out a population study which clarified the difference between the adult illness of schizophrenia occurring, very rarely, in childhood with onset always after 5 years, and the autistic and autistic-like conditions with onset almost always before 3 years of age.

AN EPIDEMIOLOGICAL APPROACH TO CLASSIFICATION

The present author, together with Judith Gould, used the methods of epidemiology in order to investigate the relationships among all autistic and autistic-like conditions (Wing & Gould, 1979).

In most epidemiological studies in this area, the investigators have adopted a particular definition of autism and have looked for subjects fitting the chosen criteria (a "top down" approach, to use the fashionable jargon). We followed a different strategy. Our aim was to find all children in one geographical area (the former London borough of Camberwell) who had any of the features described as characteristic of autism or any of the other named "syndromes" within the field of childhood "psychosis", and any who were considered to have behaviour that was strange or bizarre in any way, regardless of level of intelligence or presence of known brain dysfunction. We could then examine the patterns of impairments and behaviour for clustering of abnormalities. Children with IQ below 50 without any of the above problems were also included as a comparison group.

The details of the methods of this study are available elsewhere (Wing & Gould, 1979; Wing, 1981b) and a follow-up into adolescence and adult life of the subjects is described by Wing (1988a). Here it is sufficient to say that information on each child's history and current pattern of skills, impairments and behaviour was collected in the original study and again at follow-up.

The results showed that children with the classic picture of infantile autism could be identified. The numbers found depended on which definition was chosen. If Kanner's five criteria, listed earlier in the present paper, were applied, the prevalence rate was 2 per 10,000 children; if only the first two criteria were used, then the rate increased to 4.9 per 10,000. Although there was no difficulty in recognising the children with the full picture as described by Kanner, others were on the borderlines and there were no clear cut divisions. Some arbitrary decisions had to be made. Other named syndromes were also identified, but less easily because the published descriptions were not so clear and specific as those of Kanner. Some children could be assigned to more than one syndrome, while others had features of several but fitted none precisely. All in all, we were not impressed by the reliability of any of the named syndromes.

The Triad of Social Impairments

A different and, in our opinion, more useful way of subdividing the subjects was not anticipated before the study began, but emerged as important during the course of data collection. It gradually became more obvious that there were two main groups. The first comprised children who enjoyed social interaction for its own sake at a level appropriate for their mental age, and were interested in and stimulated by the company of other people, both children and adults. The second group were the children whose social interaction was inappropriate whatever their mental age. The various ways in which this problem can be manifested will be described later.

Impairment of social interaction was virtually always accompanied by impairment of social communication and of imaginative development, especially in its social aspects. In socially impaired children, the pretend play that normally develops in complexity and creativity from its simple beginnings in the second year of life is substituted by a narrow range of repetitive, stereotyped activities. This group of problems (known for brevity as the triad of social impairments) perhaps represents different facets of one more fundamental underlying abnormality, as discussed by Frith in her chapter.

The triad could occur in children of all levels of intelligence, but was most commonly found in association with severe mental retardation. In the area studied, 54 per cent of all children with intelligence quotients below 50 were socially impaired, nearly 2 per cent of those in the 50 to 69 range and only 0.1 per cent of those with intelligence quotents of 70 and above. Among children with the triad, 72 per cent had a history of current clinical evidence of some condition likely to be associated with brain pathology, such as maternal rubella, encephalitis, infantile spasms or other forms of epilepsy. Such findings were more common among those with severe mental retardation. Some of the children had additional handicaps such as visual or hearing impairments, and a very few had cerebral palsy or Down's syndrome, though these last two were rather rarely found with the triad. In most cases, the reported history of abnormal behaviour dated from birth or within the first three years of life, but, in 4 cases, onset was between 3 and 5 years of age.

All children with Kanner's syndrome, by definition, had the triad, as did all those with any of the named syndromes mentioned above and all children described as odd, strange, bizarre or "psychotic". The conditions in which the triad was a feature together formed a range of disorders which, for want of a better term, can be called the autistic continuum (or spectrum). This is more or less equivalent to the category of "pervasive developmental disorders" as defined in DSM III - Revised version (American Psychiatric Association, 1987).

Similar findings to those in Camberwell were reported in the Goteborg region by Gillberg et al. (1986).

CLINICAL MANIFESTATIONS OF THE TRIAD

As mentioned earlier, the manifestations of the elements of the triad vary widely. Furthermore, the triad tends to be associated with certain other problems that also vary in the way they appear in different individuals. In order to recognise the triad and the other impairments that may go with it, it is necessary to be aware of the possible variations, so these will be described. The following account is organised in the same way as the relevant section in DSM - III - Revised; that is, the manifestations of each feature are arranged in sequence from the most to the least severe. The former are most characteristic of younger and/or most handicapped individuals and the latter are found in the older and/or least handicapped people.

Impairment of Social Interaction

In its most severe form, this is manifested as aloofness and indifference to others. The child may approach others to obtain simple needs and may enjoy tickling and rough and tumble games, but will ignore the person approached once the needs are satisfied.

A somewhat less severe form is passive acceptance of approaches, but little or no spontaneous initiation of contact, apart from obtaining needs.

Some children make active but odd, one-sided, repetitive approaches to others. They have no interest in other people's responses, apart from perhaps demanding repeated stereotyped replies.

Adults who have made considerable progress can show a subtle form of impairment of social interaction, in which they appear to have learnt the rules of social life by rote rather than with true understanding.

Impairment of Social Communication

This affects non-verbal aspects even more than speech. In those most severely affected there is no interest in or attempt to communicate or to respond to communications from others.

At the next level are those who do attend to other people's attempts to communicate, albeit briefly, and who make some response.

Higher up the scale are those who initiate communication with others, but do this mainly in order to indulge their own repetitive interests and not to take part in an exchange of ideas and feelings. They may ask the same questions over and over again, or engage in long, boring monologues on their favourite topic.

At all levels, non-verbal signs of inter-personal interest, empathy and sympathy are conspicuous by their absence. Instrumental gestures such as pointing are seen in the children of moderate or higher levels of ability (Attwood, 1984).

Impairment of Imaginative Development

Many children with the triad have no pretend play at all. They use toys as meaningless objects to manipulate apparently in order to obtain simple sensations.

Some develop to the stage where they use miniatures of real objects for their correct purposes. That is, they wheel toy cars while making car noises, they pour pretend cups of tea from toy tea pots into toy cups or they feed dolls or teddy bears and tuck them up in bed. The abnormality lies in the restricted range, the repetitiveness and the lack of development into more complex pretence. The activities have usually been taught or copied from other children.

The most able socially impaired children engage in quite complex sequences of activities, such as building a miniature system of roads and bridges from any available materials, reenacting sequences of the actions of a particular character seen on television, or even inventing an imaginary character, a whole town or planet (Bosch, 1970) or a family of tiny people (Park, 1986). Again the characteristics are the repetition over and over again of the exact sequences, the lack of sharing with other children unless they are used purely as mechanical aids and the absence of interest in and insight into the thoughts and feelings of real or imaginary people. Such complex "play" activities tend to develop much later in childhood than in normal children and continue to be inappropriate in relation to chronological age.

Repetitive Stereotyped Activities

These vary from the simple to the highly complex. In those who are profoundly retarded as well as socially impaired, stereotypies tend to take the form of bodily movements such as rocking, teeth grinding, clenching and unclenching the fists, finger flicking or aimless pacing.

More complicated bodily movements can occur, such as the characteristic springing from back foot to front foot while flexing and extending the whole body. Complex movements of the head or hands and arms may also be seen.

The repetitive activities can involve particular sensory experiences, such as listening to the same passage of music or the same mechanical noise over and over again, staring at the same wallpaper pattern or display of lights, or watching spinning objects such as clothes in a washing machine or a record player turn-table, or desiring repetitive sensations of touch, taste, smell or vestibular stimulation.

Object-directed activities include continually holding the same object, amassing large collections of particular objects for no obvious purpose (dead holly leaves, chocolate wrappers, red umbrellas and odd shaped pieces of metal are examples).

More able children tend to insist upon carrying out the same sequence of actions, such as a lengthy bedtime ritual, or following the same route to familiar places. The whole family may have to fit into these routines.

At the highest level, the problems are shown in verbal or intellectual forms, such as amassing facts concerning time tables, calendars, the weather, the movement of the planets, or the characters and events in a particular series of books. As already mentioned, if "imaginative" activities develop at all, these tend to be repetitive in form, as do any attempts at "conversation" with other people.

ASSOCIATED ABNORMALITIES

All kinds of abnormalities can be associated with the triad of social impairments. Some are found in the great majority of cases, suggesting some fundamental relationship of aetiological significance, while others occur less commonly.

Language

Pragmatic aspects of language, that is, the comprehension and use of language within a social context, are always, by definition, impaired in those with the triad (Baltaxe, 1979; Frith, 1982; Tager-Flusberg, 1981).

The formal aspects of language, namely vocabulary, syntax and semantics, are delayed and deviant in most but not all socially impaired children. About half or more remain mute, with little or no comprehension. In those who speak, onset of speech is usually, but not always, delayed and its development may be halted at any level from single word utterances onwards. Where there is enough speech, echolalia, reversal of pronouns, and repetitive utterances of words, phrases, sentences or even whole conversations are characteristic.

Prosody is affected in the great majority, with peculiar phrasing and intonation that is monotonous or inappropriate. Gestures accompanying speech are usually absent, but when present may appear odd and out of context.

Motor Co-ordination

There can be any mixture of skills and deficiences in this area of function, at any level of severity. Some socially impaired children are agile in climbing and balancing, while others are clumsy and nervous of any activity requiring good balance. Some are dexterous in fine motor tasks while others have problems in this area. Skills in gross movement may be associated with poor fine co-ordination and vice-versa. Children who are agile when young often become ill co-ordinated in adolescence, when gait and posture appear odd and ungainly. Skill may vary markedly depending on the task. For example, a socially impaired person may fumble with buttons, but be able to play complex pieces on the piano without error.

Responses to Sensory Stimuli

These problems are common but not invariable. Hypersensitivity to sounds is frequent in young, socially impaired children, though it is not a universal phenomenon. It is particularly characteristic of those with classic autism.

Reactions to any type of sensory input can take the form of indifference, fascination or distress. Different sounds, for example, can elicit different responses in the same child. Even specific colours can produce positive or negative responses, such as insistence on wearing clothes that are pink in colour, combined with refusal to enter any room in which the colour yellow is present.

Cognitive Skills

Population studies of autism and related conditions have shown that most affected children are mentally retarded, with one half or more in the severely retarded range (Brask, 1972; Lotter, 1966; 1967; Wing & Gould, 1979). The most characteristic profile on testing is that of marked discrepancies between sub-test scores. Usually, purely visuo-spatial skills are better than those dependent on language. In a minority of cases, verbal scores are better than those for visuo-spatial items (Wing, 1988a), but, in such cases, comprehension of meaning is usually poor (DeMyer, 1976). Despite these marked tendencies, there is no profile that can be said to be diagnostic of social impairment in general or classic autism in particular.

The so-called "islets of ability" stand out in contrast to the retardation in other areas, but tend to be below or perhaps equal to the level expected from the individual's chronological age. In a very small proportion of socially impaired people, however, there is a truly outstanding skill well above the chronological age level, such as musical performance, numerical or calendar calculation, drawing, modelling or feats of rote memory (O'Connor & Hermelin, 1984; Selfe, 1977; 1983; Treffert, 1989).

The special skills, when they occur, are so dramatic that they tend to draw attention away from the fact that any kind of specific developmental learning disability can occur in association with social impairment, though these will only be apparent in people with a sufficiently high level of overall intelligence. These include developmental disorders of language, reading, calculation, visuo-spatial and, as already mentioned, motor skills. Asperger (1944) emphasized this aspect of the group of children with his "syndrome".

Behaviour Problems

Some socially impaired children, especially those with the passive type of social interaction, are quiet and amenable and present no behaviour problems other than their repetitive activities. The majority, however, exhibit one or more of a range of problems. These include temper tantrums, screaming, restlessness, destructiveness, creating chaos aimlessly, self-injury and unpleasant personal habits. Disturbances of sleeping, eating and excessive intake of fluids are also fairly common in the children.

Psychiatric Problems

While some socially impaired children appear generally calm and unresponsive except when moved to rage by interference with their accustomed routine or repetitive activities, others have a high level of anxiety and are fearful of a variety of harmless objects or events.

Anxiety can be manifested early in childhood, but most psychiatric problems appear in adolescence or adult life. One interesting aspect of social impairment is the association with catatonic phenomena, varying from fragments to, rarely, the full picture of catatonic stupor or excitement. Odd hand postures are the most common, and occur at all ages, but brief freezing in mid-action and inability to complete a sequence of movements can also be seen on careful observation, especially in adolescents.

Affective disorders, especially reactive depression, are also seen in adolescents and young adults. A small proportion develop what appear to be obsessional states, including hand-washing and compulsive thoughts, but it is difficult to define the borderline between these phenomena and the repetitive, stereotyped activities characteristic of those with the triad.

Schizophrenia has been reported (Petty et al., 1984) but the present author has never seen a case of this kind. Episodes of undifferentiated "psychosis" can occur in adolescents and adults (see the chapter on adults).

THE PROCESS OF DIAGNOSIS

The present author and colleagues have found that the most satisfactory and clinically useful approach to diagnosis is to establish, first, if the triad of social impairments is present and in what form, second, to identify any other impairments and abnormalities and their degree of severity and, last of all, to consider which sub-group most resembles the clinical picture in the child or adult concerned.

From the point of view of the diagnostician, identification of the presence or absence of the triad is considerably easier than diagnosing, for example, Kanner's autism, because fewer variables are involved, even though the manifestations vary widely. The more features that are required to diagnose a "syndrome" the fewer children or adults will be found who fit the picture.

From the point of view of the affected person and his or her family, whatever other problems are associated with it the presence of the triad has major implications for management, education and prognosis that are the same as for the sub-group with classic Kanner's autism, given equivalent levels of overall ability. If the diagnostician confines his interest to typical autism, the much larger group of those with the triad but not typically autistic are in danger of not receiving the help they need.

A particular problem is presented by profoundly retarded and by non-mobile people who are also socially impaired. It can be argued that people with these types of handicaps are so severely impaired in every area that the presence of the triad is irrelevant and, in any case, difficult to recognise. However, in the present author's clinical experience, it is possible to differentiate the sociable from the socially impaired at any level of ability. Furthermore, recognition of the quality of social interaction helps the carers to understand the behaviour of the handicapped person and to plan a programme of care and education.

Identification of the triad and of associated abnormalities of language, cognitive and motor skills and behaviour depends upon good history taking and careful physical and psychological assessment. Details of the child's development and present behaviour pattern cannot be obtained solely from observation in the clinic. They are collected by tactful questioning of the parents who must be listened to with patience, care and respect. The present author and colleagues have developed the Medical Research Council Handicaps, Behaviour and Skills (HBS) interview schedule to facilitate the systematic obtaining and recording of clinical information necessary for the diagnosis of the triad and associated abnormalities (Wing & Gould, 1978).

Differential Diagnosis

Differential diagnosis rests essentially upon identification of the triad. Sometimes social impairment is wrongly explained away as a secondary consequence of language or hearing disorders, but it is important to recognise that sufferers from these conditions in pure form use non-verbal ways of interacting and communicating and are interested in other people. The presence of the triad is of prime importance for management and teaching whatever other handicaps are associated with it.

Retarded children with mental ages below 20 months have no pretend play and are likely to have simple stereotypies even if they do not have the triad. The diagnosis is made by observation of the quality of their social interaction.

Severe social and physical deprivation has adverse effects upon children and affects their responses to other people, but social withdrawal from this cause is of a different kind from the aloof, or the passive, or the active but odd manifestations of social impairment and improvement tends to occur rapidly when the child is placed in a caring environment (Clarke & Clarke, 1976; Koluchova, 1972; 1976; Rutter, 1972). Of course, children with the triad can also be deprived and abused, in which case care is needed to disentangle cause and effect.

Some psychiatric conditions can cause confusion, especially if presenting in higher functioning adolescents or adults with the triad whose developmental impairment has not been previously diagnosed. Depression, obsessional conditions, anxiety states can all obscure the presence of the triad unless a history is obtained from parents or others who have known the person from childhood. Schizophrenia can also cause loss of interest in social interaction, but, again, the history and behaviour pattern found with the triad differs from that of the person with adult schizophrenia.

So-called "schizoid personality disorder" is of particular interest in this connection. The odd social interaction and circumscribed interests described as characteristic of this type of personality overlap with the features of Asperger's syndrome (Asperger, 1944; Wolff & Barlow, 1979). The early developmental history should help to differentiate the two, but the borderlines are by no means clear (Wing, 1981a).

CAN THE AUTISTIC CONTINUUM BE SUB-CLASSIFIED?

The question of sub-grouping individuals with social impairment raises a number of problems. In the Camberwell study, as already described, there were difficulties in assigning children to the named syndromes. Some combinations of impairments were more common than others, for example, aloofness, very severe communication and language impairment, comparatively good simple visuo-spatial skills and gross motor agility tended to occur together, as did active but odd social interaction, fluent though repetitive expressive speech but poor comprehension, and motor clumsiness. However, it appeared that virtually any combination of impairments could occur. Although typical Kanner's syndrome and, with somewhat less certainty, Asperger's syndrome could be recognised, they formed only a small minority of all children with the triad. Thus, as already mentioned, the rate for Kanner's syndrome in its purest nuclear form was only 2 per 10,000, and, if defined somewhat more widely, 4.9 per 10,000. The rate for Asperger's syndrome was about 1.8 per 10,000. These should be compared with the prevalence of everyone with the triad, including non-mobile children, which was 27 per 10,000, or 23 per 10,000 for the mobile group only (Wing, 1988a).

An even more difficult problem was that some children changed in their clinical pictures as they grew older, especially those of higher levels of ability. Of the 7 children who in later childhood or adolescence were classified as having Asperger's syndrome, 3 had had the picture of classic Kanner's syndrome in early childhood. Furthermore, whereas 5 of the 17 children with typical Kanner's syndrome became less typical as they grew older, 6 others, who were socially impaired but did not show the Kanner picture early on, became more and more like his descriptions as they grew older, becoming more aloof and more elaborate in their routines.

Altogether, 22 per cent of those with the triad who were still alive at follow-up changed in their style of social interaction over the years, but none became appropriately sociable.

Another major difficulty in deciding whether or not to call a child autistic is the number of definitions that have been suggested. These include Kanner's (1944) original five points and Kanner and Eisenberg's (1956) 2 points, Rutter's (1978) definition, ICD editions 9 and 10 (World Health Organisation, 1977; 1987), and DSM-III and DSM-III-Revised (American Psychiatric Association, 1980; 1987), among others.

There is little to be gained clinically from deciding whether or not a child fits one or other definition of autism. Management, education, prognosis and placement as an adult depend upon the type of social impairment, the level of ability in language, cognitive and motor skills, the presence of any associated handicaps and the child's own personality.

This should not be taken as an argument in support of those who oppose diagnosis, which they refer to as "labelling". A useful diagnosis is a formulation of the pattern of skills, handicaps and behaviour. Since the term autism is the only one that is familiar to everyone involved in this field, it is useful to refer to people with the triad as autistic or austistic-like and to emphasize that they need the types of management and education that have been developed for autistic children and adults, appropriately adapted to their levels of ability in different areas. If this wording helps to obtain the services the socially impaired person needs, it can be regarded as a constructive use of diagnostic labelling.

From the point of view of research, which is different from that of clinical work, many investigators are mainly interested in examining children or adults who fit the diagnostic criteria for the current conventionally accepted "syndromes". This presupposes that the sub-group concerned can be identified reliably and has some external validity, such as a common aetiology or location of brain pathology. A different approach that avoids these presuppositions is to examine specific impairments, regardless of diagnostic sub-group. The epidemiological studies carried out in Camberwell and Göteborg were the first to examine the phenomenon of the triad of social impairment as a developmental disorder, in all its manifestations.

This approach leaves open the question of sub-groupings. It is possible that, for example, the group described by Kanner will prove to have some kind of external validity. It is also possible that there are other ways of sub-grouping that are more appropriate. The value of any classification depends upon its suitability for the purpose for which it was devised. For instance, in clinical and educational practice, sub-grouping on quality of social interaction and level of ability is the most relevant. For work on prevention and cure, the search for sub-groups based on cause or location of brain pathology is of obvious importance.

It would be of considerable interest to discover if the various experimental findings already reported in children considered to be autistic (Baron-Cohen, Leslie & Frith, 1986; Frith, 1972, 1982; Frith & Snowling, 1983; Hermelin & O'Connor, 1970; O'Connor & Hermelin, 1978) are common to all those with the triad, given equivalent levels of cognitive and language development.

It is clear from the results of the Camberwell study (Wing & Gould, 1979) that the same kind of pre-, peri- and postnatal conditions often associated with brain dysfunction are found in the histories of all those with the triad, including typical autism. Investigations are needed of family histories designed to see if the genetic traits already shown to the associated with typical autism (Folstein & Rutter, 1987) are specific to particular sub-groups, or are found in those with the triad in any of its manifestations.

Impairment of social interaction occurs in conditions other than those in the autistic spectrum, for example in chronic schizophrenia and some forms of senile dementia. Comparative studies could show whether the similarities are superficial or have a deeper significance.

The broad view of the autistic spectrum advocated here is not a return to an uncritical lumping together of all forms of "psychosis"; it is an attempt to examine the clinical phenomena in a fresh light and to clear the way for the development of more useful methods of diagnosis and classification without losing sight of what has been achieved in the past.

REFERENCES

American Psychiatric Association. (1980). *Diagnostic and Statistical Manual of Mental Disorders (3rd ed.)*. Washington DC: Author.

American Psychiatric Association. (1987). *Diagnostic and Statistical Manual of Mental Disorders (3rd revised ed.)*. Washington DC: Author.

Anthony, E. J. (1958a). An etiological approach to the diagnosis of psychosis in childhood. *Revue de Psychiatric Infantile, 25,* 89-96.

Anthony, E. J. (1958b). An experimental approach to the psychopathology of childhood autism. *British Journal of Medical Psychology, 21,* 211-225.

Asperger, H. (1944). Die autistischen Psychopathen im Kindesalter. *Archiv für Psychiatrie und Nervenkrankheiten, 117,* 76-136.

Attwood, A. (1984). *The Gestures of Autistic Children,* Ph D Thesis. University of London.

Baltaxe, C. A. M. (1977). Pragmatic deficits in the language of autistic adolescents. *Journal of Paediatric Psychology, 2,* 176-180.

Baron-Cohen, S., Leslie, A. M., & Frith, U. (1986). Mechanical, behavioural and intentional understanding of picture stories in autistic children. *British Journal of Developmental Psychology, 4,* 113-125.

Bosch, G. (1970). *Infantile autism.* New York: Springer-Verlag.

Brask, B. H. (1972). A prevalence investigation of childhood psychoses. In *Nordic Symposium on the Comprehensive Care of the Psychotic Children.* Oslo: Barnepsykiatrisk Forening.

Clarke, A. M. & Clarke, A. D. B. (1976). Formerly isolated children. In A. M. Clarke & A. D. B. Clarke (Eds.), *Early Experience: Myth and Evidence.* London: Open Books.

Connolly, J. (1861-2). Juvenile insanity. *American Journal of Insanity, 18,* 395-403.

DeMyer, M. K. (1975). Research in infantile autism: a strategy and its results. *Biological Psychiatry, 10,* 433-452.

DeMyer, M. (1976). Motor, perceptual-motor and intellectual disabilities of autistic children. In L. Wing (Ed.), *Early Childhood Autism.* Oxford: Pergamon Press.

De Sanctis, S. (1906). Sopra alcune varieta della demenza precoce. *Rivista Sperimentale Di Freniatria E Di Medicina Legale, 32,* 141-165.

De Sanctis, S. (1908). Dementia praecocissima catatonica oder Katatonie des früheren Kindesalters? *Folia Neurobiologica, 2,* 9-12.

Earl, C. J. C. (1934). The primitive catatonic of idiocy. *British Journal of Medical Psychology, 14,* 230-253.

Folstein, S., & Rutter, M. (1987). Autism: familial aggregation and genetic implications. In E. Schopler & G. B. Mesibov (Eds.), *Neurobiological Issues in Autism.* New York: Plenum.

Frith, U. (1972). Cognitive mechanisms in autism: experiments with colour and tone sequence production. *Journal of Autism and Childhood Schizophrenia, 2,* 160-173.

Frith, U. (1982). Psychological abnormalities in early childhood psychoses. In J. K. Wing & L. Wing (Eds.), *Handbook of Psychiatry. Vol. 3:* Cambridge: University Press.

Frith, U., & Snowling, M. (1983). Reading for meaning and reading for sound in autistic and dyslexic children. *British Journal of Developmental Psychology, 1,* 329-342.

Gillberg, C. (1985). Asperger's syndrome and recurrent psychosis - a case study. *Journal of Autism and Developmental Disorders, 15,* 389-398.

Gillberg, C. (1986). Onset at age fourteen of a typical autistic syndrome. A case report of a girl with herpes simplex encephalitis. *Journal of Autism and Developmental Disorders, 16,* 569-575.

Gillberg, C., Persson, E., Grufman, M., & Themner, U. (1986). Psychiatric disorders in mildly and severely mentally retarded urban children and adolescents: epidemiological aspects. *British Journal of Psychiatry, 149,* 68-74.

Haslam, J. (1809). *Observations on Madness and Melancholy.* London: Haydon.

Hermelin, B., & O'Connor, N. (1970). *Psychological Experiments with Autistic Children.* Oxford: Pergamon Press.

Hermelin, B., & O'Connor, N. (1985). Logico-affective states and non-verbal language.

In E. Schopler & G. Mesibov (Eds.), *Communication Problems in Autism*. New York: Plenum Press.

Hulse, W. C. (1954). Dementia infantilis. *Journal of Nervous and Mental Diseases, 119,* 471-477.

Kanner, L. (1943). Autistic disturbances of affective contact. *Nervous Child, 2,* 217-250.

Kanner, L. (1949). Problems of nosology and psychodynamics in early childhood autism. *American Journal of Orthopsychiatry, 19,* 416-426.

Kanner, L., & Eisenberg, L. (1956). Early infantile autism 1943-1955. *American Journal of Orthopsychiatry, 26,* 55-65.

Koluchova, J. (1972). Severe deprivation in twins: A case study. *Journal of Child Psychology and Psychiatry, 13,* 107-114.

Koluchova, J. (1976). A report on the further development of twins after severe and prolonged deprivation. In A.M. Clarke & A.D.B. Clarke (Eds.), *Early Experience: Myth and Evidence.* London: Open Books.

Kolvin, I. (1971). Studies in the childhood psychoses: I. Diagnostic criteria and classification. *British Journal of Psychiatry, 118,* 381-384.

Lockyer, L., & Rutter, M. (1969). A five to fifteen year follow-up study of infantile psychosis: III. Psychological aspects. *British Journal of Psychiatry, 115,* 865-882.

Lotter, V. (1966). Epidemiology of autistic conditions in young children: I. Prevalence. *Social Psychiatry, 1,* 124-137.

Lotter, V. (1967). Epidemiology of autistic conditions in young children: II. Some characteristics of the parents and children. *Social Psychiatry, 1,* 163-173.

Mahler, M. S. (1952). On child psychoses and schizophrenia: autistic and symbiotic infantile psychoses. *Psychoanalytic Study of the Child, 7,* 286-305.

Maudsley, H. (1867). *The Physiology and Pathology of the Mind.* New York: Appleton & Co.

O'Connor, N., & Hermelin, B. (1978). *Seeing, Hearing, Space and Time.* London. Academic Press.

O'Connor, N., & Hermelin, B. (1984). Idiot savant calendrical calculators: maths or memory? *Psychological Medicine, 14,* 801-806.

Park, C. C. (1968). *The Siege.* Gerrards Cross: Colin Smythe.

Petty, L. K., Ornitz, M. O., Michelman, J. D., & Zimmerman, E. G. (1984). Autistic children who become schizophrenic. *Archives of General Psychiatry, 41,* 129-135.

Rutter, M. (1970). Autistic children: Infancy to adulthood. *Seminars in Psychiatry, 2,* 435-450.

Rutter, M. (1972). Psychiatric causes of language retardation. In M. Rutter & J. A. M. Martin (Eds.), *The Child with Delayed Speech.* London: Heinemann.

Rutter, M. (1978). Diagnosis and definition in childhood autism. *Journal of Autism and Childhood Schizophrenia, 8,* 139-161.

Selfe, L. (1977). *Nadia: a Case of Extraordinary Drawing Ability in an Autistic Child.* London: Academic Press.

Selfe, L. (1983). *Normal and Anomalous Representational Drawing Ability in Children.* Academic Press: London.

Tager-Flusberg, H. (1981). Sentence comprehension in autistic children. *Applied Psycholinguistics, 2,* 5-24.

Tanoue, Y., Oda, S., Asano, F., & Kawashima, K. (1988). Epidemiology of infantile autism in the Southern Ibaraki, Japan. *Journal of Autism and Developmental Disorders, 18,* 155-167.

Treffert, D. (1989). *Extraordinary People.* New York: Bantam Press.

Van Krevelen, D. A. (1971). Early infantile autism and autistic psychopathy. *Journal of Autism and Childhood Schizophrenia, 1,* 82-86.

Wing, L. (1981a). Asperger's syndrome: a clinical account. *Psychological Medicine, 11,* 115-130.

Wing, L. (1981b). Language, social and cognitive impairments in autism and severe mental retardation. *Journal of Autism and Developmental Disorders, 11,* 31-44.

Wing, L. (1988a). The continuum of autistic characteristics. In E. Schopler & G. B. Mesibov (Eds.), *Diagnosis and Assessment in Autism.* New York: Plenum.

Wing, L. (1988b). The epidemiology of autism. In A. Trillingsgard & G. Nemec (Eds.), *Tilegnet Birte Hoeg Brask: Et Skrift om Psykotiske Born.* Risskov: Psykiatrisk Bornehospital.

Wing, L., & Gould J. (1978). Systematic recording of behaviours and skills of retarded and psychotic children. *Journal of Autism and Childhood Schizophrenia, 8,* 79-97.

Wing, L., & Gould, J. (1979). Severe impairments of social interaction and associated abnormalities in children: epidemiology and classification. *Journal of Autism and Childhood Schizophrenia, 9,* 11-29.

Wolff, S., & Barlow, A. (1979). Schizoid personality in childhood: a comparative study of schizoid, autistic and normal children. *Journal of Child Psychology and Psychiatry, 20,* 29-46.

World Health Organization. (1977). *International Statistical Classification of Diseases, Injuries and Causes of Death. (9th Revision),* Geneva: World Health Organization.

World Health Organization (1987). *International Classification of Diseases. Tenth Revision Draft: Research Diagnostic Criteria,* Geneva WHO (unpublished document).

Early Symptoms in Autism

CHRISTOPHER GILLBERG

INTRODUCTION

Before discussing the issue of early symptoms in autism, one must try and make clear what is implied by the word "early". In this connection, I will mostly be concerned with symptoms and developmental problems in the under 3 years age group. However, I am aware of the possibility that autism can appear to present later and indeed occasionally does have its onset after age 3 years - but the main focus of this overview will be on the very young in an attempt to pinpoint practical guidelines for those concerned with trying to diagnose autism already in the first few years of life.

Survey of studies in the field of early symptoms

The literature on early symptoms in autism is limited. Only a handful of studies have had anything specific to say about the early clinical picture in autism (Polan & Spencer, 1959; Wing, 1969; Prior & Gajzago, 1974; Ornitz et al., 1978; Rosenthal et al., 1980; Sauvage et al., 1988). I have not been able to find more than three prospective studies (Suqiama & Abe, 1986; Sauvage et al., 1987; Gillberg et al., 1989) and neither of these can make claims for representativity.

Age of onset

The spectrum of autistic disorders (including, for instance, infantile autism and

23

Asperger syndrome) shows variation with respect to age of onset, or, at least age of onset of clinically relevant symptoms.

Autistic disorder

Even though the DSM-III-R (APA 1987) does not specify age of onset among the diagnostic criteria for autistic disorder it is generally agreed (e g Rutter 1978) that onset is usually in the first 30 months of life. Wing (1980) has speculated that onset is congenital or before age 12 months in 80 per cent of cases. Short and Shopler (1988) report that 94 per cent of parents of children with autism identify problems before age 36 months, but only 36 per cent felt there had been clearly abnormal signs before age 12 months. In a study by Volkmar et al. (1985) 55 per cent had been identified as deviant before age 12 months.

Childhood disintegrative disorder

The rare condition called Heller's dementia (Heller, 1931) and sometimes referred to as disintegrative psychosis - more recently childhood disintegrative disorder (ICD-10, 1987) - usually begins in the 2,5 - 4 years of age range. The so called pervasive developmental disorders NOS (DSM-III-R, APA 1987) refer to a group of less strictly defined "autism spectrum disorders" which probably encompass cases of Heller's dementia and with a similar age of onset range.

Asperger syndrome

Asperger syndrome, whether it is viewed as a distinct syndrome or just as a variant of "high - level - autism" (Schopler, 1985), probably is constitutional/congenital, but often doesn't cause major concern until the late pre-school or even early school years. Its main importance in this connection lies in its implication that "detection sensitivity" in the field of autism cannot be confined to infancy and the very earliest period of childhood.

Environmental perceptiveness

So long as there exist no representative prospective observational studies on early symptoms in autism, we are largely dependent on the child's closest care-giver for appropriate information. Such information, in turn, co-varies with a number of factors such as the child's position in the sibship (late discovery probably more likely in first-born children and those who are many years younger than their next youngest brother or sister) and something which might be termed "environmental perceptiveness". Parents and other care-givers vary in their degree of alertness when it comes to observing deviance in the child. A number of factors such as the age, social circumstances, educational level, personality, intelligence plus the presence/absence of age-peers and mental health of the care-giver may be relevant in this respect. Diagnosis somtimes comes late even when all these factors speak in favour of early detection and should not, without qualification, be taken - as is sometimes the case - as evidence that something is "wrong" with the parent. Just stop for a moment and consider the number of doctors who for years have reassured mothers of children with autism that there is nothing seriously wrong with their child!

Nevertheless, it is clear that most of our knowledge in the field of early symptoms in autism and autistic-like conditions, stems from the mother. Therefore, for years to come, we shall have to take the "environmental perceptiveness" into account whenever considering concepts such as "the first symptoms of autism" and so on.

EARLY SYMPTOMS IN AUTISM

I will briefly survey two recent studies from our centre which have both been concerned with symptoms under age 2 - 3 years in autism (Dahlgren & Gillberg, 1989, Gillberg et al., 1989). One of the studies is a population-based retrospective study of 26 children with autism which makes use of 2 control groups, viz a sex- and age-matched normal group and a sex-, age- and IQ-matched group. The other one is a prospective clinical study of 28 children seen by myself before their 3rd birthday, 21 of whom eventually - at follow-up years later - turned out to fulfil all the necessary criteria for autistic disorder.

The mothers in both studies were given a 130-item visual analogue questionnaire on early development and physical and psychopathological symptoms considered typical of autism. The questionnaire has been published previously (Dahlgren & Gillberg, 1989). In the retrospective study, 18 items discriminated autism from mental retardation and normality (6 of which also differentiated the mentally retarded from the normal children and the mentally retarded from those with autism). In the prospective study (possibly less representative than the retrospective one but not as likely to be biased by selective recall) 10

TABLE 1. Items discriminating autism from mental retardation and normality under age 3 yrs

| Area/item | Identified in | |
	prospective study (Gillberg et al., 1989)	retrospective study (Dahlgren&Gillberg, 1989)
SOCIAL		
<u>Appears to be isolated from surroundings</u>	+	+
Doesn't smile when expected to	+	+
Difficulties getting eye contact	+	+
Doesn't matter much whether Mum or Dad is close by or not	+	-
Doesn't like to be disturbed in own world	-	+
Contented if left alone	-	+
COMMUNICATION		
Doesn't try to attract adult's attention to own activity	+	+
Difficulties imitating movements	+	+
Late speech development	+	-
Doesn't point to objects	+	-
Doesn't understand what people say	+	-
Can't indicate own wishes	+	-
PLAY-BEHAVIOUR		
<u>Doesn't play like other children</u>	+	+
Occupies self only when alone	+	+
Plays only with hard objects	+	+
Odd attachments to odd objects	-	+
PERCEPTION		
<u>There is (or has been) a suspicion of deafness</u>	+	+
Empty gaze	+	+
Overexcited when tickled	+	+
There is something strange about his/her gaze	+	
Interested only in certain parts of objects	+	-
Exceptionally interested in things that move	+	-
Doesn't listen when spoken to	+	-
Strange reactions to sound	-	+
Doesn't seem to react to cold	-	+
Engages in bizarre looking at objects, pattern and movements	-	+
RHYTHMICITY		
There are day/periods when he/she seems much worse than usual	-	+
Severe problems over sleep	-	+

| | = | 3 items with strongest discriminatory power in prospective study |
| *italic* | = | 3 items with strongest discriminatory power in retrospective study |

of these 18 symptoms were present in more than 80 per cent of the cases. In this study another 12 items emerged which occurred in at least 80 per cent of the cases, but which had not shown up in the retrospective study. Thus, altogether 22 items emerged as typical of very young autism cases in the prospective study. All children with autism in the prospective study showed at least 15 of those 22 symptoms. An age, - sex and IQ-matched comparison group all exhibited less than 9 of these 22 symptoms. Two signs unspecifically related to late overall development occurred in several of the children with mental retardation as well as with autism and were not included in the further presentation of symptoms thought to be typical of autism early in life.

It is of some interest that in the prospective study of infantile autism we have found only one case with clear-cut regression, after a period of normal development.

Unspecific problems

Even though overall late development was considered typical both of children with mental retardation and autism, there emerged a clear tendency both in the prospective and the retrospective study for "abnormalities any kind" to have been observed earlier in autism than in mental retardation. This held among those children with autism with severe mental retardation also, provided that comparison between autism and mental retardation was made at corresponding IQ-levels. These findings are in line with those by Short and Shopler (1988).

Severe sleep problems were very common in autism but no more common in cases with mental retardation than in normal children (Table 1).

A strong tendency for periodicity was noted in the autism group.

Both sleep problems and the periodic tendency were noted only in the retrospective study which, of course, means that caution is warranted as regards generalisability of these results.

There is, of course, considerable overlap as regards early symptomatology between autism and mental retardation. According to a recent study of childhood schizophrenia (Watkins et al., 1988) there are also substantial similarities in the early histories of children with school-age onset schizophrenia and infancy onset autism. This is a controversial field, which has not attracted much attention in recent years, but which will probably again become the focus of animated discussions concerning continuities - discontinuities between autism and childhood schizophrenia.

Possibly specific symptoms

Abnormal perceptual responses represented the most important group of symptoms in the field of early abnormalities in autism (Table 1). Ten of the 26 specific symptoms belonged in this group. Regardless of whether univariate analyses or ANOVAS were performed this group stood out as clinically possibly more important than the other three (social, communication and play-behaviour). This was not an effect of there being more "perceptual items" on the questionnaire (there were about 30 each in the social, communication, play/behaviour and perception domains). It appeared that abnormal reactions to sound might be particularly typical of autism. However, abnormalities of gaze and vision seemed to be common too. It is of some interest that "overexcited when tickled" came out as a typical item. In Lorna Wing's 1970 study a lack of response to tickling was common in speaking children with autism. The results with respect to perceptual abnormalities agree with those presented by Ornitz et al. (1978) and Ornitz (1988).

Except for perceptual abnormalities, "autistic aloneness" and abnormalities of play seemed to be the most typical early symptoms in autism, but all the three areas social, communication and play/behaviour - which are considered fundamental in virtually all current diagnostic systems for autism (unlike perception which is usually not considered a necessary area of dysfunction) - were represented by several items each, both in the retrospective and the prospective studies. In a recent study by Sauvage et al. (1988), a relative lack of mimicry and an expressiveless face tended to be the most common early signs of autism, at least as judged from home movies. Whether to group such signs with the social or communicative deficits or even as secondary markers of perceptual abnormalities, is open to speculation.

It is of some interest that abnormal babble was not noted as a symptom distinguishing children with autism, mental retardation and normal children from each other.

CHECK-UPS AT THE WELL-BABY CLINIC

On the basis of the literature survey and our own studies, we have suggested screening measures (questions and observations) for the well-baby clinics to use both at age 10 and 18 months (when all Swedish children are carefully examined by both a nurse and a doctor) (Gillberg, 1985). Suggestions for questions that the nurse can ask of the parents are shown in Table 2. These questions should not be regarded as obligatory in the sense that they must be asked of all parents attending the well-baby clinic. Rather, they should be seen as a check-list if the child has anything to suggest a developmental disorder or if the parent seems concerned about the child's behaviour or development. The table also includes suggestions for what the nurse or doctor might observe at the time of the physical examination of the child.

TABLE 2. Screening for autism at the well-baby clinic at ages 10 and 18 months

---

The following questions to the mother provide a tentative framework for a check-list to be used whenever there is (even mild) suspicion of autistic-like behaviour or autism

---

Do you consider your child's eye-to-eye-contact to be normal?

Do you think that he/she listens to you or has normal hearing, or does he/she react only to particular sounds?

If there are or have been any feeding problems or abnormal behaviours in connection with feeding, what were they?

Is he/she comforted by proximity or body contact?

Does he/she oppose body contact?

Does he/she show any interest in his/her surroundings?

Does he/she often smile or laugh quite unexpectedly?

Does he/she prefer it if he/she is left alone/to himself?

Is your child, on the whole, like other children?

Examine the following features systematically

Hand stereotypies (including strange looking at or posturing of hand(s))

Avoidance of gaze contact

Stiff, staring gaze

Rejection of body contact

No or very variable reaction to strong, unexpected noise

Obvious lack of interest (e g does not show interest in peek-a-boo games)

WHO MAKES THE DIAGNOSIS?

For many years it has been common for parents to be the first to suspect and in fact even "diagnose" autism. Child psychiatrists are usually those who are expected to know enough to make a correct diagnosis, but, at least in Sweden, the empirical evidence is rather contrary to this commonly held notion. It is only in centres specializing in autism or neuropsychiatry that adequate diagnoses are established when the children are very young. In our centre, mean age at diagnosis of autism (with IQ <100) was 7.4 years 10 years ago (Gillberg, 1981). This was before we established a statewide diagnostic service. Mean age at diagnosis in cases with autism and IQ <100 was 2.6 years in 1988.

In Sweden, and in many other western countries, developmental pediatricians and child neurologists are often the doctors who first suspect that the child may be suffering from autism.

The changing panorama of core autism symptoms over time influences who sees the child. The first symptoms, according to our studies, are either so unspecific or connected with abnormal sensory responses that it would be uncommon for professionals not specifically trained in the field of autism to suspect that that might be a likely candidate for diagnosis. Also, a number of children suspected of suffering from autism under age 2 years will have received other diagnoses by the time they are 4 - 5 years of age (Gillberg et al., 1989). However, studies from our centre indicate that autism can be reliably diagnosed in infancy - and show diagnostic stability over the next few years - in something like three quarters of the cases.

"Kanner-autism" is most "Kanner-like" in the 3-7-years-old age range, and it is likely that child psychiatrists get to see children with autism in that age range.

Asperger syndrome on the other hand is perhaps most "Asperger-like" during the early school years. For children with Asperger type problems it is quite common (Gillberg, 1989) not to see any kind of specialist and for the diagnosis to be missed altogether in spite of major behavioural problems.

In children with autism and more normal levels of IQ, and in those currently diagnosed as suffering from Asperger syndrome, a correct diagnosis is rarely established in the first three or four years of life. Many come to specialist attention in the early school years when their social oddities and communication problems have made them the laughing-stock of their class or their excentric interests and failure to interact with age-peers make parents and teachers worried about the child's future. Information about high-level autism has to be spread to lay-people and teachers so that such children can be referred at an earlier age before secondary mobbing becomes the biggest problem.

CONCLUSIONS

In summary, the evidence concerning early symptoms in autism is limited indeed. Thus the suggestions I have made with respect to screening rest on a fairly shaky basis. Nevertheless, in clinical practice the method described seems to work well.

In the future, in research, rather than looking for symptoms which typify the whole of the group of autism spectrum disorders, I think we need to look carefully into the symptomatology of the various subgroups which are included under the broad heading of autistic disorder. For instance we, and others, have preliminary evidence from prospective longitudinal studies that, even though many children with the fragile-X-syndrome and tuberous sclerosis fulfill criteria for autistic disorders (and thus share many clinical features), they also show fundamental differences. Finding overall unifying features in autism will remain important for screening purposes, but differentiation as regards early symptoms according to underlying etiology will become crucial to the understanding of brain-behaviour-developmental relationships.

REFERENCES

American Psychiatric Association (1987). *Diagnostical and Statistical Manual of Mental Disorders. DSM-III-R. (3rd revised ed.).* Washington, D C: Author.

Dahlgren, S-O., & Gillberg, C. (1989). Symptoms in the First Two Years of Life. A Preliminary Population Study of Infantile Autism. *European Archives of Psychiatric and Neurological Sciences, 386,* 1 - 6.

Gillberg, C. (1981). Infantile autism - fact and fiction. *Läkartidningen 48,* 4373 - 4376 (In Swedish. Summary in English).

Gillberg, C. (1989). Asperger syndrome in 23 Swedish children: a clinical study. *Developmental Medicine and Child Neuorology, 31,* 520 - 531.

Gillberg, C. (1985). Early disturbances of social interactions - screening and diagnosis. *Läkartidningen 82,* 37 - 41 (In Swedish. Summary in English).

Gillberg, C., Ehlers, S., Lindblom, R., Bågenholm, A., Schaumann, H., Tjus, T., Dahlgren, S-O., & Blidner, E. (1989). Autism under age three years (submitted for publication).

Heller, T. (1930). Über dementia infantilis. *Zeitschrift für Kinderforschung, 37,* 661 - 667.

Ornitz, E., Guthrie, D., & Farley, A. J. (1978). The Early Symptoms of Childhood Autism. In Serban, G. (Ed.), *Cognitive defects in the development of mental illness.* New York: Brunner/Mazel, Inc.

Ornitz, E. (1988). Autism: A Disorder of Directed Attention. *Brain Dysfunction, 1,* 309 - 322.

Polan C. G., & Spencer B. L. (1959). A check list of symptoms of autism in early life. *West Virigina Medical Journal, 55,* 198 - 204.

Prior, M. R., & Gajzago, C. (1974). Recognition of early signs of autism. *Medical Journal of Australia, 3,* 183.

Rosenthal, I., Massic, H., & Wulff, K. (1980). A comparison of cognitive development in normal and psychotic children in the first two years of life from home movies. *Journal of Autism and Developmental Disorders, 10,* 433 - 444.

Rutter, M. (1978). Diagnosis and definition of childhood autism. *Journal of Autism and Childhood Schizophrenia, 8,* 139 - 161.

Sauvage, D., Hameury, L., Adrien, J. L., Larmande, C., Perrot - Beaugerie, A., Barthélémy, C., & Peyraud, A. (1987). Signes d'autisme avant deux ans. Evaluation et signification. *Annales de Psychiatrie, 2,* 338 - 350.

Sauvage, D., Faure, J. L., Adrien, J. L., Hameury, L., Barthélémy, C., & Perrot, A. (1988). Autisme et films familiaux. *Annales de Psychiatrie, 3,* 418 - 424.

Schopler, E. (1985). Convergence of learning disability, higher - level autism and Asperger's syndrome. *Journal of Autism and Developmental Disorders, 15,* 359 - 360.

Short, A. B, & Schopler, E. (1988). Factors Relating to Age of Onset in Autism. *Journal of Autism and Developmental Disorders, 18,* 207 - 216.

Suqiama, T., & Abe, T. (1989). The Prevalence of Autism in Nagoya, Japan: A Total Population Study. *Journal of Autism and Developemental Disorders, 19,* 87 - 96.

Volkmar, F. R., Cohen, D. J., & Paul, R. (1986). An evaluation of DSM-III criteria for infantile autism. *Journal of the American Academy of Child Psychiatry, 25,* 190 - 197.

Watkins, J. M., Asarnow, R. F., & Tanguay, P. R. (1988). Symptom development in childhood onset schizophrenia. *Journal of Child Psychology and Psychiatry, 29,* 865 - 878.

Wing, L. (1971). Perceptual and language development in autistic children: a comparative study. In M Rutter (Ed.), *Infantile Autism: Concepts, Characteristics and Treatment* (pp 173 - 197). London: Churchill-Livingstone.

Wing, L. (1980). *Early childhood autism. 2nd ed.* L Wing (Ed.), Oxford: Pergamon Press.

World Health Organization. (1987). ICD-10:1986 Draft of Chapter V, Categories F00-F99 Mental, Behavioural and Developmental Disorders. Geneva: Author.

Autism and "Theory of Mind"

UTA FRITH

Research is a painfully slow process, but from time to time there is a breathtaking acceleration. After many years of experimentation we have suddenly found a window through which we can glimpse a new view of autism. This new view is little explored as yet, but it has come to be known by the catch phrase "theory of mind". Finding the window was not sheer luck however. We were led towards it by a number of converging paths.

It all started with the idea that a developmental disorder such as autism could be caused by a specific cognitive dysfunction (Hermelin & O'Connor, 1970). This idea is an enormous advance on motivational explanations which essentially are along the lines of "autistic children COULD if they WOULD". The question "Why won't they?" has to be asked as well. One obvious answer, namely, if something is hard for you to do then you probably avoid doing it, - leads us straight back again to consider cognitive problems. Cognitive psychology provides models for analyzing what people can do into component processes. Some of these components are innate devices designed to make life easy. Clearly, if certain biological problems occur, one or more of these components might become faulty. By means of carefully designed experiments it should be possible to pinpoint such faulty components. In this way we can explain why some individuals can not do certain things, or can learn them only in a roundabout way and with great effort. In the case of autism we hope to find out which components, with which dysfunctions, are responsible for distorted development, and result in the observable symptoms.

By the Eighties many researchers had come to realize that the experimental study of basic psychological abilities such as language, memory, and perceptions - while extremely interesting and important -, would not result in an explanation of the social-affective problems that are so central to the syndrome of autism (e. g. Fein et al., 1986). Poor language, poor memory, and poor perceptions could all contribute to general social impairment. However, this would be equally true for children who suffer from mental retardation without autism. The question had to be asked afresh: what is it that we need to explain in autism?

One way out of the dilemma was to study more directly the emotions of autistic children. After all, Kanner suggested originally that autism is a disturbance of affective contact. This way was taken by Peter Hobson for instance, who found that autistic children were noteably impaired in their recognition to the emotional content of faces, gestures and voices (Hobson, 1986a, 1986b). Another solution was to study in detail the difficulties in verbal and nonverbal language in order to define more precisely what makes communication so peculiar in autistic individuals of all abilities. This line of research was pursued, for instance by Baltaxe (1977) but has since stimulated many other investigators as well. As a result we now have an increasing body of empirical facts about pragmatics deficits in autistic children. Yet a third approach was the detailed study of the social interaction of autistic children. There was an obvious need to identify what makes their affective contact so abnormal in ordinary social situations. Investigators such as Sigman and her colleagues (1986, 1987) looked at the quality of social interaction in very young autistic children, and found highly specific difficulties in shared attention behaviour. For instance, autistic children are much less likely than other children to spontaneously bring or show a toy to another person.

The burgeoning work on the social and affective problems in autistic children has extended our knowledge into previously uncharted domains. However, it was not from here that the impetus came for focussing on "theory of mind". True, we now knew better WHAT it was that needed to be explained, but we were no further in HOW to explain it. Cognitive psychology had provided tools, but only now was it ready to provide a detailed enough framework for progress in theorizing. In many areas including animal psychology, psycholinguistics, and developmental psychology, theories were being proposed, not just about the classical problems of these subjects, but about the phenomenon of theory-building itself.

It was long apparent to cognitive psychologists that the knowledge and skills that intelligent beings aquire depend on structures and systems in the mind, which must to some extent be innate. These systems facilitate learning and organize what has been learned in such a way that knowledge can applied flexibly. Karmiloff-Smith (1988) in a recent review of her work gives many examples of children's theorizing. They have firm ideas, for instance, about mechanics when attempting to balance blocks, but also about syntactic structures. Thus, young children make such intriguing mistakes as "he goed" instead of "he went", presumably because they realize that there is a rule for forming the past tense (verb plus -ed). Furthermore, Karmiloff-Smith showed that the force of theory is such that children ignore data that do not fit (the parent saying "he went"), or even invent data that do not exist. By means of a theory children can relate new and old facts and generalize from one piece of learning to other pieces. These theories are often primitive, but they are working systems and capable of being modified and developed just like scientific theories.

When Carey (1985) summarized her work on children's spontaneous concepts concerning people, animals, and living things in general, she concluded that by age ten children have reasonably adult-like theories of a (naive) biology. However, astonishingly, already by age 5, they have explicit theories of a (naive) psychology. They think and talk about state of mind, and show great propensity to explain behaviour in terms of underlying intentions. The precocious preference for psychologizing is amply documented in a recent review by Miller and Aloise (1989). As adults too we like to explain what other people do, what animals do, and even what machines do in terms of psychological motives. We find ourselves shouting at stupid computers and accuse machines of being "against us". Of course, the attribution of intentions to machines is only an occasional lapse, a misguided application of an activity that is pervasive and fundamental in all our social interactions. There is no doubt that we use an elaborate folk psychology of mental activities (Rips & Conrad, 1989).

Ironically, the interest in theory of mind originated not from human psychology, but from the study of primate intelligence. In 1978 Premack and Woodruff published a groundbreaking paper which was entitled "does the chimpanzee have a theory of mind?". Some of the most fascinating work that was reported in this paper explored a very "human" characteristic, namely the ability to deceive. The evidence presented was based on ingenious experiments where animals learned to recognize keepers acting as "goodies" and "baddies". The question was whether the animals would go as far as actively helping the goodie and hindering the baddie at critical moments. Would they for instance be able to work out whether the baddie knew that a closed box contained food? Could he be deceived? In order to deceive someone successfully one must take into account what this person knows or does not know. This is precisely what a theory of mind allows one to do.

A theory of mind allows one to "mind-read". That is, one can infer somebody's mental state on the basis of such intangible, yet everyday notions as BELIEFS and WISHES. Obviously, we are not always successful in our naive psychologizing. Indeed, we often do injustice to others by imputing wrong motives, and we can misinterpret our own motives too. However, the differences between successful and unsuccessful "mentalazing", to use a term coined by John Morton (1986), are negligible when we consider the opposite, namely trying to explain somebody else's behaviour on the basis of a (physical) state of affairs. Let us consider an example: Claire reluctantly cancels an appointment and decides to stay at home on Monday "because of the bus strike". Does this explanation imply that we believe the bus strike is physically responsible for Claire's behaviour? Surely not, by any reasonable notion of physical causes and effects. In fact, the phrase is only shorthand for inferences that are based on very active mentalizing. Claire's decision is explained by the fact that she BELIEVED that there would be a strike and by the fact that she WANTED to avoid being stuck in traffic jams. This explanation has nothing to do with the physical state of affairs in the world. It is independent of whether of not there actually is a strike. Our explanation of Claire's decision to stay at home is an example of mind-reading and it still holds even when unbeknown to Claire the strike is unexpectedly cancelled.

The philosopher Dennet (1978) in a commentary on Premack and Woodruff's paper pointed out that the acid test for the existence of a "theory of mind" in primate as well as in man would be to demonstrate attribution of a false belief. Claire's belief that there is a strike when in fact it has unexpectedly been cancelled is a false belief. Reality and mental representation of reality diverge. This does not disturb us. On the contrary, we now have the basis for considering a "psychological" test question: Will Claire's friend Linda (the one she was going to meet for lunch), who has privileged information that the strike will be cancelled, telephone her to tell her about it? If she does, then we can explain why: Linda very much wants to see Claire. She is also aware of Claire's now wrong belief and of the consequences. She can on this basis infer that Claire would stay at home unnecessarily. Therefore Linda will inform Claire. This complicated reasoning is not only made possible, but made childlishly easy by the existence of a theory of mind. Given this theory, mental states such as beliefs are kept track of when circumstances change and are taken into account when we predict and explain behaviour.

While the debate continued whether or not chimpanzees have a theory of mind, Wimmer and Perner (1983) asked at what age young humans first show incontrovertible evidence of such a theory. They divised a well controlled paradigm using a story that could be acted out with puppets. Using the acid test that requires attribution of a false belief they found this to be beyond the competence of children under the age of three. However, from about four ALL children became highly competent at predicting behaviour on the basis of a false belief and, furthermore, between age 6 and 8, they started to show the ability to take account of a belief about a false belief (Perner & Wimmer, 1985). It is a small step from here to a fully developed theory of mind that allows us to understand such convoluted problems as: "Plain, chubby Pat is secretely in love with David - whom she treats brusquely - and who thinks he is in love with beautiful but feckless Laura"; or, "MI5 agent 007 gets the false message that his partner has defected to the other side and consequently thinks that the enemy will now know his secret identity". It is readily apparent that such problems, far from being comprehensible only to the sophisticated few, are the stuff of soap operas and popular novels.

It was Wimmer and Perner's (1983) paper that arrived on my desk after I had been wondering for some time how to apply the new insights of Premack and his colleagues to the study of autistic children. I had been wondering because a very striking characteristic of normally intelligent autistic individuals is their inability to deceive and their disarming innocence in social encounters. Now, suddenly, there was a paradigm that could be applied to study autistic children with a view to investigate their understanding of such commonplace social skills as lying, teasing and flattering, all of which seem to be outside their competence. It seemed to me at the time that autistic children with a mental age of three and above should easily pass Wimmer and Perner's false belief test. On the other hand I expected difficulties even for the most able children when it came to more complex and sophisticated test problems. The idea then was simply to see to what extent mental retardation alone, rather than autism, could explain the social naivety of autistic people. For this reason, clearly, other handicapped children who were not autistic, had to be tested, as well as young normal and autistic children. Down's syndrome children were an obvious control group.

At exactly this time two very fortunate things happened. The first was that Simon Baron-Cohen had just embarked on his Ph. D. thesis with a view of studying autistic children's understanding of self. He was immediately enthusiastic about carrying out the Wimmer and Perner experiment, slightly adapted, with autistic, normal and Down's syndrome children. He proved an excellent experimenter and collected the truly startling results that able and older autistic children failed the simple false belief task that three- to four-year olds and Down's syndrome children passed with ease. My own skeptiscism was such that I had to witness the experiment before I fully believed it!

The second fortunate thing was the formidable theoretical input of Alan Leslie who just then was formulating a first sketch of a new cognitive developmental theory. Alan Leslie's interest in autism was captured by the regular discussions in our Unit seminars that were led by John Morton. Here the topic of autism was considered from many different viewpoints, the cognitive, the neuropsychological, the developmental and the linguistic. Now, what really caught Alan Leslie's imagination was the constellation of some typical but hitherto not especially prominent features of autism: the lack of pretend play, the lack of irony and the lack of deception. It was exactly these sorts of abilities that he had wished to link together in normal development. The possibility that all of them might be specifically impaired led him to apply his theory to autism. For a start, the failure of autistic children on the false belief task could actually be predicted from the theory.

Meanwhile, in a different discipline, namely linguistics, an exciting cognitive theory was being developed by Dan Sperber and Deidre Wilson (1986). This theory, the theory of relevance, attempts to explain how human communications is possible. Since autism is universally associated with a disorder of communication, and since limited and literal understanding is a major symptom, relevance theory has obvious application to autism. Relevance theory takes as a starting point the idea that normal cognitive processes are amenable to a cost/benefit analysis. The underlying mental mechanisms are tuned in such a way that they seek to obtain the greatest possible effect at the lowest possible cost. This principle can account for the fact, inexplicable from any other point of view, that we can understand what people "really" mean when they talk to us or give us some nonverbal sign. In order to comprehand the full intended meaning of an utterance, - not just its literal meaning-, the theory proposes that the listener must, amongst other things, compute the speaker's intention. A deliberate sideways glance, for example, means quite different things in different contexts which apparently we have no trouble interpreting. Intention is of course a classic example of a mental state, and clearly, mental state computation is a vital part of the comprehension process. There is then a close link to theory of mind since inferences about speaker's and listener's mental states are vital components in the explanation of successful communication.

With these contemporary developments in related but different disciplines and with this constellation of co-workers one can indeed speak of good fortune. Thus, a whole chain of coinciding circumstances led to the new approach to autism. But, is it really justified to talk about the work on theory of mind in autism as a new approach, as a new point of view that is beginning to change our understanding of this disorder? In order to answer this question it will be necessary to take stock of the main experiments and to see what exactly they allow us to conclude. I shall therefore describe briefly the experiment that originated with Wimmer and Perner's paradigm and then summarize some other experiments that arose from the application of Leslie's meta-representational theory. This theory is descirbed fully elsewhere (Leslie, 1987, 1988a, b; Leslie & Frith, in press). Suffice it to say that meta-representations concern the ability to distance ourselves from our own perceptions and memories. This distancing is achieved by forming a new layer of second-order representations that themselves represent first-order representations. The difference is equivalent to one of "perceiving something" and of "knowing that one is perceiving something".

Second-order representations are crucial for imagination and pretense, for sophisticated social relationships that require a theory of mind, and also for understanding the intention behind every communication. Therefore, if there is a failure in forming and using meta-representations there would also be a failure in imaginative activities, in two-way social interaction and in verbal and non-verbal communication. This constellation of problem areas is, of course, Wing's (1988a; 1988b) triad of impairments. It is this triad which alone is common to the whole spectrum of autistic disorders and discriminates socially impaired from socially unimpaired handicapped children (Wing & Gould, 1979). There is reason to suppose that the ability to form meta-representations comes about because there is an innate cognitve mechanism available precisely for this purpose. If this mechanism were linked to a specific brain process, then we could hypothesize that a circumscribed abnormality in the operation of just this process is responsible for the triad of impairments. This would be a way of linking a biological cause via a cognitive process to the behavioural symptoms of autism (Frith, 1988).

The breakthrough then consists not in demonstrating yet another deficit in autistic children, however interesting, but rather it consists in providing a link between previously unconnected impairments and in suggesting a specific dysfunction in a single mechanism. Over and above these theoretically important advances there is also an advance in our understanding of the social-affective and communicative disturbances which are so evident to anyone who is in close contact with an autistic individual. The concept of theory of mind enables us to see autism as a kind of blindness, a mind-blindness, that is, an inability to conceive of states of mind and of mind itself. On the other hand, the concept also enables us to understand our own propensity to believe that our mental states self-evidently explain our behaviour. How did this propensity come about and why is it there? These questions are yet to be answered, but a start has been made. Many fascinating ideas from human and animal psychology have recently been put together in a volume by Byrne and Whiten (1988). Humphrey (1984) in an essay on consciousness vividly discussed what it means from an evolutionary point of view NOT to be mind-blind:

"If I ask myself WHY I am doing something, like as not my answer will be framed in conscious mental terms: I am doing it BECAUSE I am aware of this or that going on inside me. 'Why am I looking in the larder? Because I'm feeling hungry.....Why am I raising my right arm? Because I wish to .....Why am I sniffing this rose? Because I like its smell.....'." (Humphrey goes on to suggest:) "So, once upon a time there were animal ancestral to man who were not conscious. That is not to say that these animals lacked brains. They were no doubt percipient, intelligent creatures, whose internal control mechanisms were in many respects the equals of our own. But it is to say that they had no way of looking in upon this mechanism. They had clever brains but blank minds" (p. 48).

THE SALLY - ANNE EXPERIMENT

The first experiment (Baron-Cohen, Leslie & Frith, 1985) which was entitled "Does the autistic child have a theory of mind?" is itself a useful and direct illustration of what we mean by theory of mind and why the attribution of a false belief should be a critical test of having or not having the rudiments of such a theory.

It goes like this: Sally has a basket, Anne has a box. Sally puts a marble into her basket. She goes out for a walk. (Sally disappears under the table.) Now, Anne, - naughty Anne-, takes the marble out of the basket and puts it into her own box. It is time now for Sally to come back from her walk. She now wants to play with her marble. Where will Sally look for her marble? (This is the critical test question. There are then two control questions, namely, where did Sally put the marble in the first place? and, where is the marble really?).

In order to answer the critical question correctly: Sally will look in the basket -, it is necessary to keep track of Sally's mental state, not just of the real state of affairs. True, the marble is now in the box, but Sally does not know this, because she was away when the marble was hidden in the new place. Clearly, the relevant mental state of Sally is a false belief. The normal three-to-four-year-old has no difficulty in attributing a false belief to somebody else. In everyday life children often hide something and are delighted when another child looks in the old place. They know about tricking people. Of course, it is precisely this that autistic children do not do in real life. In our experiment too they behaved very differently from normal and from Down's syndrome children.

Autistic children, that is, about 80 % of the group of able children that were initially tested, systematically pointed to the wrong place. They pointed to Anne's box where the hidden object really was but not to Sally's basket where Sally must have believed it was. These children had average non-verbal mental ages of around 9 and verbal mental ages of around 5 years. Although they correctly remembered where Sally had put the marble herself, and although they fully admitted that Sally was not present when Ann hid the marble in a different place, they nevertheless expected Sally to look straightaway in the new place. When they were asked in different ways in some later experiments where real people took the part of Sally and Anne and where the marble was a coin, they performed in exactly the same way (Leslie & Frith, 1989). For instance, the question "where does Sally think the marble is?" would be answered wrongly, i. e. as if Sally had witnessed the transfer. Likewise the question "does Sally know where the marble is now?" would be answered wrongly "yes". In fact we concluded that the meaning of the words "to know" and "to believe" must be totally obscure to autistic children.

THE PICTURE-SEQUENCE EXPERIMENT

It would be dangerous to rely on one paradigm when such striking group differences are found. Also, we wanted to have a method which did not rely so heavily on comprehending the critical test question. There was another point that we wished to clarify. Was it the case that autistic children simply failed to put together certain facts in a logical order so that they could not draw the correct inference? "If Sally did not see the transfer then she could not know about it" is the kind of inference that has to be made quite apart from understanding belief.

Clearly, if we wish to show that it is the concept of belief that is truly the cause of the difficulty, then we must rule out problems with logical inference. We attempted to do this by producing certain control conditions. We made up picture sequences that hang together by virtue of the protagonist's mental state (very much like the Sally - Anne story), and we compared these with picture sequences that hang together by virtue of mechanical-physical causes, as well as those which hang together by virtue of being well known social routines. The task and materials are described fully in Baron-Cohen et al. (1986).

Essentially, the task was to put the four pictures of each story into the correct order "so as to make a story". The first picture was put into place and the remaining three were ostentatiously mixed up. The child then had to complete the sequence in the correct order and afterwards was asked to "tell the story".

The average number of correct placements in sequence proved to be a sensitive measure. The result of interest is that autistic children had almost 100 % success with mechanical-causal sequences, but only chance success with mental-state sequences. With normal 5-year old control children the pattern was quite the opposite, and their best performance was with mental state stories. We can now hypothesize that the failure of autistic children with the concept of mental states is specific in the sense that the failure is not due to general problems with logical inference. After all, inferences had to be drawn in those conditions too where mental state attribution was not involved and where autistic children excelled.

This claim is strengthened by the results from the way that the children told the story after they had put the pictures in order. Wordings with mental state terms (e. g., know, think, believe) were used rarely by autistic children, that is, there were instances of such terms in only about 20 % of the narratives, while there were instances in about 80 % of the narratives of young normal and Down's syndrome children. On the other hand, autistic children's wordings for the mechanical-causal stories were often sophisticated enough to include phrases (e. g. because, made happen).

THE SMARTIES TUBE EXPERIMENT

Josef Perner who originally devised the false-belief paradigm on which the Sally - Anne experiment was based, contributed another strikingly simple paradigm in which the child has to attribute a false belief to himself as well as to another person. It was our good fortune yet again that a collaboration was possible (Perner, Frith, Leslie & Leekam, in press). The Smartie-tube experiment is based on the fact that British children are very familiar with the typical colour, shape, and presentation of a well known brand of sweets. Indeed, when shown a smarties tube all children we asked, including the autistic ones, said it contained "smarties" or "sweets". After this question the experimenter opened the tube to reveal that it contained only an uninteresting little pencil. The lid was put back, and the child was asked again what the tube contained ("a pencil"). Now, a little incident was staged where the second experimenter appeared announcing that the next child was ready to be tested. At this point the child was told: Your friend (Johnny) will be next. He hasn't seen this box. When he comes in, I will take out the box just like this and ask: what's in there? What will Johnny say?

The answer - taking into account Johnny's ignorance - has to be "smarties" or "sweets". However, the answer produced by the majority of autistic children was "a pencil". This answer reflects their own knowledge and it also reflects reality. However it does not make allowances for somebody else's state of knowledge. Again, we must conclude that autistic children behave as if they did not take account of mental states in their inferences and therefore it can be said that they do not possess or make use of a theory of mind.

THE NODDING AND FLAPPING BEE EXPERIMENT

In this experiment, also described by Perner et al. (in press), we asked the question whether autistic children would provide a missing piece of information which they knew about but somebody else did not. It needs a theory of mind in order to compute the right thing to say. In accordance with the principle of relevance it would be wrong to impart information that the other person has alrady. The experiment revolved around the demonstration of a fairly interesting and novel toy, a mechanical bee. The bee could perform two separate actions: to flap its wings and to nod its head. The experimenter introduced the toy to the child and to a second experimenter who purported to be very interested to learn "what the bee can do". The first experiment demonstrated the bee flapping its wings. Naturally, this was greeted with the appropriate delight by the second experimenter, if not by the child. The first experimenter then began to talk of "another thing" the bee could do. At exactly this point the second experimenter left the room, on a pretext, saying "wait for me, I'll be back in a minute". The first experimenter however did not wait and immediately proceded to show the second action, namely, how the bee nodded its head. Now, the second experimenter returned and realizing that she had come too late, turned directly to the child and asked "what can the bee do?"

The pragmatically correct answer which is given by normal children aged 3 to 4 is to mention the actions which the questioner had missed. The child might mention both actions, of course, but the nodding action which is the one the questioner really wants to know about (inferred on the grounds that she has not seen it) should be mentioned first. We tried a number of different situations with different toys and different types of missing information so as to rule out chance results. What we found in autistic children was highly unreliable responding. That is, on one trial it might seem that they properly supplied the missing information, on another trial they repeated the information that was already known. In fact, this pattern suggests that their replies to the question were not systematically guided by considering the questioner's mental state.

WHAT THEORY OF MIND MEANS FOR COMMUNICATION

The experiment with the nodding and flapping bee provides a link between lack of theory of mind and the particular failure to communicate in autistic individuals. The failure to communicate in autistic children is by no means a total failure. After all, autistic people readily answer questions to which they know the answer, and furthermore there are those who willingly relate every detail concerning their special interests. We can now be more specific about the nature of the communication failure that is so characteristic of even able autistic individuals.

Communication in the full sense involves taking account of mental states. In the example of the mechanical bee demonstration, the communication required involves taking account of what the questioner already knew and what she did not know about. To be relevant the answer had to provide the information that the questioner did not have. Take the example of the ordinary question "can you tell me the time?" The relevant answer here is not "yes, I can", but rather "the time is.....". We know what to say because we are automatically guided by the principle of relevance. In other words, we compute that the questioner wants to know the time and that is why he is asking. We rule out the possibility that the questioner already knows the time. So, if he replied to our statement of the time "but I just wanted to know if you could tell me the time", we would treat it as a joke.

In the case of an autistic person such involuntary "jokes" can occur quite often and they can go both ways, because the conversation partner of an autistic person often has quite the wrong idea about what he is asked and what he is told about. John, on his first school camp, was supervised taking a shower and was told "not put the shampoo on your head". Result: He took the bottle and balanced it on his head! Instead of the smooth working of the principle of relevance, there are constant hitches which reveal on later analysis that communication was not based on shared assumptions. An autistic boy at his first meeting her asked the speech therapist, Maureen Aarons: "Do you notice something different about me?" It turned out that this question referred to the fact that he recently had a haircut. Of course, such a question is quite inappropriate to ask a person who has never seen him before. This kind of error can make one realize just how different the mind of a bright autistic child is from that of a normal child.

While novel information is not spontaneously supplied by the autistic person, old information is unnecessarily repeated. The first point has the practical consequence that one should not rely on the autistic person conveying important information but instead check systematically. It would be wise to assume that autistic people behave unconsciously as if everybody knew just the same as they themselves know, and as if what people knew was just a mirror of the world outside. Such an expectation would have been helpful in the smarties experiment to explain why the child responds as if he believed that the next child KNEW that there was a pencil in the box. The second point has the practical consequence that one can better understand why autistic people often engage in extremely boring, repetitive talk. This is because they do not take into account that the partner already has the information, and that ordinarily, - on the principle of relevance -, one would not trouble each other to convey the same thing again. Showing boredom is therefore not sufficient to stop the monologue and more direct means are required. The analysis of language and communication competence in autism provides many examples that can be explained in the framework of Sperber and Wilson's theory of relevance (see Frith, 1989b).

The nonverbal behaviour of autistic children too is capable of being analysed in terms of its communicative competence. Attwood, Frith and Hermelin (1988) reported an experimental and observational study of autistic children's manual gestures. It was found in this investigation that autistic children were well able to understand and to spontaneously produce instrumental gesture. These are gestures such as "go away", "be quiet", or "look up". The object of the communication is to affect a direct change in behaviour.

Quite different are expressive gestures. These convey for instance such messages as "I am embarrassed" or "I love you". The object of expressive gestures is not so much to affect a change in behaviour but to affect a change in mental state. Primarily, however, they express a mental state and they express this state, a feeling about something or somebody, quite deliberately. In this way they are very different from instrumental gestures and also from unintentional give-away body language. If autistic children lack a theory of mind they should not show deliberately expressive gestures. This was precisely what we found, in strong contrast to Down's syndrome children. The study of gestures therefore underlines the statement that autistic children show a failure of communication when and only when, mental states are the object of communication. They do not seem to have a wish to communication just for the sake of conveying a mental state, or manipulating somebody else's mental state. They show perfect ability and motivation to communicate if it is for an instrumental purpose.

As partners of autistic people we would do well to adapt our everyday theory of mind for the special case of the mind of the autistic individual. We might for instance set up the expectation that autistic people behave on the basis that their own mental state is a shared mental state. If there are no differences between different people's mental states, then the wish to communicate would be reduced. However, it is important to remember that autistic people do not really behave on this basis, because this would imply an awareness of mental states. One can only make the assumption that mental states are shared, consciously or unconsciously, when one has a concept of mental states. The experimental evidence makes this very doubtful for autistic people. Rather, it seems that their lack of theory of mind does not even let them consider that mental states exist, let alone that they may be shared. My suggestion of adaption is strictly for practical purposes, but I think we can more easily adapt our own theory of mind for our interaction with autistic individuals, than train them to form a flexible theory of mind of their own.

WHAT THEORY OF MIND MEANS FOR SOCIAL-EMOTIONAL EXPERIENCES

It is useful to have an illustration of how attributing beliefs to others is an automatic and emotionally significant activity. It is a very common activity in our daily life, for instance when we consider whether we upset someone by being late for an appointment, or whether we let someone else know that we feel upset. But it is also basic to our understanding of plays, novels and films.

A scene in a well known Hollywood comedy illustrates the importance of attributions of beliefs in general and the appreciation of different beliefs in particular. The scene is an opulent drawing room. We see a portrait of an old lady hanging over the fireplace. We witness this portrait being replaced by the picture of a giant white rabbit. The lady of the house and a visitor, - who is a psychiatrist -, now walk into the room.

The psychiatrist sees the picture, and, sure enough, he asks the lady who the picture represents. The lady without looking at the picture answers that it is a portrait of her mother. Naturally a ridiculous conversation ensues.

The audience of the film appreciates that the lady believes, falsely, that the old portrait is still in place and that the psychiatrist does not know that there previously WAS a portrait of the mother. The comedy depends on recognizing these different beliefs and computing their consequences.

Imagine what it is like not having any clear idea of such everyday concepts as knowing, thinking, and believing. What would it be like without such concepts such as wishing, imaging, feeling, wanting, remembering, and perceiving? So far, we have empirically investigated only knowing and believing and we can say that a conscious awareness of these mental states in themselves or in others cannot be taken for granted in autistic children. It is likely that other mental states too will not be a part of their conscious experience. Of course, there is no doubt that autistic children HAVE mental states. What is in doubt is that they know that they have them.

The most concise way of describing the social-affective disturbance of autistic individuals is to say that they lack empathy. This is readily seen as an outcome of lack of theory of mind. Lack of empathy essentially consists in not taking into account somebody else's reactions and feelings to emotionally significant events. We can now see a reason for this disturbing symptom. The reason quite clearly is not "coldness" or emotional flatness, or some motivational failure, but not having a proper concept of emotions in the first place. An analogue to blindness would be closer than an analogue to emotional disorder. While normally we "read" the mind of others and can often accurately predict how they will react and behave, the autistic person cannot "mind-read" in this sense.

Voice, gesture, eye gaze, facial expressions and the wider context of similar experiences are ordinarily cues that are meaningful to us because we can interpret them in terms of their relevance to mental states. In the case of autistic children, Hobson (1986a, b), showed that there is a surprising degree of impairment in the identification of emotional expressions. From the point of veiw of a primary inability to conceive of mental states including emotions, this is only to be expected. However, the cognitive dysfunction hypothesis allows us to predict further: if autistic individuals were taught the meaning of the various cues (smile is happy etc.) then they would still be unable to understand why people often hide their true emotions and, for instance, smile when they are not happy. In normal social interaction we take non-verbal cues no more literally then we do verbal messages. It would be difficult to see how this distinction could be successfully maintained without taking into account a great deal of context, and without a working theory of mind.

It would now also be possible to answer some difficult questions concerning the moral development of autistic children and their ability to judge right and wrong. If they lack a theory of mind it should be very difficult for them to make any judgements that take into account intent. They should not understand "malice aforethought", nor "but she only meant well". One would expect that autistic people would judge a misdeed on the basis of its immediate effect, rather than on the basis of its motive. Deception would not be understood nor, presumably, would the opposite, namely the good intention behind an accidental mishap. This area has not yet been tackled by research, but clearly it should prove a useful way of testing predictions from the point of view of theory of mind.

One important development of the notion of theory of mind which has not yet been tackled is the child's awareness of self. Self-consciousness can readily be seen as an outcome of awareness of mind. There is no reason to distinguish the ability to reflect on other people's mental states and on our own. This reflective ability is self-awareness in the case when we consider our own states of mind. To know that we know and to think about our own thinking are accomplishments that presuppose higher order processing ability. Here it is not enough to represent in the mind what is going on in the outside world, but we must also represent the fact that we can represent the world. We can paraphrase Descartes' famous dictum "I think therefore I am" in the following much less elegant way: "I know that I think therefore there is my self".

According to our hypothesis it would follow that the autistic person would have a different and non-reflective sense of self. This self would presumably include an awareness of self as a bodily object, but it might not include an awareness of self as a mental subject.

One important consequence which, at first sight is not obvious, would be devastating failure of a specific type of memory. One would not expect a failure of all kinds of memory, but only of that type of memory that involves a representation of oneself having had the experience, at a particular time in a particular place. Perner (in press) points out the importance of this type of memory in the development of experiential awareness and relates it to Tulving's (1985) concept of autonoetic, that is, self-conscious, memory. According to Tulving it is one thing to retrieve stored facts by means of searching through associations, and another to retrieve them by means of reviewing one's personal experience. In one case one may recall, for instance, that Verona is a town in northern Italy, with a Roman arena, in the other case, one may recall having been to Verona in the blazing hot sun and thinking about visiting the arena. Perner, however, makes a further distinction. He emphasizes that it is crucial to distinguish between memory for personally experienced events (usually called episodic memory) and memory for the personal experience of the event. The classic literary treatment of personal experience remembered must surely be Proust's remembrance of things past. In his famous madeleine episode, Proust expresses the experience of the experience of the remembered event.

Following the logic of the argument that autism leads to a failure in self-consciousness we can hypothesize that autistic individuals would show problems with autonoetic memory. Although this hypothesis has yet to be tested, Boucher and Lewis (1989) report some intriguing results which would support it: Very able autistic children, while being able to recall story detail very well, failed strikingly when asked "what did you do when you came to see me?" The difference can be explained if we assume that recalling such episodes in one's past normally depends on having coded the event as a personal experience and recalling the personal experience of the event. This coding may be facilitated by having available a second order representation of one's own mental state at the time the memory was formed.

METAREPRESENTATION AND THEORY OF MIND

Weakness or absence of a theory of mind can explain very precisely the many diverse behavioural symptoms of autism that concern social-emotional failure and communication failure and I have explored these explanations and their practical consequences at some length (Frith, 1989a). However, we need to explain the absence of a theory of mind as well.

At the beginning of this paper I have talked of various strands from different research areas that contributed crucially to our new understanding of autism. The strand that I have left until last is probably the most important. It is Alan Leslie's developmental theory of first- and second-order representations. This theory made it possible to suggest an explanation of autistic children's failure to form and use a theory of mind. It also suggests an explanation for autistic children's failure in imaginative pretend play (Baron-Cohen, 1987).

Briefly, first-order representations are what the mind makes of real states in the world, and second-order representations are what the mind makes of these first-order representations. Second-order representations are therefore one step removed from reality and can be held concurrently with first-order representations. In this way there is no contradiction between realizing that at cup is empty and pretending (playfully) that it is full. Pretending that the empty cup is full is an example of a thought process that would not be possible without second-order representation.

The single and innate mechanism that according to Leslie is the essential prerequisite to the development of the capacity to form second-order representations is the decoupling of first-order representations from their relationship with the real world. Once first-order representations are decoupled, they are free to be used in all sorts of ways and to become the subject matter of our inner experience. It is conceivable that the decoupling mechanism is faulty and that this is the component we have been looking for in order to explain the specifically abnormal social-emotional and communicative developement of autistic children.

Leslie's theory not only predicted the failure of theory of mind tasks, such as the Sally - Anne test, which otherwise was totally unexpected, but it also accounted for autistic children's failure to follow imaginative plots in fiction. Forming and using a theory of mind depends not just on the experience of people and what they do, but crucially depends on an awareness of mental states. An awareness of mental states can only be achieved by using second-order representations. In this way a real state of affairs (the marble is in the box) is not contradictory to Sally's belief (the marble is in the basket). The theory also accounts for autistic children's literalness, e. g., their failure to understand and use irony. Here again, a statement such as "you are in good shape today" does not contradict the stated knowledge that the person addressed actually has a hangover and is consequently in particularly poor shape. In all these examples it can be seen that second-order representations are a powerful tool to deal with potentially contradictory information.

Let us briefly consider what is involved in understanding that somebody is pretending a cup is full and teddy can sip tea from it. It is not a true state of affairs, but a state in somebody's imagination. Looked at in this way understanding pretence involves taking account of mental states and it is indeed remarkable that all normal two-year-olds comprehand when others are pretending. It is perhaps less remarkable that this capacity flowers into a full theory of mind which allows the child to manipulate and no doubt take advantage of other people's attitudes, beliefs and feelings about things.

Perhaps the first evidence of a primitive theory of mind is even earlier than we thought so far. It is possible that the "shared attention" behaviour shown already by some children when under one year of age presupposes some awareness of another person's mental state: When the child looks towards the mother for no apparent reason and gives her a beaming smile, it could well be that he does it "just" to show her his affection. This would be an example of a deliberately expressive gesture. If this was so, then the lack of "shared attention" behaviour in young autistic children, as observed for instance by Sigman and her colleagues (reviewed in 1987), would fall into place: we might be able to identify it as the very first reliable symptom of autism, a first sign of "mind-reading" failure.

A fault in the decoupling mechanism would be a very simple explanation of the "cause" of the triad of impairments. In reality however, matters are rarely simple. There are many other ways in which metarepresentational ability could be inefficient, weak or faulty. There is the strong possibility that we must distinguish between degrees of failure. This would enable us to account for the clinical phenomenon that autism can apparently be mild in some people and severe in others. Yet another hypothesis to be considered is that the failure that underlies the triad of impairments is due simply to excessive developmental delay. If this were the case, we could explain why a minority of older and highly able autistic children seem to be able to understand pretence (Lewis & Boucher, 1989), and false belief (Baron-Cohen, 1989). It is possible that these individuals have acquired the ability to form and use second-order representations at a late age. Nevertheless, the period in development has passed for this ability to have its proper impact on the potential formation of a theory of mind.

There is clearly a great deal of work to be done before we can decide between these and other options. Nevertheless the outlook is good, because the theory is at the same time strong enough to be falsified by empirical data and flexibel enough to be modified as more information becomes available. What is particularly exciting is that for the first time we can offer an hypothesis about cognitive dysfunction that is capable of being linked to an hypothesis about brain dysfunction. While we cannot map specific behaviour directly onto brain processes, we believe we can map behaviour onto deeply underlying cognitive processes. The idea of an identifiable biological mechanism that must be faulty in autism is no longer remote given that there is an identifiable cognitive mechanism that we can recognize as faulty. It will only be a matter of time before such techniques as PET-scanning can be applied while the subject is engaged in specially designed "theory of mind" tasks. When this happens we might see which brain areas are most active when the mind is engaged in thinking about thinking. In this mind-boggling mirror we might gain not only more understanding about autism, but we might also gain more understanding about ourselves.

ACKNOWLEDGEMENTS

I would like to thank Chris Frith, Alan Leslie, Francesca Happe and Simon Baron-Cohen for their critical reading of this chapter and for their helpful suggestions.

REFERENCES

Attwood, A., Frith, U., & Hermelin, B. (1988). The understanding and use of interpersonal gestures by autistic and Down's Syndrome children. *Journal of Autism and Developmental Disorders, 18,* 241-257.

Baltaxe, C. A. M. (1977). Pragmatic deficits in the language of autistic adolescents. *Journal of Pediatric Psychology, 2,* 176-180.

Baron-Cohen, S. (1987). Autism and symbolic play. *British Journal of Developmental Psychology, 5,* 139-148.

Baron-Cohen, S. (1989). The autistic child's theory of mind: a case of specific developmental delay. *Journal of Child Psychology and Psychiatry, 30,* 285-297.

Baron-Cohen, S., Leslie, A. M., & Frith, U. (1985). Does the autistic child have a "theory of mind"? *Cognition, 21,* 37-46.

Baron-Cohen, S., Leslie, A. M., & Frith, U. (1986). Mechanical, behavioural and intentional understanding of picture stories in autistic children. *British Journal of Developmental Psychology, 4,* 113-125.

Boucher, J., & Lewis, V. (1989). Memory impairments and communication in relatively able autistic children. *Journal of Child Psychology and Psychiatry, 30,* 99 - 122.

Byrne, R., & Whiten, A. (1988). *The Machiavellian Ape.* Oxford: Oxford University Press.

Carey, S. (1985). *Conceptual change in childhood.* Cambridge, MA: MIT press.

Dennett, D. C. (1978). Belief about belief. *Behavioural and Brain Sciences, 4,* 568-570.

Fein, D., Pennington, P., Markovitz, P., Braverman, M., & Waterhouse, L. (1986). Toward a neuropsychological model of infantile autism: are the social deficits primary? *Journal of the American Academy of Child Psychiatry, 24,* 198-212.

Frith, U. (1988). Autism: possible clues to the underlying pathology: Psychological Facts. In L. Wing (Ed.), *Aspects of Autism, Biological Research.* London: Gaskell, Royal College of Psychiatrics.

Frith, U. (1989a). *Autism: Explaining the enigma.* Oxford: Blackwell.

Frith, U. (1989b). A new look at language and communication in autism. *British Journal of Disorders of Communication, 24,* 123 - 150.

Hermelin, B., & O'Connor, N. (1970). *Psychological experiments with autistic children.* Oxford: Pergamon Press.

Hobson, R. P. (1986a). The autistic child's appraisal of expressions of emotion. *Journal of Child Psychology and Psychiatry, 27,* 321-342.

Hobson, R. P. (1986b). The autistic child's appraisal of expressions of emotion: a further study. *Journal of Child Psychology and Psychiatry, 27,* 671-680.

Humphrey, N. (1984). *Consciousness Regained: Chapters in the Development of Mind.* Oxford: Oxford University Press.

Karmiloff-Smith, A. (1988). The child is a theoretician, not an inductivist. *Mind and Language, 3,* 183-195.

Leslie, A. M. (1987). Pretence and representation: the origins of "theory of mind". *Psychological Review, 94,* 412-426.

Leslie, A. M. (1988a). Some implications of pretence for mechanisms underlying the child's theory of mind. In J. Astington, P. Harris, & D. Olson (Eds.), *Developing Theories of Mind.* Cambridge: Cambridge University Press.

Leslie, A. M. (1988b). The necessity of illusion: perception and thought in infancy. In L. Weiskrantz, (Ed.), *Thought without language.* Oxford: Oxford University Press.

Leslie, A. M., & Frith, U. (1988). Autistic children's understanding of seeing, knowing and believing. *British Journal of Developmental Psychology, 4,* 315-324.

Leslie, A. M., & Frith, U. (1989). Prospects for a neuropsychology of autism: Hobson's choice. *Psychological Review* (in press).

Lewis, V., & Boucher, J. (1988). Spontaneous, instructed and elicited play in relatively able autistic children. *British Journal of Developmental Psychology, 6,* 325-339.

Miller, P. H., & Aloise, P. A. (1989). Young children's understanding of the psychological causes of behaviour: a review. *Child Development, 60,* 257 - 285.

Morton, J. (1986). Developmental continency modelling. In P. L. C. Van Geert (Ed.), *Theory Building in Developmental Psychology.* North Holland: Elsevier.

Perner, J., Frith, U., Leslie, A. M., & Leekam, S. (1989). Exploration of the autistic child's theory of mind: knowledge, belief and communication. *Child Development* (in press).

Perner, J. (1989). Experiential awareness and children's episodic memory. In W. Schneider & F. E. Weinert (Eds.), *Interactions among Aptitudes, Strategies and Knowledge in Cognitive Performance.* New York: Springer Verlag.

Rips, L. J., & Conrad, F. G. (1989). Folk psychology of mental activities. *Psychological Review, 96,* 187 - 207.

Sigman, M., Mundy, P., Sherman, T., & Ungerer, J. (1986). Social interactions of autistic, mentally retarded and normal children and their caregivers. *Journal of Child Psychology and Psychiatry, 27,* 647-656.

Sigman, M., Ungerer, J. A., Mundy, P., & Sherman, T. (1987). Cognition in autistic children. In D. J. Cohen, A. Donnellan & R. Paul (Eds.), *Handbook of Autism and Pervasive Developmental Disorders.* New York: Wiley.

Sperber, D., & Wilson, D. (1986). *Relevance: Communication and Cognition.* Oxford: Blackwell.

Tulving, E. (1985). Memory and consciousness. *Canadian Psychology, 26,* 1 - 12.

Wing, L. (1988a). The autistic continuum. In L. Wing (Ed.), *Aspects of Autism: Biological Research.* London: Gaskell and Royal College of Psychiatrics.

Wing, L. (1988b). The continuum of autistic characteristics. In E. Schopler & G. B. Mesibov (Eds.), *Diagnosis and Assessment of Autism.* New York: Plenum Press.

Wing, L., & Gould, J. (1979). Severe impairments of social interaction and associated abnormalities in children: Epidemiology and classification. *Journal of Autism and Developmental Disorders, 9,* 11-30.

Social or Cognitive or Both?
Crucial Dysfunctions in Autism

LYNN WATERHOUSE and DEBORAH FEIN

Although the word "autism" means social withdrawal, and although the syndrome of autism is defined with social withdrawal as a core deficit, the nature of social withdrawal in autism has yet to be clearly understood. What has become clear is that the social impairment is much more complex and more various than can be adequetely summed up by the behavioral label of "social withdrawal" (Wing, 1981).

Not only is the range of social impairments poorly understood but the cause of social impairment in autism are not understood. Some theorists claim that social impairment is caused by a cognitive disorder. Others claim that arousal, reward and motivation mechanisms are impaired in autism. Still others claim that social impairment arises from a disorder in a putative brain system controlling affect and sociability. There are two problems which must be addressed before the causal question can be explored.

ROADBLOCKS FOR CURRENT RESEARCH IN AUTISM

The two roadblocks which limit understanding of the social impairment in autism are (1) the failure of current research to recognize the heterogeneity of social deficit in autism, and (2) the lack of a unified and adequate understanding of the biological basis of human sociability.

Roadblock one. First, the true heterogeneity of the social deficit in the population diagnosed as autistic/PDD must be accepted by the research community. Despite empirical evidence which suggests that the range of social impairment in autism is quite wide (Fein & Waterhouse, in press; Waterhourse, 1988; Waterhouse et al., 1989; Wing, 1981), a majority of researchers continue to conceptualize the social deficit in the syndrome as a unitary pattern and continue to search for a single social core deficit across all autistic children.

In fact, individuals meeting diagnostic criteria for autism may be attached to their mothers or may not be, thay may be somewhat sociable or may not be sociable at all. Autistic individuals may express a wide range of positive and negative emotions or may express little emotion. They may make eye contact with others or may completely avoid eye contact. Autistic individuals may smile appropriately at times, may smile inappropriately, or may never smile at all. They recognize themselves in mirrors or photographs or may not. This range of expression of social behaviors may be tied to the individual's mental age or may not be. Furthermore, there may or may not be a discontinuity between the social impairments in autistic individuals and those of children with serious language disorders or severe personality disorders. It is this wide range of variation in social deficit that the research community has avoided addressing.

Human beings are designed by evolution to be extraordinarily sensitive to one another's signals. Smells, movements, patterns of facial expression, sounds and touch are all capable of eliciting exqusitely marked reactions in others. We all react to other individuals both abstractly - i. e., through the filters of imagination, of expectations and conceptualizations based on prior learning and directly - i. e., through the preconscious, etiologically prewired assessment of smells, movement, patterns of facial expression, sounds and touch.

Individuals diagnosed as autistic fail to send or respond to some signals of this sort, and may send uninterpretable or unpredictable signals or misinterpret the complex pattern of signals from others. We call abnormalities in sending signals a social deficit. If we infer abnormality in feeling states internal to autistic individuals we call this an affective deficit. When autistic individuals fail to adequately interpret the complex pattern of signals from others we call this a social cognitive deficit.

Clinicians experience the behavior of autistic individuals as socially impaired both directly and abstractly. The direct experience of another individual's social abnormality depends in large part on a preconscious awareness. The abstract experience of the social abnormalities of autism by clinicians is fueled by prior training, by ideas about social deficit generated in clinical practice, and by imaginative interpretation of what the social deficit consists of for the inner experience of the autistic individuals.

Unfortunately, neither the direct ethological sense of another human's social behavior, nor the abstract assessment within the clinician's theoretical framework can generate an analysis of the components which make an individual's social behavior odd, wrong or bizarre. Simply put, whether we directly interact with a socially impaired individual or whether we attempt to understand their odd behavior within an ideational framework, we cannot generate an analysis of what components make the behavior bizarre. While diagnostic systems, particularly the new DSM-III-R criteria which were developed in large part by Lorna Wing, may help to differentiate variations in impairment, the criteria are not designed to sample aspects of behavior which may reveal the basis of deviance.

Therefore, because neither a "gut" clinical direct response to another individual nor our trained framework systems will suffice to explore variation in social impairment, new approaches are needed. At present we are working on adapting a system of behavior analysis from primate work in order to examine the sequences, nature, and possible meaning of micro segments of social behavior in autistic individuals. We hope that this may help to explicate in a more formal fashion the elements and patterns which generate the heterogeneity of social behavior impairment in autism. It is clear, however, that such research can only serve to document differences, it cannot explain the causes of those differences.

Roadblock two. The second roadblock to current research in autism is the simple fact that so little is known about the biological basis of human social behavior. Few people today believe that parents-as-environment cause autism and most researchers believe that social impairments in autism have been engendered by organic deficits. The key question is what might those organic deficits be?

Nearly every brain area (except perhaps the occipital lobes) has been hypothesized to be the dysfunctional site. The plethora of notions should serve as a tipof to take a step back from this sort of theorizing. We do not have a reasonable model of the components of social behavior and we do not have a model of brain function underlying those components of social behavior. In fact, it is reasonable to assume that many brain areas subserve social behavior because nearly all aspects of being a social individual depend on multiple cognitive and affective functions. It is also clear that there is no brain tissue/physiology division social vs cognitive.

There are three general positions that have been taken concerning the biological basis of social behavior as it relates to social impairment in autism. The first position is that normal social behavior depends on a large constellation of brain systems working well, and that a deficit in any subsystem will impair the expression of normal social behavior. Clearly both affective and cognitive components are involved in social behavior and are interrelated in very complex ways. Etiologists have argued in fact that social behavior is such a complex task that other human skills are "smaller" in scope than is our sociability. It may be that most of the measureable language and perception skills that we label as "cognitive" - and that may be spared in some autistic individuals - do not require as complex a temporal interplay of sensory analysis, integration of drive states, recall of episodic memory and complex sequential motor patterning all within the same response as does social behavior.

The more components the system requires in order to function the more places, of course, it can go wrong. More important, even when only one element in a complex system is initially impaired the impairment may come to affect the rest of the system. This can open a window for flattening a developmental program to a nullity or conversely may open a developmental program to a range of extreme pathological variation. From this point of view many distinct neurological deficits in the domains of perception, affect, cognition or attention could produce the ultimate deficits in sociability and social cognition observed in autism. In sum this position claims that the social behavior depends on the adequate functioning of many brain systems, such that a deficit in any single subsystem will impair the expression of normal social behavior.

Another viewpoint is that older, earlier, or more basic mental prosesses are disordered in autism and disruptions in one of these specific systems may have the consequence of disturbing sensory analysis, social motivation, social learning, and ultimately social behavior. In this argument, if, for example, attention mechanisms are impaired information carrying content important for social interaction (i. e. language) will not be properly attended to, learned and acted upon. Dawson et al. (1989) and others have concluded that failure of attentional regulation to new events and experiences is a basic system disruption in autism. In this view irregular (Courchesne et al., 1985) or unbalanced (Dawson et al., 1989) or overfocused attention may lead to inadequate or improper social learning and consequently a withdrawal from social interaction as too complex to manage.

Another single limitation theory is that of Panksepp and Sahley (1987) who theorized that autistic children have abnormally high levels of brain opiods. This condition, they theorize, effectively nullifies the reinforcing effects of social behavior. If we normally are rewarded by experiencing pleasure through the release of endogenous opiates when we engage in socially relevant actions then having abnormally high levels of these substances would mean that there was no special reward for engaging in social behavior.

The third position which can be taken is that it may be the very newest "fanciest" cognitive skills which have been disturbed in autistic individuals. Baron-Cohen et al. (1985) have proposed that autistic individuals do not have the particular sort of imagination necessary to generate the notion of the mind of another individual.

Presumably, the ability to imagine the existence of the mind of another individual would be a very human brain function - this newest function may be an end state of frontal function specific to human social interaction, and failure in this system would be like taking the star off the top of the Christmas tree. In this model it is assumed that other older more basic and primitive areas of brain functioning such as reward and attention in relation to sociability are intact but that the newest and fanciest subsystem - imagination generating the imagined mind of another human being - is not.

Whether to model social deficits in autsm as stemming from a single old brain system deficit, (in affect, attention, arousal or motivation), or a single new brain system deficit (in cognitive skills), or as a stemming from a complex array of deficits in a variety of brain systems or single deficit in a complex array - this is the basic question for current research on the social impairment in autism.

However, until we as researchers can accept the actual heterogeneity of social impairment in autism and see it as part of a larger continuum which can be explored for individual differences, and until we can accept the real state of limited knowledge of the neural basis of human social behavior, most research may turn out to be theoretically fanciful, empirically inadequate or tautological.

PRO TEM SOLUTIONS

Given that more has to be done to accept and explore variation in the social deficits in autism, and given that the biological basis for social behavior is not yet well understood, what can be done now to redefine the central task in order to conduct productive research at present? There are at least five pro tem solutions possible. The first three obviate the need for accepting heterogeneity, which of course remains a problem - and the last two address heterogeneity in two different ways.

Pro tem solution one: Look for a behaviorally defined single social deficit. This strategy asserts that impaired sociability is the core deficit of autism and accepts the fact that "cognitive" function may vary widely in autistic individuals. Further these researchers assume that there is a single social behavior that all autistic individuals share to a degree not found in any other group of individuals.

An example of this kind of theorizing is found in the model proposed by Sigman (Ungerer & Sigman, 1981; Loveland & Landry, 1986). In this theory autistic individuals fail to engage in joint attention with another human being on a task at hand. The failure of joint attention leads to a central failure in interaction whether in symbolic play, object play or direct social communicative interaction. The danger, of course, for exploring a particular pattern of behavior as the unifying social deficit is that the piece of behavior selected may turn out to be artifactual or epiphenomenal and thus may not be a good place to hang one's research hat in trying to understand the entire spectrum of social impairment in autism.

Pro tem solution two: Looking for biologically defined underlying dysfunction. Heterogeneity in social deficit and cognitive deficit may be seen as constrained if a single unifying biological dysfunction is discovered. In the medical model for disease a single biological deficit may lead to a vast array of behavioral manifestations. This sort of reasoning from brain to behavior accepts as a working premise that there can be a wide variety of aberrant expressed behaviors stemming from a single organic locus of deficit especially in the case of post lesion developmental progression.

Several abnormal loci have been found in series of autistic children. The problem has always been that these loci have not been demonstrated to be relevant to social impairment per se nor have they been shown to be unique to autism (Balottin et al., 1989). While it can be accepted that at single brain locus may have diverse behavioral outcomes, the sine qua non for the brain behavior link is nonetheless a clear tie between a set of possible behavioral syndromes and a specific brain locus. This has yet to be accomplished for the autistic spectrum.

These single locus deficit models may implicate a neurotransmitter systems (as in the opiod theory) or a specific anatomical site, such as the temporal lobe (Hauser et al., 1975; Heltzer & Griffin, 1981). Regardless of the type of claim, they will remain unsatisfying until tightly linked to a specific pattern of abnormal social behavior, or, at least, to a limited set of such patterns.

Pro tem solution three: Developing a behavioral construct as a casual model. This solution essentially argues that brain system impairment may be various and many aspects of autistic functioning in behavior may be varied, however, there is a particular psychological system which is impaired in some specific way. This posited psychological construct is then unifying to the syndrome. Baron-Cohen (1988) and Baron-Cohen et al. (1985) in arguing for a failed theory of mind in autistic individuals have posited a psychological conceptual base to the disorder which lies deeper than the surface of behavioral functioning and must be inferred through special research paradigms.

Pro tem solution four: Accept the heterogeneity of theories as inferentially homologous to the heterogeneity of social deficit in the autistic population. In this strategy all models and theories could be accepted theoretically as possibly descriptive of some subset of the whole autistic population (Fein & Waterhouse, in press). In other words, the various notions of opiod disruption, attentional deficit, metacognitive deficit, and a host of other models may all be accepted as possible for some subset of autistic individuals.

However, simply because there are many models of mechanisms underlying social deficits and because there are many observed types of social deficit in autism, this doesn't mean that each of the many models is equally likely to be correct for a specific subset of autistic individuals. This having been said, it is nonetheless true that the range of variation in social deficit in autism does suggest that more than one model, and maybe many models of mechanisms will be necessary to explain the complete range of deficit which has been observed. Worse still, the range of variation may require explanations that recognize overlap of dysfunction in the course of development. Modeling this sort of interactive overlapping dysfunction will undoubtedly be extremely difficult. This, however, should not deter us from exploring multiple explanatory models.

Pro tem solution five: Redefine a major term in this equation - whether the term be autism or sociability. Efforts to explore the wider boundaries of autism as a syndrome (Wing, 1981; Waterhouse et al., 1989) have not been met with enthusiasm. One form that negative reaction has taken is that of purifying the disorder by asserting a narrow band definition with a unitary underlying cause such as a genetic basis (Folstein & Rutter, 1988). Another form of reaction to expanding the sense of the autistic spectrum is the assertion that efforts to widen understanding of the social deficits in autism/PDD are dangerous for research because a wider net will catch too many of the wrong sort of fish (Volkmar et al., 1988). Purifying and constricting concepts of the disorder actually are likely to lead to a cleaner understanding of one subgroup of the group of individuals who can be considered to be socially impaired but will not further the larger understanding of the whole range and continuum of social impairment that the general category autism/PDD encompasses. By making an effort to purify the disorder by selecting a smaller and more homogeneous group of individuals with a shared etiology the danger is that excluded subgroups with the larger group will be viewed as "non-autistic" and subsequently not important for further study. Another danger is the unproven assumption that selecting a behaviorally more homogeneous group will acctually result in a group more homogenous in etiology.

Another type of redefinition can be worked out - that of explaining or exploring the basic framework of human social behavior in a more theoretical fashion (Waterhouse, 1988) has argued that a review of a variety of theories concerning the origin of human social behavior yields an understanding of three sets of mechanisms crucial for human social behavior: (1) the physical contact of pair bonding; (2) the face to face behavior systems of imitation and identification and (3) the abstract memory based system of symbol use. An associated redefinition of human social behavior argues that all specific social behaviors have the goal of coregulating a wide variety of adaptive behaviors in order for the survival and success of the species. This claim has two parts: 1. that social behavior underwrites the basic processes of coregulation of all other human activities and 2. that coregulation - the coupling of two or more individuals' behaviors - is vital to species success.

In this model the three systems or three mechanisms of coregulation which determine social behavior are theorized to operate at three different proximities of requisite human contact. Pair bonding in the mother - child nursing couple and male - female sex couple requires direct physical contact and the ability to smell and feel one another. Reward and arousal systems are crucial to these functions. Imitation and identification require that individuals be within visual range of one another in order to copy one another and to identify each other. Complex motor programs and pattern analysis are needed skills for both imitation and identification. Finally, symbolic coregulation allows the physical separation of individuals in time and space and is adaptive for planning activities in the future or in another location. The application of this tripartite notion of social behavior as coregulation to autistic social deficit suggests that as all three sets of mechanisms come into play in the first 12 - 18 months of life in human beings that these emergent systems will unfold together but may be disrupted to unfold in a separable, dissociable, or fragmented fashion.

Certainly most aspects of coregulation must have a basis in neurological function and all aspects of coregulation require a degree of learning over the course of development. In this model the question "What is the neurological basis for human social behavior?" cannot have an answer because there would be likely to be quite a wide variety of neurological bases for the variety of coregulatory submechanisms all of which build together to generate what we call "social behavior".

The question of this paper concerns what underlies social deficits in autism. We believe that there are many types of expressed social deficits in autism - too many to claim that any single deficit (whether cognitive, affective, motivational or attentional) can be considered to be the unitary cause of the disorder which is labeled as autism. Moreover, we do not believe that brain systems respect these distinctions, that is "affective" versus "cognitive". This is a distinction that has been made by researchers. The brain does not seem to work along lines which can be neatly separated into components which could be called "social" or "cognitive". Whether there are an integrated set of social coregulatory functions which may be disrupted in some identifiably separable fashion or not we don't know as yet. We do feel that the solution for understanding social deficits in autism will depend on a multiple set of disrupted brain mechanisms and will depend on seeing the social deficit in autism as a wide variety of distinct and overlapping deficits which lead to a continuum of social disorder, a portion of which we have identified at present as "autism".

REFERENCES

Baron-Cohen, S. (1988). Social and pragmatic deficits in autism: cognitive or affective? *Journal of Autism and Developmental Disorders, 18,* 379-402.

Baron-Cohen, S., Leslie, A. M., & Frith, U. (1985). Does the autistic child have a "theory of mind?". *Cognition, 21,* 37-46.

Courchesne, E., Lincoln, A. J., Kilman, B. A., & Galambos, R. (1985). Event-related brain potential correlates of the processing of novel visual and auditory information in autism. *Journal of Autism and Developmental Disorders, 15,* 55-76.

Dawson, G., Finley, C., Philipps, S., Galpert, L., & Lewy, A. (1989). Reduced P3 amplitude of the event-related brain potential: its relation to language ability in autism. *Journal of Autism and Developmental Disorders, 18,* 493-504.

Fein, D. (1987). Social functioning in the autistic child. The League School Symposium, Boston, May 1987.

Folstein, S. E., & Rutter, M. L. (1988). Autism: familial aggregation and genetic implications. *Journal of Autism and Developmental Disorders, 18,* 3-30.

Hauser, S. L., De Long, G. R., & Rosman, P. (1975). Pneumographic findings in the infantile autism syndrome. *Brain, 98,* 677-688.

Heltzer, B. E., & Griffin, J. L. (1981). Infantile autism and the temporal lobe of the brain. *Journal of Autism and Developmental Disorders, 11,* 317-330.

Loveland, K., & Landry, S. (1986). Joint attention and language in autism and developmental language delay. *Journal of Autism and Developmental Disorders, 16,* 335-349.

Panksepp, J., & Sahley, T. L. (1987). Possible brain opioid involvement in disrupted social intent and language development of autism. In E. Schopler & G. B. Mesibov (Eds.), *Neurobiological Issues in Autism.* New York: Plenum Press.

Ungerer, J., & Sigman, M. (1981). Symbolic play and language comprehension in autistic children. *Journal of the American Academy of Child Psychiatry, 20,* 318-337.

Waterhouse, L. (1988). Aspects of the evolutionary history of human social behavior. In L. Wing, (Ed.), *The Biological Aspects of Autism.* London: British Society for Psychiatry.

Waterhouse, L., Wing, L., & Fein, D. (1989). Reevaluating the syndrome of autism in the light of empirical evidence. In G. Dawson & S. Segalowitz (Eds.), *Autism: The State of the Field.* New York: Guilford.

Wing, L. (1981). Language, social and cognitive impairments in autism and severe mental retardation. *Journal of Autism and Developmental Disorders, 11,* 31-44.

The Etiology of Autism

SUZANNE STEFFENBURG and CHRISTOPHER GILLBERG

INTRODUCTION

Leo Kanner, in 1972 claimed that from his "first publication to the last" he had spoken of autism "in no uncertain terms as innate" (Kanner, 1972). Yet, Time magazine in 1960 had quoted the same Kanner as saying "that children with infantile autism were the offspring of highly organized professional parents, cold and rational, who just happened to defrost long enough to produce a child". Kanner was ambivalent about the etiology of autism, and in this he was not alone. Since his time there have been a great many etiological theories which have basically assumed that the infant was normal at birth and attribute its development of symptoms to poor nurturing, particulary poor mothering. The literature on parents was reviewed in 1978 by McAdoo and DeMyer who concluded that as a group, parents of autistic children 1) display no more signs of mental or emotional disorder than parents whose children have "organic" disorders, with or without psychosis, 2) do not have extreme personality traits such as coldness, obsessiveness, social anxiety or rage, and 3) do not possess specific deficits in infant and child care. Since then, no sound studies making use of adequate controls have been published which provide support for the notion that parents of autistic children have been "socially" involved in the etiology or pathogenetic mechanisms of their child's disorder. Instead, evidence has accumulated (Folstein & Rutter, 1977; Steffenburg et al., 1989) in favour of hereditary factors operating in certain cases of autism. It could be that "old" observations about a connection between "cold" parents and children with autism in certain families were correct. However, the appropriate interpretation might be that "Asperger-type" problems in the parent are linked genetically and not socially to autism (Wolff et al., 1988; Gillberg, 1989).

There are several other myths in the field which would seem to implicate environmental - social factors in the genesis of autism. One such myth is that autistic children are from the upper social classes (Kanner 1943, 1949). There are at least eleven epidemiological studies of autism (Brask, 1970; Ritvo et al., 1971; Wing, 1980a; Gillberg & Schaumann, 1982; Bohman, 1983; Andersson & Wadensjö, 1981; Ritvo et al., 1989; Steffenburg & Gillberg, 1986; Steinhausen & Breulinger, 1986; Bryson et al., 1988; Tanoue et al., 1988) and all have shown autism to be almost equally distributed over social strata. Only Lotter's epidemiological study (Lotter, 1966), the first population-based survey in the field, has shown a slight excess of children with autism from the upper social classes. Schopler, Andrew and Strupp (1979) have provided evidence that the reason for the social class bias is a social class referreral bias in some studies of autism.

Another myth has been generated from the "first and only child" theory (Despert, 1951, Pitfield & Oppenheim, 1964; Kanner, 1954; Rimland, 1965; Deykin & MacMahon, 1980). Two considerations are of major importance: a) there is no study suggesting that a majority of autistic children are first-born, and b) there are several epidemiological studies that have not come up with results in support of the "first born notion" (Lotter,1966; Wing, 1980b; Gillberg, 1984).

HOW COMMON IS AUTISM?

There have been several population-based studies of autism (Lotter, 1966; Wing & Gould, 1979; Gillberg, 1984; Bohman et al., 1983; Steffenburg & Gillberg, 1986) which have all yielded population rates for autism of 4.0-6.7 per 10 000 children, "nuclear" ("Kanner-autism") cases accounting for half to three-quarters of these. There does not seem to be any major difference in frequency between urban and rural areas. This finding combined with the low and comparatively stable base rate does not argue in favour of a psycho-social model for the development of autism.

Just recently, results from five epidemiological studies (Tanoue et al., 1988; Bryson et al., 1988; Cialdella & Mamelle, 1989; Gillberg & Steffenburg, 1989; Suqiama & Abe, 1989) indicate that autism might be more common than previously demonstrated by the earlier population studies. The new Swedish study shows an increase in the rate of autism among children with severe mental retardation as well as among those with normal levels of intelligence. No clear increase appears in the group with mild - moderate mental retardation. These findings imply better detection rather than an actual increase in the rate of autism per se. Further, about half of the increase was accounted for by children born to "exotic" immigrants, of whom there were very few when the previous Swedish studies were performed. The "new" studies suggest a prevalence rate for autism of c. 10 in 10,000 children.

NEUROBIOLOGICAL FINDINGS ASSOCIATED WITH AUTISM

Table 1 lists the various neurobiological associations which have so far been documented in more than one case of autism. The heterogenous group of disorders shown suggests that autism represents a behavioural syndrome with multiple etiologies.

TABLE 1. Neurobiological findings associated with autism

Neurobiological findings associated with autism	Important reference
1 Boy:girl ratio	Wing, 1981
2 Mental retardation	Rutter, 1983
3 Epilepsy	Ohlsson et al., 1988
4 Infantile spasms	Riikonen & Amnell, 1981
5 Pubertal deterioration	Gillberg & Steffenburg, 1987
6 Fragile - X (q27) chromosome abnormality	Wahlström et al., 1986
7 Other sex chromosome abnormalities	Gillberg & Wahlström, 1985
8 Tuberous sclerosis	Lotter, 1974
9 Neurofibromatosis	Gillberg & Forsell, 1984
10 Hypomelanosis of Ito	Gillberg & Åkefeldt, 1989
11 PKU	Friedman, 1969, Lowe et al., 1980
12 Lactic acidosis	Coleman & Blass, 1985
13 Purine disorder	Coleman et al., 1985
14 Intrauterine rubella infection	Chess et al., 1971
15 Postnatal herpes infection	DeLong et al., 1981, Gillberg, 1986
16 Rett syndrome	Witt-Engerström & Gillberg, 1987
17 Hydrocephalus	Schain & Yannet, 1960; Fernell & Gillberg, 1989
18 Moebius syndrome	Ornitz et al., 1978, Gillberg & Steffenburg, 1989
19 Reduced optimality in pre- and perinatal periods	Gillberg & Gillberg, 1983; Bryson et al., 1989
20 Concordance monozygotic twins	Folstein & Rutter, 1977 Steffenburg et al., 1989
21 Duchenne muscular dystrophia	Komoto et al., 1984
22 Williams syndrome	Reiss et al., 1985

In this table the first 20 findings have been documented in population-based or other large scale studies of autism.

Sex Ratios

Boys outweigh girls in all studies of autism at a ratio of 1.4-4.8 to 1 (Lotter, 1966; Brask, 1970; Torrey, Hearsch, & McCabe, 1975; Wing, 1981a; Bohman et al., 1983; Gillberg, 1984; Steinhausen & Breulinger, 1986). A high boy:girl ratio in a given medical condition suggests a biological link, presumably genetic or partially genetic (Omenn, 1973).

IQ in Autism

The population-based studies agree that the great majority of children with autism are also mentally retarded. 75 - 90 per cent of all autistic children are clearly mentally retarded, suggesting a neurobiological primary deficit in the child. Another piece of evidence suggesting the same thing is the overwhelming association of autism with severe cognitive handicap.

IQ Trends in Boys and Girls

Many authors, most notably Lorna Wing (1981), have documented that among the severely mentally retarded children with autism, girls are almost as frequent as boys, and that bright girls with autism are exceedingly rare. In short, these trends could be interpreted to mean that genetic factors are relatively more important in boys, and that severe brain damage (affecting the sexes with about the same frequency) is of major importance for the development of autism in girls.

In Asperger syndrome, the relative male:female ratio is particularly high, (Gillberg & Gillberg, 1989). Asperger syndrome is currently conceptualized as a (at least partially) genetic disorder. It is appropriate in this connection to note that Asperger syndrome is possibly considerably more common than "autism proper" (Gillberg & Gillberg, 1989; Wing, 1989, personal communication).

Cognitive Profile

Frith and her group have conducted a series of thought-provoking experiments with normal children and children with Down's syndrome and autism in order to test the hypothesis that in autism there might exist a syndrome-specific deficit in the ability to conceive of other people as having "minds" or "mental states". Their latest publication in this field (Attwod, Frith & Hermelin, 1988) concerns 22 children and adolescents who were shown to be relatively unimpaired with respect to "non-verbal" instrumental gestures (e g raising a hand with palm outwards, in order to stop somebody approaching) but totally lacking in the use of gestures expressing inner feelings or response to mental states in others. The results support the hypothesis. Indirect support for this neuropsychological deficit model was also found in a study of 10 high-functioning men with autism (residual state) - four of whom had originally been diagnosed by Leo Kanner - who did not show overt neurological symptoms (Rumsey & Hamburger, 1988). These men performed poorly on the word comprehension and picture arrangement subtests of the Wechsler Adult Intelligence Scale, both of which involve "social imputation" skills and conceptual thinking rather than rote memory processes (which tended to be unimpaired). In this context it is of some interest that "idiots savants" with exceptional rote memory skills almost always have autism, whereas "savants" skilled in other areas may or may not have autism (O'Connor & Hermelin, 1988). Further details are provided in the chapter on "Theory of Mind" by Frith in this book.

Epilepsy in Autism

The occurrence of epilepsy in autism has been clearly documented in four population-based studies (Lotter, 1974; Wing & Gould, 1979; Gillberg & Steffenburg, 1987; Ohlsson, Steffenburg & Gillberg, 1988). In particular there seems to be unequivocal support for the notion of an association between infantile spasms and infantile autism (Riikonen & Amnell, 1981; Ohlsson et al., 1988). The study by Ohlsson et al. (1988) showed psychomotor epilepsy to be the most common seizure type in preadolescence. The follow-up study by Gillberg and Steffenburg (1987), in which 29 per cent of cases with autism and 46 per cent of cases with autism-like conditions developed seizures before age 16 - 23 years, showed pubertal onset of seizures to be particularly common. Fifty per cent of all cases of epilepsy appeared for the first time around age 13 - 14 years. Fifty per cent of these cases of pubertal onset epilepsy were of the psychomotor variant.

Deterioration in Adolescence

One population-based study (Gillberg & Steffenburg, 1987) has provided empirical support for the notion launched by Rutter - on the basis of a mixed hospital series of autism and similar cases (Rutter, 1970) - that a considerable number of children with autism undergo deterioration at the time of puberty. So far, no precipitating factor other than puberty has been identified. This in itself argues for endocrine/neurochemical dysfunction in autism.

Chromosomal and Other Genetic Disorders

The fragile X (q) (273) chromosome abnormality is a contributing pathogenetic factor in 5 - 16 per cent of all autism cases (Watson, Lechman, Annex, Breg, Boles, Volkmar & Cohen, 1984; Gillberg & Wahlström, 1985; Wahlström, Gillberg, Gustavsson & Holmgren, 1986). Boys are affected relatively more often than girls, but recently several groups (e g Gillberg et al., [1988]) have shown that the fragile - X chromosomal defect probably plays a role in female autism as well.

Other chromosomal abnormalities particularly involving the sex chromosomes are possibly over-represented in autism (Gillberg & Wahlström, 1985).

Tuberous sclerosis is perhaps the best documented genetic disorder known to be associated with autism (Lotter, 1974; Wing & Gould, 1979; Coleman & Gillberg, 1985). About 5 per cent of all autism cases probably have tuberous sclerosis.

Neurofibromatosis and hypomelanosis of Ito are other neurocutaneous disorders which have also recently been suggested to be associated with autism (Gillberg & Forsell, 1984, Gillberg & Åkefeldt,1989).

Metabolic Disorders

Some children with autism have concomitant metabolic disorders (Coleman & Gillberg, 1985). Connections between PKU and autism and between autism and PKU have been described by many authors (e g Friedman, 1969; Knobloch & Pasamanick, 1975; Bliumina, 1975; Lowe, Tanaka, Seashou, Young & Cohen, 1980). Animal studies have shown that experimental hyperphenylalaninemia - imitating PKU - interferes with myelinization in the brain. The cerebellum might be specifically affected (Huether, Neuhoff & Kaus, 1983).

Abnormalities of purine metabolism (Coleman et al., 1976) and lactic acidosis (Coleman & Blass, 1985) have also been associated with autism.

Infectious Diseases

Chess, Korn and Fernandez (1971) have provided convincing evidence that autistic symptomatology in childhood can result from intrauterine rubella infection. Rubella is a contributing pathogenetic factor in 5 - 10 per cent of all autism cases. Postnatal herpes virus infection (De Long, Beau & Brown, 1981; Gillberg, 1986) can also produce full blown Kanner-type autism. It is possible that congenital cytomegalovirus infection can also lead to autism (Stubbs, Ash & Williams, 1984)

Other Disorders Associated with Autistic Symptomatology

It is now clear that a large number of children with Rett syndrome (Hagberg, Acardi, Dias & Ramos, 1983) have been primarily diagnosed as suffering from infantile autism or childhood psychosis (Witt-Engerström & Gillberg, 1987). Rett syndrome provides a striking illustration of how "the autistic syndrome" will eventually turn out to consist of a number of syndromes with varying etiology.

Other disorders and diseases which may be connected with autism in a more than chance fashion are hydrocephalus, Moebius syndrome, Duchenne muscular dystrophia and the de Lange syndrome (see Coleman & Gillberg, 1985 for a review).

Twin Studies

Two population-based twin studies (Folstein & Rutter, 1977; Steffenburg, Gillberg C, Hellgren, Gillberg I C, Jakobsson & Bohman, 1989) suggest that in some cases autism or some factor closely related to autism has been inherited. It is possible that the fragile - X chromosome abnormality accounts for an important minority of these cases.

Other Genetic Studies

There is an increased rate of autism in siblings of autism cases (Folstein & Rutter, 1988). This increase is in the range of 50 - 150 times compared with the general population and could indicate the operation of genetic factors in some cases. Multiple incidence families with several cases of autism are not quite uncommon. It seems likely that there is a subgroup of clearly genetic autism. This subgroup may show overlap with other genetic disorders such as tuberous sclerosis and the fragile-X-syndrome, but the possibility of a "purer" genetic subgroup cannot be ruled out.

Just recently, De Long and Dwyer (1989) reported an increased rate of affective disorders in the families of relatively brighter children with autism.

Reduced Optimality in the Pre- and Perinatal Period

There is abundant evidence that although there is no one specific pre- or perinatal event which always causes autism, in a large proportion of cases there are "reductions of optimality" in the intrauterine, intrapartal or the perinatal period (Gillberg & Gillberg, 1983, Bryson et al., 1989). Bleedings in pregnancy, in particular, seem to have been prevalent in autism cases in several independent investigations. In Gothenburg, the reduced pre- and perinatal optimality concept has been used in a number of population-based studies (Table 2).

TABLE 2. Reduced optimality* in total population groups of normal children and children with various handicaps according to the method described in Gillberg and Gillberg (1983). All evaluations of medical records done blind in respect of child's diagnosis.

Group	n	Reduced optimality score	S. D.	Reference
Normal	55	2.2	1.8	Gillberg et al., 1986
	130	2.3	1.7	Gillberg et al., 1989
	51	2.6	1.3	Gillberg & Rasmussen, 1982
Teenage psychosis	55	3.0	2.0	Gillberg et al., 1986
Mental retardation	130	3.4	1.8	Gillberg et al., 1989
Deficits in attention, motor control and perception	42	4.1	2.0	Gillberg & Rasmussen, 1982
Autism	25	5.6	2.5	Gillberg & Gillberg, 1983

* The same checklist of 29 obstetrical/perinatal conditions was used in all 5 groups. Possible reduced optimality scores range from 0-29.

The pooled results from these studies indicate that "normal" children have low reductions, children with teenage psychosis slightly (though significantly) higher, mental retardation higher still, and motor-perceptual problems about twice the level of the normal groups. Children with autism had greater reductions of optimality than all these groups. The autism group, in fact, was close to a representative group of cases with cerebral palsy (Kyllerman, 1982).

Neuropathological Studies of Autism

A very limited number of satisfactory autopsy studies on the brains of children with typical autism is available. Recently, Ritvo, Freeman, Scheibel, Duong, Robinsson, Guthrie & Rit (1986) reported that cerebellar changes, in particular those affecting the Purkinje fibres, may be a common denominator in autism.

Neuroradiological Studies

Studies using PEG and CAT-scans on autistic children indicate that major brain tissue damage is relatively common and that central (internal) atrophy may be more than just an incidental finding in many cases (e g Gillberg & Svendsen, 1983; Jacobsen, LeCouter, Howlin & Rutter, 1988). A study by Prior in Australia (Prior, Tress, Hoffman & Boldt, 1984) on high-functioning autistic children has suggested that CAT-scan-abnormalities may not be typical of non-retarded autistic children. However, the number of children in that study was small indeed (N=9) and the results have not been borne out by other researchers yet (cf Gillberg, Steffenburg & Jakobsson, 1987; Jacobsen et al., 1988). Recently Gaffney, Kuperman, Tsai, Minchin and Hassanein (1987) found enlargement of the fourth ventricle in several children and adolescents with autism, using midsagittal MRI scans. Abnormalities in the brainstem and/or cerebellum could account for the findings. This is similar to what the Rutter group (Jacobsen et al., 1988) reported. Courchesne et al. (1988) also used MRI scans and compared scans of "high level" autistic subjects with "normal controls". The high-functioning autistic children showed results indicating neocerebellar maldevelopment/damage.

These studies, using MRI, along with some of the autopsy findings from the mid-1980s indicating cerebellar Purkinje cell abnormality and the considerable literature indicating brainstem/vestibular damage in autism, show that our efforts at disclosing the neural basis for autism must also be directed to parts of the central nervous system not previously considered important in connection with social and cognitive deficits. The cerebellar changes, if upheld by further studies, could directly impair cognitive functioning, or they could occur concomitantly with damage to other areas in the nervous system whose dysfunction directly underlies the social and cognitive defects seen in autism.

An interesting study of regional cerebral metabolic rates for glucose determined by PET (position emission tomograhpy) technique (Horwitz, Rumsey, Grady & Rapoport, 1988) has shown that, as a group, adult men with autism and relatively high IQs showed indications of a functional impairment of the interaction between frontal/parietal regions and the neostriatum, and the neostriatum and thalamic regions that subserve directed attention. This study did not find any indications of disturbed cerebellar/neocortical interrelationships. However, as the authors point out, minimal cerebellar functioning was required in the study. A recent PET-study by Rutter and his group (Herold, Frackowiak, LeCouteur, Rutter & Howlin, 1988) yielded no evidence of abnormalities of the kind seen in the Horwitz et al. study.

Neurophysiological Studies

There is compelling neurophysiological evidence that the temporal lobes and the brainstem might be dysfunctional in relatively large groups of patients with autism.

EEG studies (Sarvis, 1960; Hauser, DeLong Rosman, 1975; DeLong et al., 1981; Riikonen & Amnell, 1981) have indicated temporal lobe pathology in selected patients with autism. Partial complex "psychomotor" seizures indicative of underlying temporal lobe dysfunction seem to be particularly common in autism.

The Ritvo group (1988) compared children, adolescents and adults with sex- and age-matched healthy volunteers. The group with autism was shown to have signs of abnormal retinal function in almost half the cases.

Studies of vestibular function (Ornitz, 1974), autonomic regulation (Bonvallet & Allen, 1963; James & Barry, 1980) and of auditory brainstem responses (ABR) (e g Gillberg, Rosenhall & Johansson, 1983) have combined to produce evidence of brainstem dysfunction in autism.

A study of oculomotor function in relatively high functioning children with autism suggests abnormalities that are different from those seen in schizophrenics and implicate brainstem/vestibular/ cerebellar dysfunction rather than impaired attention (Rosenhall, Johansson & Gillberg, 1988).

Neurochemical Studies

A relatively limited number of neurochemical studies of autism have so far produced essentially three major leads for further hypothesis testing (see Coleman & Gillberg, 1985 for a review): (a) serotonin is raised in the body fluids of a substantial subgroup of autistic patients, but this could be due to concomitant mental retardation rather than to autism per se; (b) dopamine may be dysfunctional in many patients with autism. This has been suggested by cerebrospinal fluid and urine studies from independent laboratories and can probably not be attributed merely to co-variation with mental retardation - however, one recent study in this field was negative (Minderaa et al., 1989) (c) endorphin fraction II levels might be raised in the central nervous system in at least some patients with autism, in particular those with self-injurious behaviour. There is also preliminary evidence suggesting low CSF-beta-endorphin levels (Gillberg et al., 1989) in autism, but conflicting results by other groups are currently in press. This area was recently surveyed by Sahley and Panksepp (1987).

Previous reports of specific patterns of urinary peptide excretion in autistic children were not upheld in a well-designed study of adults with autism and mentally retarded and normal comparison cases (Le Couteur, Trygstad, Evered, Gillberg & Rutter, 1988).

IS ASPERGER DISTINCT FROM AUTISM?

Asperger syndrome is currently mostly considered to be a variant of autism in people of very good, normal or almost normal intelligence (Tantam, 1988). Some recent findings (e g Bowman, 1988) suggest that genetic factors are important in Asperger syndrome. A genetic component common to "Asperger" and "Kanner" syndromes might be in operation. This hypothesis is supported in a recent family study from our centre (Gillberg, 1989). In that study one family contained two boys who showed all the characteristics of Asperger syndrome and another boy, who had suffered prenatal brain damage, who was typically "Kanner autistic".

CONCLUSIONS

To summarize, it is clear that autism can be the final common expression of various contributary/etiological factors. Some biological factors/medical conditions have an exceptionally high risk of accompanying autistic symptomatology. Family and twin studies suggest that genetic factors are in operation in some cases. Disease entities or pre- and perinatal damage leading to destruction/dysfunction in certain brain areas can cause autism in others.

So far it has not been possible to clearly disentangle whether many of the chromosomal, neurochemical, neuropsychological and brain imaging findings in autism could be attributed to autism per se or to the often concomitant mental retardation. However, a number of recent studies have shown high-level autism cases to have brain damage/dysfunction also. Seventeen children with classical Kanner autism and three children with Asperger syndrome, all of whom had full-scale IQs above 65, were subjected to a comprehensive neurobiological assessment (Gillberg et al., 1987) including CAT scan, auditory brainstem response, EEG, chromosomal cultures, cerebrospinal fluid, blood and urine examinations and a thorough physical examination. Fifteen of the 20 children had a definite abnormality on at least one of these examinations. There seems to be no good rationale for insisting on the organic/non-organic dichotomy when the evidence is that behaviour in both entities is similar (Garreau et al., 1984). Also the number of "non-organic" cases will decrease constantly as our neurobiological examination tools become increasingly more sophisticated. Nevertheless, subdivision of cases into various groups according to the associated biological pathology may prove very useful, and it is possible, indeed highly probable, that autism will eventually be collapsed into quite a number of "autistic syndromes". There is no known unitary brain pathology common to all autism cases. However, this does not detract from the possibility that specific neural circuitry or circuitries in the central nervous system may be dysfunctional in all cases with core autistic symptoms (Damasio & Maurer, 1980; Ornitz, 1983; Coleman & Gillberg, 1985). It could be that important "cross-roads" in the nervous system are damaged. Or it could be a matter of ascending attentional systems being haphazardly put out of order or disconnected by processes similar to those seen in epilepsy leading to cortical centres being "illuminated" in a kaleidoscopic fashion with certain centres being gradually "locked-in" (Courchesne, 1987). In summary, there is overwhelming evidence that infantile autism has major biological roots. There is no scientific evidence that purely psychological or psychosocial stressors or circumstances can lead to autism.

One of the pathophysiologic theories in the field of autism implicates brainstem-mesolimbic system dysfunction as a possible cause of central autistic symptoms. Ascending dopaminergic/endorphinergic nerve fibers arising in the brainstem/diencephalon may be dysfunctional or damaged. The target cell areas of these neurons in the mesolimbic areas may then be secondarily dysfunctional and, in a growing child, underdeveloped. It is fairly well established that sensory input is necessary in young children for the development of what we might term "end interpretation loci". If the mesolimbic areas are bilaterally dysfunctional, central autistic symptomatology, such as severe incapacity in the field of recognizing the emotional significance of objects and social relationships, could result (Coleman & Gillberg, 1985). If other areas are damaged or dysfunctional as well, additional symptoms would ensue. The mesolimbic cortex could of course also be specifically and primarily affected by damage of dysfunction in which case central autism symptoms but no signs of brainstem pathology - clinically or at neurophysiological testing - would appear. Primary brainstem or mesolimbic damage or dysfunction could result from a number of different causes such as the fragile-X syndrome, intrauterine rubella infection, tuberous sclerosis and perinatal brain damage. Cerebellar abnormalities, if present, could easily be fitted into this model.

Any theoretical model for the biological basis of autism needs to keep in touch with recent developments in basic neurobiology. Strict localization theories in many instances now seem obsolete in the face of ever-growing evidence that functional neural systems in the brain are interconnected in so many ways as to make one biological model for the development of a behavioural syndrome with multiple etiologies rather unlikely.

Nevertheless, no one familiar with modern research in the field of autism can possibly espouse psychogenic causal theories any more. Autism as a biologically determined behavioural disorder should no longer be a matter of dispute (Gillberg, 1988). It is high time that autism be regarded as an administrative rather than a specific disease label. Autism, like mental retardation is not a disease, but an umbrella term, covering a variety of disease entities with certain common behavioural features.

REFERENCES

Andersson, L., & Wadensjö, K. (1981). Early childhood psychosis in Malmöhus län - a descriptive study. Research report. *Social Welfare Authorities County of Malmöhus län* .

Attwood, A., Frith, U., & Hermelin, B. (1988). The understanding and use of interpersonal gestures by autistic and Down's syndrome children. *Journal of Autism and Developmental Disorders, 18,* 241 - 257.

Bliumina, M. (1975). A schizophrenic-like variant of phenylketonuria. *Zhurnal Neropathogii i Psikiatrii, 75,* 1525 - 1529.

Bohman, M., Bohman, I. L., Björck, P., & Sjöholm, E. (1983). Childhood psychosis in a northern Swedish county: some preliminary findings from an epidemiological survey. In M. H. Schmidt & H. Remschmidt (Eds.), *Epidemiological Approaches in Child Psychiatry,* Stuttgart: Georg Thieme.

Bowman, E. P. (1988). Asperger syndrome and Autism: The Case for a Connection, *British Journal of Psychiatry, 152,* 377 - 382.

Bonvallet, M., & Allen, M. B. D. (1963). Prolonged spontaneous and evoked activation following discrete bulbar lesions. *Electroencephalography and Clinical Neurophysiology, 15,* 969.

Brask, B. H. (1970). A prevalence investigation of childhood psychosis. *Paper given at the 16th Scandinavian Congress of Psychiatry.*

Bryson, S., Smith, I., & Eastwood, D. (1989). Obstetrical Optimality in Autistic Children. *Journal of the American Academy of Child and Adolescent Psychiatry, 27,* 418 - 422.

Chess, S., Korn, S. J., & Fernandez, P. B. (1971). *Psychiatric Disorders of Children with congenital Rubella.* New York: Brunner/Mazel.

Cialdella, Ph., & Mamelle, N. (1989). An Epidemiological Study of Infantile Autism in a French Department (Rhône): a Research Note. *Journal of Child Psychology and Psychiatry, 30,* 165 - 175.

Coleman, M., Landgrebe, M. A., & Landgrebe, A. R. (1976). Purine autism. Hyperuricosuria in autistic children: does this identify a subgroup of autism? In M. Coleman (Ed.), *The Autistic Syndromes* (pp 183 - 195). Amsterdam: North Holland.

Coleman, M., & Blass, J. P. (1985). Autism and lactic acidosis. *Journal of Autism and Developmental Disorders, 15,* 1 - 8.

Coleman, M., & Gillberg, C. (1985). *The Biology of the Autistic Syndromes.* New York: Praeger.

Courchesne, E. (1987). A neurophysiological view of autism. In E. Schopler & G. Mesibov (Eds.), *Neurobiological Issues in Autism.* New York: Plenum Press.

Courchesne, E., Yeung-Courchesne, R., Press, G. A., Hesselink, J. R., & Jernigan, T. L. (1988). Hypoplasia of cerebellar vermal lobules VI and VII in autism. *New England Journal of Medicine, 318,* 1349 - 1354.

Damasio, A. R., & Maurer, R. G. (1978). A neurological model for childhood autism. *Archives of Neurology, 35,* 777 - 786.

DeLong, G. R., & Dwyer, J. T. (1988). Correlation of Family History with specific autistic subgroups: Asperger's syndrome and bipolar affective disease. *Journal of Autism and Developmental Disorders, 18,* 593 - 600.

DeLong, G. R., Beau, S. C., & Brown, F. R. (1981). Acquired reversibel autistic syndrome in acute encephalopathic illness in children. *Archives of Neurology, 38,* 191 - 194.

Despert, J. L. (1951). Some considerations relating to the genesis of autistic behaviour in children. *American Journal of Orthopsychiatry, 21,* 335.

Deykin, E., & MacMahon, G. (1980). Pregnancy, delivery and neonatal complications among autistic children. *American Journal of Diseases of Children, 134,* 860 - 864.

Fernell, E., & Gillberg, C. (1989). Behaviour problems in children with infantile hydrocephalus (submitted).

Folstein, S., & Rutter, M. (1977). Infantile autism: a genetic study of 21 twin pairs. *Journal of Child Psychology and Psychiatry, 18,* 297 - 321.

Folstein, S., & Rutter, M. (1987). Familial aggregation and genetic implications. *Journal of Autism and Developmental Disorders, 18,* 3 - 30.

Friedman, E. (1969). The autistic syndrome and phenylketonuria, *Schizophrenia, 1,* 249 - 261.

Gaffney, G. R., Kuperman, S., Tsai, L., Minchin, S., & Hassanein, K. M. (1987). Midsagittal resonance imaging of autism. *British Journal of Psychiatry, 151,* 831 - 833.

Garreau, B. C., Barthelemy, C., Sauvage, D., Leddet, I., & Lelord, G. (1984). A comparison of autistic syndromes with and without associated neurological problems. *Journal of Autism and Developmental Disorders, 14,* 105 - 111.

Gillberg, C. (1984). Infantile autism and other childhood psychoses in a Swedish urban region. Epidemiological aspects. *Journal of Child Psychology and Psychiatry, 25,* 35 - 43.

Gillberg, C. (1986). Onset at age 14 of a typical autistic syndrome. A case report of a girl with herpes simplex encephalitis. *Journal of Autism and Developmental Disorders, 16,* 569 - 575.

Gillberg, C. (1988). The neurobiology of infantile autism. *Journal of Child Psychology and Psychiatry, 129,* 245 - 256.

Gillberg, C. (1989). Asperger syndrome in 23 Swedish children: a clinical study. *Developmental Medicine and Child Neurology, 31,* 520 - 531.

Gillberg, C., & Forsell, C. (1984). Childhood psychosis and neurofibromatosis - more than a coincidence. *Journal of Autism and Developmental Disorders, 13,* 1 - 8.

Gillberg, C., & Gillberg, I. C. (1983). Infantile autism: a total population study of reduced optimality in the pre-, peri- and neonatal period. *Journal of Autism and Developmental Disorders, 13,* 153 - 166.

Gillberg, C., & Gillberg, I. C. (1989). Another note on the relationship between population-based and clinical studies: the question of reduced optimality in autism. *Journal of Autism and Developmental Disorders* (in press).

Gillberg, C., Ohlsson, V-A., Wahlström, J., Steffenburg, S., & Blix, K. (1988). Monozygotic female twins with autism and the Fragile-X-syndrome (AFRAX). *Journal of Child Psychology and Psychiatry, 29,* 447 - 452.

Gillberg, C., & Rasmussen, P. (1982). Perceptual, motor and attentional deficits in seven-year-old children. Background factors. *Developmental Medicine and Child Neurology, 24,* 752 - 770.

Gillberg, C., Rosenhall, U., & Johansson, E. (1983). Auditory brainstem responses in childhood psychosis. *Journal of Autism and Developmental Disorders, 13,* 181 - 195.

Gillberg, C., & Schaumann, H. (1982). Social class and infantile autism. *Journal of Autism and Developmental Disorders, 12,* 223 - 228.

Gillberg, C., & Steffenburg, S. (1987). Outcome and prognostic factors in infantile autism and similar conditions. A population based study of 46 cases followed through puberty. *Journal of Autism and Developmental Disorders, 17,* 271 - 285.

Gillberg, C., & Steffenburg, S. (1989). Is autism more common now than 20 years ago? (Submitted).

Gillberg, C., & Steffenburg, S. (1989). Autistic behaviour in Moebius syndrome. *Acta Paediatrica Scandinavica, 78,* 314 - 316.

Gillberg, C., Steffenburg, S., & Jakobsson, G. (1987). Neurobiological findings in 20 relatively gifted children with Kanner type autism and Asperger's syndrome. *Developmental Medicine and Child Neurology, 29,* 641 - 649.

Gillberg, C., & Svendsen, P. (1983). Childhood psychosis and computed tomographic brain scan findings. *Journal of Autism and Developmental Disorders, 13,* 19 - 32.

Gillberg, C., & Wahlström, J. (1985). Chromosome abnormalities in infantile autism and other childhood psychoses. A population study of 66 cases. *Developmental Medicine and Child Neurology, 27,* 293 - 304.

Gillberg, C., Wahlström, J., Forsman, A., Hellgren, L., & Gillberg, I. C. (1986). Teenage psychoses - epidemiology, classification and reduced optimality in the pre-, peri- and neonatal periods. *Journal of Child Psychology and Psychiatry, 27,* 87 - 98.

Gillberg, C., & Åkefeldt, A. (1989). Autism and hypomelanosis of Ito (in preparation).

Gillberg, C., Terenius, L., Hagberg, B., Witt-Engerström, I., & Eriksson, I. (1989). Beta-endorphins in child neuropsychiatric disorders. *Brain and Development* (in press).

Hauser, S. G., DeLong, G. R., Rosman, N. (1975). Pneumographic findings in the infantile autism syndrome: A correlation with temporal lobe disease, *Brain, 98,* 667 - 688.

Hagberg, B., Aicardi, J., Dias, K., & Ramos, O. (1983). A progressive syndrome of autism, dementia, ataxia and loss of purposeful hand use in girls: Rett syndrome. Report of 35 cases. *Annals of Neurology, 14,* 471 - 479.

Herold, S., Frackowiak, R. S. J., Le Couteur, A., Rutter, M., & Howlin, P. (1988). Cerebral blood flow and metabolism of oxygen and glucose in young autistic adults. *Psychological Medicine, 18,* 823 - 831.

Horwitz, B., Ramsey, J., Grady, C., & Rapoport, S. (1988). The cerebral metabolic landscape in autism. Inter-correlations of regional glucose utilization. *Archives of Neurology, 45,* 749 - 755.

Huether, G., Neuhoff, V., & Kaus, R. (1983). Brain development in experimental hyperphenylalaninaemia: Disturbed proliferation and reduced cell numbers in the cerebellum. *Neuropaediatrics, 14,* 12 - 19

Jacobsen, R., LeCouteur, A., Howlin, P., & Rutter, M. (1988). Selective subcortical abnormalities in autism. *Psychological Medicine, 18,* 39 - 48.

James, A. L., & Barry, R. J. (1980). A review of psychophysiology in early onset psychosis. *Schizophrenia Bulletin, 6,* 506 - 525.

Kanner, L. (1943). Autistic disturbances of affective contact. *Nervous Child, 2,* 217 - 250.

Kanner, L. (1949). Problems of nosology and psychodynamics in early childhood autism. *American Journal of Orthopsychiatry, 19,* 416.

Kanner, L. (1954). To what extent is early childhood autism determined by constitutional inadequacies? In D. Hooker & C. C. Hofe (Eds.), *Genetics and the inheritance of neurological and psychiatric patterns.* Baltimore: Williams and Wilkins.

Kanner, L. (1972). Proceedings of the Annual Meeting of the National Society of Autistic Children (avaiable from NSAC, 1234 Massachusetts Avenue, N W, Suite 1017, Washington, D C, 20005).

Knobloch, H., & Pasamanick, B. (1975). Some etiologic and prognostic factors in early infantile autism and psychosis. *Journal of Paediatrics, 55,* 182 - 191.

Komoto, J., Udsui, S., Otsuki, S., & Terao, A. (1984). Infantile autism and Duchenne muscular dystrophy. *Journal of Autism and Developmental Disorders, 14,* 191 - 195.

Kyllerman, M. (1982). Dyskinetic cerebral palsy. University of Göteborg, Thesis.

Le Couteur, A., Trygstad, O., Evered, C., Gillberg, Ç., & Rutter, M. (1988). Infantile autism and urinary excretion of peptides and protein-associated peptide complexes. *Journal of Autism and Developemental Disorders, 18,* 181 - 190.

Lotter, V. (1966). Epidemiology of autistic conditions in young children -I. Prevalence. *Social Psychiatry, 1,* 124 - 137.

Lotter, V. (1974). Factors related to outcome in autistic children. *Journal of Autism and Childhood Schizophrenia, 4,* 263 - 277.

Lowe, T. L., Tanaka, K., Seashore, M. R., Young, J. G., & Cohen, D. J. (1980). Detection of phenylketonuria in autistic and psychotic children. *Journal of the American Medical Association, 243,* 126 - 128.

Mc Adoo, W. G., & De Myer, M. (1978). Personality characteristics of parents. In M. Rutter & E. Schopler (Eds.), *Autism: A Reappraisal of Concepts and Treatment.* (pp 251 - 269). New York: Plenum Press.

Minderaa, R. B., Andersson, G. M., Volkmar, F. R., Akkerhuis, G. W., & Cohen, D. J. (1988). Neurochemical study of dopamine functioning in autistic and normal subjects. *Journal of the American Academy of Child and Adolescent Psychiatry, 28,* 190 - 194.

O'Connor, N., & Hermelin, B. (1988). Low intelligence and special abilities. *Journal of Child Psychiatry, 29,* 391 - 396.

Ohlsson, I., Steffenburg, S., & Gillberg, C. (1988). Epilepsy in autism and autistic-like conditions: a population-based study. *Archives of Neurology, 45,* 666 - 668.

Omenn, G. (1973). Genetic issues in the syndrome of minimal brain dysfunction. In S. Waltzer & P. Wolff (Eds.), *Minimal Cerebral Dysfunction in Children* (pp 5-17). New York: Grune & Stratton.

Ornitz, E. M. (1978). Neurophysiologic Studies in Autism: In M. Rutter & E. Schopler (Eds.), *A Reappraisal of Concepts and Treatment* (pp 117 - 139). New York: Plenum Press.

Ornitz, E. M. (1983). The functional neuroanatomy of infantile autism. *International Journal of Neuroscience, 19,* 85 - 124.

Ornitz, E. M., Brown, M. B., Mason, A., Putnam, A. (1974). Effect of visual input on vestibular nystagmus in autistic children. *Archives of General Psychiatry, 31,* 369 - 375.

Pitfield, M., & Oppenheim, A. (1964). Child rearing attitudes of mothers of psychotic children. *Journal of Child Psychology and Psychiatry, 5,* 52 - 57.

Prior, M. R., Tress, B., Hoffman, W. L., & Boldt, D. (1984). Computed tomographic study of children with classic autism. *Archives of Neurology, 41,* 482-484.

Reiss, A. L., Feinstein, C., Rosenbaum, K. N., Borengasser-Caruso, M. A., & Goldsmith, B. M. (1985). Autism associated with Williams syndrome, *Journal of Paediatrics, 106,* 247 - 249.

Riikonen, R., & Amnell, G. (1981). Psychiatric disorders in children with earlier infantile spasms. *Developmental Medicine and Child Neurology, 23,* 747 - 760.

Rimland, B. (1965). *Infantile Autism.* London: Methuen.

Ritvo, E. R., Cantwell, D., Johnson, E., Clements, M., Bennbrook, F., Slagle, P., Kelly, P., & Ritz, M. (1971). Social class factors in autism. *Journal of Autism and Childhood Schizophrenia, 1,* 297 - 310.

Ritvo, E. R., Creel, D., Realmuto, G., Crandall, A. S., Freeman, B. J., Bateman, J. B.,

Bahr, R., Pingree, C., Coleman, M., & Purple, R. (1988). Electroretinograms in autism - a pilot study of b-wave amplitudes. *American Journal of Psychiatry, 145,* 229 - 232.

Ritvo, E. R., Freeman, B. J., Scheibel, A. B., Duong, T., Robinson, H., Guthrie, D., & Ritvo, A. (1986). Lower purkinje cell counts in the cerebella of four autistic subjects: Initial findings of the UCLA-NSAC Autopsy Research Report. *American Journal of Psychiatry, 143,* 862 - 866.

Ritvo, E. R., Freeman, B. J., Pingree, M. S., Mason-Brothers, A., Jorde, L., Jenson, R., McMahon, W., Petersen, B., Mo, A., & Ritvo, A. (1989). The UCLA-university of Utah Epidemiologic Survey of Autism: Prevalence, *American Journal of Psychiatry, 146,* 194 - 199.

Rosenhall, U., Johansson, E., & Gillberg, C. (1989). Oculomotor findings in autistic children. *Journal of Otolaryngology, 102,* 435 - 439.

Rumsey, J. M., & Hamburger, S. D. (1988). Neuropsychological findings in high-functioning men with infantile autism, residual state. *Journal of Clinical Experimental Neuropsychology, 10,* 201 - 221.

Rutter, M. (1983). Cognitive deficits in the pathogenesis of autism. *Journal of Child Psychology and Psychiatry, 24,* 513 - 531.

Rutter, M. (1970). Autistic children. Infancy to adulthood. *Seminars in Psychiatry, 2,* 435 - 450.

Sahley, T. L., & Panksepp, J. (1987). Brain opioids and autism - an updated analysis of possible linkages. *Journal of Autism and Developmental Disorders, 17,* 201 - 216.

Sarvis, M. A. (1960). Psychiatric implications of temporal lobe damage. *Psychoanalytic Study of the Child, 15,* 454 - 481.

Schain, R., & Yannet, H. (1960). Infantile autism: an analysis of 50 cases and a consideration of certain relevant neuropsychological concepts. *Journal of Paediatrics, 57,* 560 - 567.

Schopler, E., Andrew, C. E., & Strupp, K. (1979). Do autistic children come from upper-class parents? *Journal of Autism and Developmental Disorders, 9,* 139 - 152.

Steffenburg, S., & Gillberg, C. (1986). Autism and autistic-like conditions in Swedish rural and urban areas: a population study. *British Journal of Psychiatry, 149,* 81 - 87.

Steffenburg, S., Gillberg, C., Hellgren, L., Andersson, L., Gillberg, I. C., Jakobsson, G., Bohman, M. (1989). A Twin Study of Autism in Denmark, Finland, Iceland,

Norway and Sweden. *Journal of Child Psychology and Psychiatry, 30,* 405 - 416.

Steinhausen, H - C., & Breulinger, M. 1986. A community survey of infantile autism. *Journal of the American Academy of Child Psychiatry, 25,* 186 - 189.

Stubbs, E. G., Ash, E., & Williams, C. P. (1984). Autism and congenital cytomegalovirus infection. *Journal of Autism and Developmental Disorders, 14,* 183 - 189.

Suquiama, T., & Abe, T. (1989). The Prevalence of Autism in Nagoya, Japan: A Total Population Study. *Journal of Autism and Developmental Disorders, 19,* 87 - 96.

Tantam, D. (1988). Asperger's syndrome. *Journal of Child Psychology and Psychiatry, 29,* 245 - 255.

Tanoue, Y., Oda, S., Asano, F., Kawashima, K. (1988). Epidemiology of infantile autism in Southern Ibaraki, Japan: Differences in prevalence rates in Birth Cohorts. *Journal of Autism and Developmental Disorders, 18,* 155 - 166.

Torrey, E. F., Hersch, S. P., & McCabe, K. D. (1975). Early childhood psychosis and bleeding during pregnancy: A prospective study of gravid women and their offspring. *Journal of Autism and Childhood Schizophrenia, 5,* 287 - 297.

Wahlström, J., Gillberg, C., Gustavsson, K-G., & Holmgren, G. (1986). Infantile autism and the Fragile-X-syndrome. A Swedish population multicenter study. *American Journal of Medical Genetics, 23,* 403 - 408.

Watson, M. S., Leckman, J. F., Annex, B., Breg, W. R., Volkmar, F. R., & Cohen, D. J. (1984). Fragile-X in a survey of 75 autistic males. *New England Journal of Medicine, 310,* 1462.

Wing, L., & Gould, J. (1979). Severe impairments of social interaction and associated abnormalities in children: Epidemiology and classification. *Journal of Autism and Developmental Disorders, 9,* 11 - 29.

Wing, L. (1980a). Childhood autism and social class: A question of selection. *British Journal of Psychiatry, 137,* 410 - 417.

Wing, L. (1980b). *Early childhood autism.* 2nd Edn. Oxford: Pergamon Press.

Wing, L. (1981). Sex ratios in early childhood autism and related conditions. *Psychiatry Research, 5,* 129 - 137.

Wing, L. (1981). Language, social and cognitive impairments in autism and severe mental retardation. *Journal of Autism and Developmental Disorders, 11,* 31 - 44.

Witt-Engerström, I., & Gillberg, C. (1987). Autism and Rett syndrome. A preliminary epidemiological study of diagnostic overlap. *Journal of Autism and Developmental Disorders, 17,* 149 - 150.

Wolff, S., Narayan, S., & Moyes, B. (1988). Personality characteristics of parents of autistic children: a controlled study. *Journal of Child Psychology and Psychiatry, 29,* 143 - 154.

Recent Neurobiological Findings in Autism

LUKE Y. TSAI

INTRODUCTION

Neurobiological studies of autism have found that many autistic individuals suffer from organic brain disorders, ranging from 30 to 100%, depending on whether the children were selected from psychiatric or pediatric-neurologic cohorts (Fish & Ritvo, 1979). Neurological abnormalities including hypotonia or hypertonia, disturbance of body schema, clumsiness, choreiform movements, pathological reflexes, myoclonic jerking, drooling, abnormal posture and gait, dystonic posturing of hands and fingers, tremor, ankle clonus, emotional facial paralysis, and strabismus have been reported in 30 to 75% of several series of autistic patients (reviewed by Tsai, 1987a). There are also studies that show autistic children exhibiting high incidence of congenital minor physical anomalies (Campbell et al., 1978). Furthermore, a wide variety of established neurologic disorders have been reported in some cases of autism, including cerebral palsy, maternal rubella, toxoplasmosis, tuberous sclerosis, cytomegalovirus infection, demyelinating disease, lead encephalopathy, meningitis, encephalitis, severe brain hemorrhage, phenylketonuria, and many types of epilepsy (reviewed by Ornitz, 1983). Based on these findings, it is now well accepted that autism results from dysfunction in certain parts of the central nervous system (CNS) that affects language, cognitive and intellectual development, and the ability to relate. The findings also suggest that autism may be the final common pathway of a diverse range of organic brain conditions. It has become widely recognized that there is heterogeneity within autistic syndrome. This is particularly true when the subgroups are divided based on neurobiological measures (e.g. hyperserotonemic autism versus hyposerotonemic autism) or disease entitites (e.g. fragile-X autism versus non-fragile-X autism). The number of subgroups will continue to increase when our examination methods and diagnostic classifications increase in sophistication. The proliferation of subgroups should be viewed positively because it allows us to identify truly homogeneous subgroups of autistic children with a defined disease entity or brain condition. It may allow us to obtain important clues about the etiology of autism. The list of empirical studies of brain conditions which are or may be associated with autism is quite extensive. Within the limits of this presentation, the present paper reviews mainly those studies published since 1980 when the DSM-III became a widely used diagnostic system. It focuses primarily on findings obtained from studies of pre-, peri-, and neonatal complications, neurochemical studies, neuropathological studies, studies based on brain imaging, and neurophysiological studies. Recent findings of another important empirical research, genetic implications, will be described in another chapter (by Hagerman).

PRE-, PERI-, AND NEONATAL FACTORS IN AUTISM

Obstetrical and Postnatal Complications

It has been suggested that pre- or perinatal insults to the brain are the biological causation of autism for individuals whose autistic symptoms are manifested from birth, and that postnatal cerebral infections or injuries have been suggested as the etiology for those whose autism is manifested after a period of apparently normal development. Several investigators report that pre-, peri-, and neonatal complications appear with increased frequency in the histories of autistic patients (reviewed by Tsai, 1987). Several unfavorable pre-, peri-, and neonatal factors (particularly older mother, first- and fourth- or later born, bleeding after the first trimester, use of medication, and meconium in amniotic fluid) appear to be more frequent in autistic subjects than in their siblings or control subjects.

It seems that, in some instances, unfavorable pre-, peri-, and neonatal factors may be associated with autism. However, the data do not indicate a unifying pathologic process in autism. This lack of specificity suggests either that various types of obstetric and/or postnatal complications may cause autism (Deykin & MacMahon, 1980) or that there is (are) yet unidentified unifying obstetric and/or postnatal variable(s) responsible for all cases of autism, or that factors (e.g. genetic) other than obstetric and postnatal complications may also be responsible for the subsequent development of autism. In future studies it will be necessary to consider all of these aspects.

Immunological Studies

Chess and her associates reported increased frequency of autism in individuals with congenital rubella (Chess et al., 1971; Chess, 1977). The findings led Deykin and MacMahon (1979) to evaluate a number of infectious agents (e.g. measles, rubella, mumps, and chickenpox) as possible etiological factors of autism. They found no more than 5% of autism associated with prenatal rubella or influenza infection. Their investigation also revealed that the presence of other infectious agents during pregnancy was equally low for the autistic children and their normal siblings. Three other studies (Finegan & Quarrington, 1979; Gillberg & Gillberg, 1983; Mason-Brothers et al., 1987) also found a low rate of maternal infections during pregnancy in both the autistic and control groups.

With ever improving understanding of basic immunological mechanisms, as well as advancing research technology, there is a promising avenue along which researchers may some day identify certain infectious agent(s) that is (are) responsible for a subgroup of autism. Young and his associates studied the cerebrospinal fluid (CSF) immunoglobulin levels in 15 autistic children. They found no abnormalities of glucose, protein, cells, or folate. They concluded that the hypothesis of slow virus playing a role in autism could not be supported (Young et al.,1977).

In an attempt to retrospectively diagnose prenatal rubella, Stubbs (1976) gave rubella vaccine challenge to 15 autistic children and 8 controls matched for age. The rubella vaccine challenge did not differentiate autistic children from the controls. However, 5 of the 13 autistic children had undetectable hemagglutination-inhibition antibody titers despite previous vaccine, whereas all control subjects had detectable titers. Stubbs (1976) speculated that these autistic children might have an altered immune response or an immune defect.

Stubbs and his associate (1977) further postulated that the type of immune defect would be of the thymic-derived lymphocytes (T cells) and would be expressed either as (a) weak manifestation of cell mediated immunity or (b) deficient antibody response to T-dependent antigens. Cellular immune function was assessed in vitro by phytohemagglutinin (PHA) stimulation of lymphocyte cultures obtained from 12 autistic children and 13 control subjects. The autistic group showed a depressed lymphocyte transformation response to PHA when compared to the controls. The authors concluded that these autistic children had a relative T-cell deficiency which might be caused by viral infections.

Warren et al. (1986) reported findings of several immune-system abnormalities in 31 autistic patients, including reduced responses in the lymphocyte blastogenesis assay to PHA, concanavalin A, and pokeweed mitogen; decreased number of T lymphocytes; and an altered ratio of helper to suppressor T cells. In a further study of the activity of the natural killer (NK) cell (a large granular lymphocyte and a likely part of basic defense mechanism against virus-infected cells and malignancy) they found that about 40% of their autistic subjects had significally reduced NK cell activity (Warren et al., 1987).

Based on the observation that reactivity to human myelin basic protein measured by a migration inhibition factor had been implicated in a number of CNS disorders such as multiple sclerosis, the Guillan-Barre syndrome, and acute disseminated encephalomyelitis; Weizman et al. (1982) investigated the cell-mediated immune response to human myelin basic protein using the macrophage migration inhibition factor test in 17 autistic patients and 11 control subjects with other mental disorders. Thirteen out of the 17 (76%) autistic subjects exhibited inhibition of macrophage migration, while none of the controls had such response. The results were interpreted as a cell-mediated autoimmune response to brain antigen in some autistic individuals. Westall and Root-Bernstein (1983), however, suggested that "the lympocytes were probably a secondary response to increased serotonin levels stablizing myelin basic protein fragments against normal breakdown". They called for attention to be paid to the serotonin binding sites in future studies of autism. This suggestion seemed to gain some support from Todd and Ciaranello (1985) who reported that about one-third of the autistic children in their study had an unusual antibody circulating in their blood and spinal fluid. This antibody appeared to attack the receptor for serotonin.

In a further study to test for the presence of a generalized anti-brain antibody response in autistic patients, Todd and his associates (1988) failed to find such a response. They concluded that "if antibody-mediated autoantigen recognition is important in, or related to, established infantile autism, only a few antigens are involved".

All of these findings seem to suggest that depressed immune function, autoimmune mechanism, or faulty immune regulation may be associated with the etiology of autism. However, the exact cause-effect relationship remains unsettled. Clearly, more extensive studies are needed.

NEUROPATHOLOGICAL STUDIES

There are only a few studies of brain neuropathology in autism. Initial postmortem brain studies of seven cases revealed negative findings (Darby, 1976; William et al., 1980). Bauman & Kemper (1985) recently reported major cellular and structural changes in the amygdala, cerebellum, and hippocampus of a 29-year-old retarded autistic person, who died of drowning. The changes included increased cell packing densities, reduced size of neurones, and a lamina dissicans in entorhinal cortex.

Another more recent report seems to provide some support for these changes. Decreased Purkinje cell densities were found in the cerebella of four autistic patients studied by Ritvo and his associates (Ritvo et al., 1986). As these studies examined only limited brain structures of few subjects, the meaning of the findings is not clear. Nevertheless, they provide some direction (i.e. posterior cerebral fossa) for *in vivo* neuroanatomical imaging studies of autism.

BRAIN IMAGING STUDIES

Computerized Tomographic (CT) Scan Studies

CT studies have identified gross abnormalities (e.g. porencephalic cyst) in a minority of autistic patients (Balottin et al., 1989; Damasio et al., 1980; Gillberg & Svendsen, 1983). However, no uniform abnormality has been found. Most CT studies of autistic subjects look for subtle abnormalities by using quantitave measures.

An early study (Hier et al., 1979) reported a high incidence of abnormal anterior or posterior cerebral asymmetry in autistic children. Since then, four additional studies have failed to confirm this finding (Damasio et al., 1980; Tsai et al., 1983; Gillberg & Svendsen, 1983; Rumsey et al., 1988).

Damasio et al. (1980) reported ventricular asymmetries in autistic patients with neurological disease. This finding could not be replicated with less biased measures in idiopathic cases of autism (Rosenbloom et al., 1984). Enlargement of lateral and third ventricles was seen in a minority of physically healthy autistic patients (Campbell et al., 1982; Caparulo et al., 1981; Rosenbloom et al., 1984). However, two other studies did not find such abnormality (Creasey et al., 1986; Prior et al., 1984). Creasey et al. (1986) also reported that there was no significant group difference in volumes of CSF, white matter, gray matter, the caudate nuclei, lenticular nuclei, or the thalami. Bauman et al. (1985) reported a finding of increased fourth ventricular width and cerebellar atrophy in the autistic children. This finding, however, has not been confirmed by a more recent study of 15 healthy autistic men (Rumsey et al., 1988).

Magnetic Resonance Imaging (MRI) Studies

MRI uses the innate magnetic properties of hydrogen and phosphorus to provide a completely new technolgoy for the study of the human brain. It permits better delineation of the posterior fossa structures than does CT and scanning at planes other than the transverse plane used in CT. Coronal images permits a better evaluation of temporal horn abnormality than CT. MRI is rapidly displacing CT as the method of choice of obtaining detailed anatomical information about the brain.

Because many autistic subjects require sedation to remain still for scanning, only a few head MRI studies have been carried out in the autistic subjects. Minshew et al (1986) found that the cerebellum and fourth ventricle were normal in all 10 autistics with IQs of 70 or greater. However, three of the 6 patients with IQs of 70 to 85 had abnormalities: enlarged lateral ventricles in 2 and decreased cortical volume with increased subarachnoid space and normal ventricles in 1. Gaffney and his associates studied the head MRI of 14 autistic patients aged 4 to 22 years with IQs of 60 or greater. Six of the 14 patients had brain lesions seen on the MRI scans, including heterotopic gray matter, basal ganglia abnormalities, dilated lateral and fourth ventricle, and right temporal lobe cyst. There was no single, circumscribed lesion common to all the autistic patients. Midsagittal MRI scans showed the fourth ventricle being significantly larger and the entire brainstem to be significantly smaller in the autistic group, compared to the control group. In the coronal scans, the cerebella of the autistic patients were proportionally smaller and the fourth ventricles proportionally larger. Axial MRI scans showed no difference in the fourth ventricles, vermes, cerebella, and cerebella-pontine complexes between the groups (Gaffney et al., 1987, 1988; Gaffney & Tsai 1987; Gaffney, Tsai et al., 1987). Courchesne and his colleague recently reported that the neocerebella vermal lobules VI and VII were significantly smaller in the group of 18 autistic patients, compared to the normal controls (Courchesne et al., 1988). Garber et al., (1989) recently reported that the measurements of the midsagittal area and volume of the fourth ventricle did not differ between 15 autistic patients and 15 normal control subjects.

The abnormalities of the cerebellum are consistent in *in vivo* MRI findings as well as in microscopic post-mortem findings described earlier. Although the link between the cerebellar abnormalities and autism is yet to be determined, MRI technology has provided an exciting new avenue for future *in vivo* study of the brain. Furthermore, MRI provides information more than just anatomy. It can also be used as an *in vivo* spectrometer to distinguish among a large array of physiological compounds such as ATP, phosphocreatinine, and nonorganic phosphate. It is anticipated that in the near future, MRI will enable researchers to use hydrogen spectra to monitor changes in such major brain neuroregulators as GABA and other amino acids (Elliot & Ciaranello, 1987).

Positron Emission Tomography (PET) Studies

Another exciting new technology is positron emission tomography (PET) which provides three-dimensional images of a variety of biochemical processes. PET allows the measuring of brain energy metabolism, regional blood volumes, blood flow, tissue drug levels, and receptor binding. Application of PET to the study of childhood mental disorders has been slow because the amount of radiation exposure with current techniques is unacceptable for research with children.

In one recent study, Rumsey and her associates reported substantially elevated utilization of glucose throughout many parts of the brain of 10 autistic men (mean age of 26 years), as compared with control (Rumsey et al., 1985). More recently, Heh et al., (1989) used PET to examine cerebellar and vermal glucose metabolism in 7 adult autistic patients and 8 age-matched controls. The results showed no significant difference in mean cerebella glucose metabolism between the two groups, though all mean glucose rates of the autistic patients were either equal to or greater than those of the control subjects. Although the meaning of these findings remains to be determined, it appears that PET should become increasingly important for researchers studying autism.

NEUROCHEMICAL STUDIES

The results obtained from neuropathological and brain imaging studies suggest that the cerebral defect in autism is microscopic or functional, without major gross neuroanatomic pathology. The etiological implication of such a conclusion is that autism results from disturbances in the late stages of CNS development (Ciaranello et al., 1982). As neurochemical factors are very important in terms of initiating and maintaining the terminal stages of CNS development, it is necessary to examine the neurochemical correlates in autism.

Serotonin

Serotonergic activity in the brain has been linked to body temperature, pain, sensory perception, sleep, sexual behavior, motor function, neuroendocrine regulation, appetite, learning, memory, and immune response (reviewed by Young et al., 1982). Many studies have consistently reported that about one-third of autistic individuals have hyperserotonemia (reviewed by Anderson et al., 1987). There are three possible explanations of the hyperserotonemia: 1) enhanced platelet uptake, storage, or platelet volume, 2) increased synthesis, and 3) decreased catabolism.

It is well agreed that the major source of serotonin (5-hydroxytryptamine) (5-HT) in whole blood derives from platelet-stored amine. Plasma serotonin reported in the literature is mostly a measure of platelet 5-HT, or the release of serotonin from platelet during collection and/or processing. Recently, Geller et al. (1988) reported that there was no significant difference in platelet volumes between autistic patients and controls. Nor did the platelet volumes and blood serotonin concentration correlate.

Although previous studies found that the platelets handling of 5-HT appeared to be normal in autism (Anderson et al., 1985; Boullin et al., 1982), recent works, however, have indicated that the role of the platelet may need to be reexamined (Rotman et al., 1980; Katsui et al., 1986; Safai-Kutti et al., 1985). Furthermore, the autistic probands and their first-degree-relatives have strong familial resemblance. There is positive correlation of both platelet-rich plasma 5-HT and platelet-poor (free) plasma 5-HT between the autistic proband and their first-degree relatives (Cook et al., 1988; Kuperman et al., 1985).

The studies of 5-HT synthesis in autism have focused on the measurement of urinary 5-hydroxyindoleacetic acid (5-HIAA) either with or without tryptophan loading. The results have been conflicting. An earlier study reported a lower excretion rate in autistic subjects as compared to normals (Sutton et al., 1958). Another study found higher 5-HIAA excretion in autistic patients (Hanley et al., 1977). Several studies did not find any difference between autistic and normal subjects (Minderaa et al., 1987; Partington et al., 1973; Schain & Freedman, 1961).

Several studies have reported that the functioning of the principle catabolic enzyme monoamine oxidase (MAO) appeared to be normal in autism (Boullin et al., 1976; Campbell et al., 1976; Cohen et al., 1977b; Launay et al., 1987; Minderaa et al., 1987).

So far no consistent correlations have been found yet between blood serotonin levels and any autistic behaviors or symptoms. On the other hand, hyperserotonemia has also been found in some children who are severely retarded. Thus, the mechanism and importance of hyperserotonemia in autism remains unclear.

Dopamine

The brain dopaminergic system is considered to affect several functions and behaviors, including cognition, motor function, eating and drinking behaviors, sexual behavior, neuro endocrine regulation, and selective attention (Young et al., 1982). The studies of dopamine in autism have focused on the measurement of the homovanillic acid (HVA), the main metabolite of dopamine. The CSF level of HVA was found to be higher in the more severely impaired children, especially those with greater locomotor activity and more severe stereotypies (Cohen et al., 1974, 1977a). These studies, however, found that autistic children did not differ from other diagnostic groups in CSF level of HVA. Leckman et al (1980) also failed to find a difference in CSF HVA between "child psychosis (largely autism)" and "perceptual cognitive disorder" diagnostic groups.

Gillberg et al. (1983a) found elevated CSF HVA in 18 of their 22 psychotic children. When the sample was later expanded to 37 subjects (25 of whom had autism), the authors continued to find increases of CSF HVA in the autistic subjects (Gillberg & Svennerholm, 1987). These authors also found indications of a disturbed ratio of dopamine versus norepinephrine metabolites in autism. One study found a high correlation between HVA and 5-HIAA in the CSF samples of autistic patients (Elliot & Ciaranello, 1987).

Two studies found no difference for plasma HVA between autistic children and controls (Launay et al., 1987; Minderaa et al., 1989).

Several studies reported elevated free HVA levels in urine (Barthelemy et al., 1988; Garnier et al., 1986; Lelord et al., 1978), but the finding has not been confirmed by other investigators (DeVillard & Dalery 1979; Launay et al., 1987; Minderaa et al., 1989).

HVA concentrations have not been shown to correlate with any autistic behaviors or symptoms (Elliot & Ciaranello, 1987).

Epinephrine and Nor-Epinephrine

Epinephrine (E) and nor-epinephrine (NE) are often discussed concurrently because of their similar effects on behavior. They are associated with cardiovascular function, respiratory function, appetite, activity level, arousal, attention, anxiety, response to stress, movement, sleep, memory, and learning (Young et al., 1982).

Plasma NE has been reported to be elevated in autistic subjects (Lake et al.,1977). Launay et al. (1987), however, reported that both E and NE in platelets were significantly lower in the autistic group as compared with the controls.

Urinary excretion of NE and its major metabolite 3-methoxy-4-hydroxyphenylethylen glycos (MHPG) was decreased in autistic subjects, compared with normal controls (Young et al., 1982). Launay et al. (1987) found no significant difference between the autistic group and controls. Barthelemy et al., (1988) reported that autistic children showed high NE, low MHPG urinary level.

Three recent studies found no difference in CSF MHPG between autistic patients and controls (Gillberg et al., 1983; Gillberg & Svennerholm 1987; Young et al., 1982).

Dopamine-b-hydroxylase (DBH)

Conflicting results have been reported on the study of dopamin-b-hydroxylase (DBH), the enzyme that controls the conversion of dopamine to NE. Goldstein et al. (1976), and Lake et al. (1977) found a decreased DBH activity in autistics as compared to controls, whereas Young et al. (1980) found no difference. Recently, Garnier et al. (1986) also reported no difference in DBH activity between controls and autistic subjects as a group. However, the authors noted a significant increase of DBH activity in non-retarded autistics as compared to retarded autistic patients.

The real meaning of blood DBH activity is unclear, since normal human beings also exhibit wide range of DBH activity without evident effect.

Cathecol-O-methyl transferase (COMT) and MAO

Two metabolic enzymes, catechol-o-methyl transferase (COMT) and MAO, may change NE activity. Giller et al. (1980) found no difference in COMT activity in cultured fibroblasts and in red blood cells between autistic children and controls. MAO activity also appeared to be normal in autistic patients (Boullin et al., 1976; Lake et al., 1977; Young et al., 1982).

Peptides

In 1980, Trygstad et al. described a number of different urinary peptides profile patterns each said to be characteristic of a different behavioral abnormality. The characteristic profile for autism was initially shown in 20 patients with a variation of + 30 % for each peak. In a further study of 24 autistic children, Gillberg et al. (1982) reported that more than half the autistic children showed the pattern said to be characteristic of autism. However, in an attempt to replicate such a finding from 69 urine samples obtained from three groups of young male adults (autistic, mentally handicapped, and normal), no consistent patterns of urinary chromatographic profile were identified (Couteur et al., 1988).

In 1986, Reichelt et al. reported findings from a work which was an extension of the earlier study of Trygstad et al. (1980). The authors used somewhat different procedures and identified three G-25 gel filtration patterns among the autistic subjects. Type A is a relatively normal peak from 600 to 900 ml and a stepwise peak increase from 1100 to 1600 ml with a large late peak. Type B1 is a large peak from 600 to 900 ml and two small peaks at 1100-1500. Type B2 has only a large 600-900 ml peak and the two peaks from 600 to 900 ml are confluent or elute as one peak without a late peak. In those with Type A pattern, all but one had a period of normal development, whereas in Types B1 and B2 patients the disorder was present from the early neonatal period. Unfortunately, the diagnostic specificity of the G-25 chromatographic patterns is rather low because they cannot differentiate autism subgroups from other psychiatric disorders.

Nevertheless, the findings are intriguing and further study may develop patterns with high specificity. Any isolation and identification of any factors present in the chromatographic fractions may contribute to the understanding of the pathogenesis of autism.

Brain Opioids

The endorphin hypothesis was proposed based on the analogy between opiate addiction and autism (Kalat, 1978) and the similarity between opiate-induced psychosocial distortion in animals and clinical manifestations of autism (Panksepp, 1979). Weizman et al. (1984) found that compared with schizophrenic children or normal controls, autistic subjects had relatively low concentration of an endorphinlike substance (i e H-endorphin) in the blood. Gillberg et al. (1985) reported that the mean CSF endorphin fraction II levels was higher in autistic children in comparison to normal children. As the major opioid peptide in fraction II of human CSF is methionine enkephalinlys, a peptide deriving from proenkephalin A. Weizman et al. (1988) suggested that this opioid could not indicate the CSF content of b-endorphin.

Rose et al. (1985) reported elevated CSF immunoreactive ß-endorphin (ir-ß-EP) in autism and a correlation between the beneficial effect of fenfluramine treatment and suppression of CSF ir-ß-EP levels. Weizman et al. (1988), however, found that the mean value of plasma ir-ß-EP level was significantly lower in autistics compared to age- and sex-matched schizophrenics and healthy controls. The authors speculated that the reduced ir-ß-EP levels in autistics might account for some of the clinical manifestations of autism such as hypersensitivity to sensory stimuli, mood lability, panic reactions to minor changes, unexplained crying, and restlessness. Gillberg and his associates recently also found evidence of low ß-endorphin in the CSF of 30 autistic children (personal communication, 1989).

It seems that the actual identity of the brain opioids needs to be ascertained, so that the cause-effect mechanism can be established.

NEUROPHYSIOLOGICAL STUDIES

Given the limited success of neuropathological investigation, as well as neuroanatomical imaging in identifying localized brain lesion(s) in autism, neurophysiological techniques may play a more vital role in pursuing such goals. A comprehensive review of the neurophysiologic studies of autism has recently been carried out by the present author (Tsai, 1987b).

There are two rather disparate neurophysiologic hypotheses of autism. The first, which considers a primary cortical dysfunction in autism, emphasizes the autistic symptoms of language and communication, and assumes an underlying specific cognitive disorder that is presumably of cortical origin (Rutter, 1978). More specifically, this hypothesis considers that autism results from a disorder of hemispheric lateralization, that is, that the neural substrates in the left hemisphere necessary for sequential forms of information processing fail to develop (Blackstock 1978; Prior 1979; Tanguay 1977).

A second hypothesis proposes a primary brainstem dysfunction in autism. This hypothesis has been developed through observation of the impaired ability of autistic children in modulating their own responses to sensory input and consequently their own motor output (Ornitz, 1974, 1983). This hypothesis suggests a rostrally directed sequence of pathophysiologic influences originating in the brainstem and diencephalic structures, particularly the reticular formation of pontine and midbrain, substantia nigra, and the nonspecific nuclei of thalamus (Ornitz, 1985).

The cortical-dysfunction hypothesis of autism has received some support from computerized quantitative EEG studies that indicate abnormal pattern of cerebral lateralization (Cantor et al., 1986; Dawson et al., 1982; Ogawa et al., 1982; Small, 1975). Several studies of event-related brain potential have found that autistic individuals have, on the average, smaller auditory P3b response (a component occurs 300-900 ms after stimulus which representing purely cognitive functions; reviewed by Courchesne, 1987). Recently, Courchesne and his associates uncovered another long-latency evoked-potential component (i. e., Nc, appears 200 to 300 ms after stimulus and is associated with attention and memory processes) seemed to be consistently very much smaller (i.e., less negative in potential) in the nonretarded autistic group (Courchesne, 1987; Courchesne et al., 1989). More recently, Dawson et al. (1988) found that compared to normal controls, the autistic subjects in their study had a significantly smaller P3b amplitude to phentic stimuli ("Da") for vertex (Cz) and left hemisphere (LH) recording sites; impaired language ability was related to greater P3b amplitude for right hemisphere (RH) recording site, but no group differences in P3b amplitude were found for the chord stimulus (piano) at any recording site. These findings suggest that autistic people may have a diminished or altered capacity for selectively channeling information for further internal attention and processing, as well as that differential hemispheric involvement in the attentional deficits.

The hypothesis of brainstem dysfunction in autism is supported to a limited extent by indirect evidence from autonomic responses (Hutt et al., 1975; MacCulloh & Williams, 1971) and sleep studies (Ornitz et al .,1973a, 1973b), as well as evidence from vestibular nystagmus studies (reviewed by Ornitz, 1985). Several auditory brainstem evoked-potential (ABEP) studies described subgroups of autistic subjects with one or another abnormal response component, particularly prolonged brainstem transmission time (BSTT) (Fein et al., 1981; Gillberg et al., 1983b; Rosenbaum et al., 1980; Skoff et al., 1980; Student & Sohmer, 1978; Taylor et al., 1982). However, several other studies did not find the relatively high incidence of abnormality in BSTT in the autistic patients (Novick et al., 1980; Rumsey et al., 1984; Tanguay et al., 1982). Rumsey et al. (1984) even found shortened BSTT in 4 autistic subjects. Courchesne and his associates found all their 14 autistic patients had "clinically and neurophysiologically" normal ABEP (Courchesne, 1987). Thus, the results of ABEP studies have been equivocal.

SUMMARY AND COMMENT

Neurobiological investigations in autism have found various abnormalities. However, no single measure of the abnormalities has been consistently found, and the etiological implications of the findings are far from clear. The inconsistent findings may arise from a number of factors. These include the use of different diagnostic criteria for patient selection, failure to control developmental factors (many studies included both children and adults), lack of suitable control groups (most studies used normal rather than mentally retarded controls and hence fail to control concomitant mental retardation that existed in the majority of autistic subjects), failure to control concomitant medical disorders (particularly CNS pathologies), as well as medications that may significantly affect subject's neurochemical and/or neurophysiological responses, and lack of collaborative studies and hence fail to use uniform measuring and reporting procedures. Nevertheless, the lack of consistent and specific findings can also be viewed as supportive evidence of many different subgroups within autistic syndrome. Future neurobiological research in the field of autistic syndrome should focus on the question of specificity and selectivity within each of the subgroups.

Neurobiological and behavioral understanding of the fundamental properties of the human brain is growing at an exponential rate. It is an exciting time to be doing neurobiological research in the field of autism. A variety of promising new leads and new technologies already offer directions, and there is much hope for the future in terms of searching for the answer of cause and treatment of autism.

REFERENCES

Andersson, G. M., Schlicht, K. R., & Cohen, D. J. (1985). Two-dimensional high-performance liquid chromatographic determination of 5-hydroxyindoleactic acid and homovanillic acid in urine. *Analytical Biochemistry, 144,* 27 - 31.

Andersson, G. M., Freedman, D. X., Cohen, D. J., Volkmar, E., Hoder, L., McPhedran, P., Minderaa, R. B., Hansen, C. R., & Young, J. G. (1987). Whole blood serotonin in autistic and normal subjects. *Journal of Child Psychology and Psychiatry, 28,* 885 - 900.

Balottin, U., Bejor, M., Cecchini, A., Martelli, A., Palazzi, S., & Lanzi, G. (1989). Infantile autism and computerized tomography brain-scan findings: Specific versus nonspecific abnormalities. *Journal of Autism and Developmental Disorders, 19,* 109 - 117.

Barthelemy, C., Bruneau, N., Cottet - Eymard, J. M., Domenech-Jouve, J., Garreau, B., Lelord, G., Muh, J. P., & Peyrin, L. (1988). Urinary free and conjugated catecholamines and metabolites in autistic children. *Journal of Autism and Developmental Disorders, 18,* 583 - 591.

Bauman, M., & Kemper, T. L. (1985). Histoanatomic observations of the brain in early infantile autism. *Neurology, 35,* 866 - 874.

Bauman, M., LeMay, M., Bauman, R. A., & Rosenberger, P. B. (1985). Computerized tomographic (CT) observations of the posterior fossa in early infantile autism. *Neurology, 35,* (Suppl 1) 247.

Blackstock, E. G. (1978). Cerebral asymmetry and development of early infantile autism. *Journal of Autism and Developmental Disorders, 8,* 339 - 353.

Boullin, D., Bhagavan, H. N., O'Brien, R. A., & Youdim, M. B. H. (1976). Platelet monoamine oxidase in children with infantile autism. In M. Coleman (Ed.), *The Autistic Syndromes.* New York: Elsevier.

Boullin, D., Freeman, B. J., Geller, E., Ritvo, E., Rutter, M., & Yuwiler, A. (1982). Toward the resolution of conflicting findings. *Journal of Developmental Disorders, 12,* 97 - 98.

Campbell, M., Friedman, E., Green, W. H., Small, A. M., & Burdoch, E. I. (1976). Blood platelet monoamine oxidase in schizophrenic children and their families. *Neuropsychobiology, 2,* 239 - 246.

Campbell, M., Geller, B., Small, A. M., Petti, T. A., & Ferries, S. H. (1978). Minor physical anomalies in young psychotic children. *American Journal of Psychiatry, 135,* 573 - 575.

Campbell, M., Rosenbloom, S., Perry., R., George, A., Kricheff, I., Andersson, L., Small, A., & Jennings, S. (1982). Computerized axial tomography in young autistic children. *American Journal of Psychiatry, 139,* 510 - 512.

Cantor, D. S., Thatcher, R. W., Hrybyk, M., & Kaye, H. (1986). Computerized EEG analyses of autistic children. *Journal of Autism and Developmental Disorders, 16,* 169 - 187.

Caparulo, B., Cohen, D. J., Rothman, S., Young, J., Shaywitz, S., & Shaywitz, B. (1981). Computed tomographic brain scanning in children with developmental neuropsychiatric disorders. *Journal of the American Academy of Child Psychiatry, 20,* 338 - 357.

Chess, S. (1977). Follow-up report on autism in congenital rubella. *Journal of Developmental Disorders, 7,* 69 - 81.

Chess, S., Korn, S. J., & Fernandez, P. B. (1971). *Psychiatric disorders of children with congenital rubella.* New York: Brunner/Mazel.

Ciaranello, R. D., Van den Berg, S., & Anders, T. F. (1982). Intrinsic and extrinsic determinants of neuronal development: Relation to infantile autism. *Journal of Autism and Developmental Disorders, 12,* 115 - 145.

Cohen, D. J., Shaywitz, B. A., Johnson, W. K., & Bowers, M. (1974). Biogenic amines in autistic and atypical children: cerebrospinal fluid measure of homovanillic acid and 5-hydroxyindole acetic acid. *Archives of General Psychiatry, 31,* 845 - 853.

Cohen, D. J., Caparulo, B. K., Shaywitz, B. A., & Bowers, M. (1977a). Dopamine and serotonin metabolism in neuropsychiatrically disturbed children. *Archives of General Psychiatry, 34,* 545 - 550.

Cohen, D. J., Young, J. G., & Roth, J. A. (1977b). Platelet monoamine oxidase in early childhood autism. *Archives of General Psychiatry, 34,* 534 - 537.

Cook, E. H., Leventhal, B. L., & Freedman, D. X. (1988). Free serotonin in plasma: Autistic children and their first-degree relatives. *Biological Psychiatry, 24,* 488 - 491.

Courchesne, E. (1987). A neurophysiological view of autism. In E. Schopler & G. B. Mesibov (Eds.), *Neurobiological Issues in Autism* (pp 285 - 234). New York and London: Plenum Press.

Courchesne, E., Lincoln, A. J., Yeung-Courchesne, R., Elmasian, R., & Grillon, C. (1989). Pathophysiologic findings in nonretarded autism and receptive developmental language disorder. *Journal of Autism and Developmental Disorders, 19,* 1 - 17.

Courchesne, E., Yeung-Courchesne, B. A., Press, G. A., Hesselink, J. R., & Jernigan, T. L. (1988). Hypoplasia of Cerebellar vermal lobules VI and VII in autism. *New England Journal of Medicine, 318,* 1349 - 1354.

Couteur, A. L., Trygstad, O., Evered, C., Gillberg, C., & Rutter, M. (1988). Infantile autism and urinary excretion of peptides and protein-associated peptide complexes. *Journal of Autism and Developmental Disorders, 18,* 181 - 190.

Damasio, H., Maurer, R. G., Damasio, A. R., & Chui, H. C. (1980). Computerized tomographic scan findings in patients with autistic behavior. *Archives of General Psychiatry, 37,* 504 - 510.

Darby, J. C. (1976). Neuropathologic aspects of psychosis in children. *Journal of Autistic Children and Schizophrenia, 6,* 339 - 352.

Dawson, G., Warrenburg, S., & Fuller, P. (1982). Cerebral lateralization in individuals diagnosed as autistic in early childhood. *Brain Language, 15,* 353 - 368.

Dawson, G., Finley, C., Phillips, S., Galpert, L., & Lewy, A. (1988). Reduced P3 amplitude of the event-related brain potential. Relationship to language ability in autism. *Journal of Autism and Developmental Disorders, 18,* 493 - 504.

Deykin, E. Y., & MacMahon, B. (1989). Pregnancy, delivery, and neonatal complications among autistic children. *American Journal of Diseases of Children, 134,* 860 - 864.

Elliott, G. R., & Ciaranello, R. D. (1987). Neurochemical hypotheses of childhood psychoses. In E. Schopler & G. B.Mesibov (Eds.), *Neurobiological Issues in Autism.* New York and London: Plenum Press.

Fein, D., Skoff, B., & Mirsky, A. F. (1981). Clinical correlates of brainstem dysfunction in autistic children. *Journal of Autism and Developmental Disorders, 11,* 303 - 315.

Finegan, J-A., & Quarrington, B. (1979). Pre-, peri-, and neonatal factors and infantile autism. *Journal of Child Psychology and Psychiatry, 20,* 119 - 128.

Fish, B. & Ritvo, E. (1979). Psychoses of childhood. In J. D. Noshpitz (Ed.), *Basic Handbook of Child Psychiatry,* New York: Basic Books.

Gaffney, G., & Tsai, L. (1987). Magnetic resonance imaging of high level autism. *Journal of Autism and Developmental Disorders, 17,* 433 - 438.

Gaffney, G., Kuperman, S., Tsai, L., Minchin, S., & Hassanein, K. M. (1987). Midsagittal magnetic resonance imaging of autism. *British Journal of Psychiatry, 151,* 831 - 833.

Gaffney, G., Kuperman, S., Tsai, L., & Minchin, S. (1988). Morphological evidence for brainstem involvement in infantile autism. *Biological Psychiatry, 24,* 578 - 586.

Gaffney, G., Tsai, L., Kuperman, S., & Minchin, S. (1987). Cerebellar structure in autism. *American Journal of Diseases of Children, 141,* 1330 - 1332.

Garber, H. J., Ritvo, E. R., Chiu, L. C., Griswold, V. J., Kashanian, A., Freeman, B. J., & Oldendorf, W. H. (1988). A magnetic resonance imaging study of autism. Normal fourth ventricle size and absence of pathology. *American Journal of Psychiatry, 146,* 532 - 534.

Garnier, G., Comoy, E., Barthelemy, C., Leddet, I., Garreau, B., Muh, J. P., & Lelord, G. (1986). Dopamine-beta-hydroxylase (DBH) and homovanillic acid (HVA) in autistic children. *Journal of Autism and Developmental Disorders, 16,* 23 - 29.

Geller, E., Yuwiler, A., Freeman, B. J., & Ritvo, E. (1988). Platelet size, number, and serotonin content in blood of autistic childhood schizophrenic, and normal children. *Journal of Autism and Developmental Disorders, 18,* 119 - 126.

Gillberg, C., & Gillberg, I. C. (1983). Infantile autism: a total population study of reduced optimality in the pre-, peri-, and neonatal period. *Journal of Autism and Developmental Disorders, 13,* 153 - 166.

Gillberg, C., & Svendsen, P. (1983). Childhood psychosis and computed tomographic brain scan findings. *Journal of Autism and Developmental Disorders, 13,* 19 - 32.

Gillberg, C., & Svennerholm, L. (1987). CSF monoamines in autistic syndromes and other pervasive developmental disorders of early childhood. *British Journal of Psychiatry, 151,* 89 - 94.

Gillberg, C., Trygstad, O., & Foss, I. (1982). Childhood psychosis and urinary excretion of peptides and protein-associated peptide complexes. *Journal of Autism and Developmental Disorders, 12,* 229 - 241.

Gillberg, C., Rosenhall, U., & Johansson, E. (1983). Auditory brainstem responses in childhood psychosis. *Journal of Autism and Developmental Disorders, 13,* 181 - 195.

Gillberg, C., Svennerholm, L., & Hamilton-Hellberg, C. (1983). Childhood psychosis and monoamine metabolites in spinal fluid. *Journal of Autism and Developmental Disorders, 13,* 383 - 396.

Gillberg, C., Terenius, L., & Lönnerholm, G. (1985). Endorphin activity in childhood psychosis. *Archives of General Psychiatry, 42,* 780 - 783.

Giller, E. L., Jr., Young, J. G., Breakfield, X. O., Carbonari, C., Braverman, M., &

Cohen, D. J. (1980). Monoamine oxidase and catechol-O-methyltransferase activities in cultured fibroblasts and blood cells from children with autism and the Gilles la Tourette syndrome. *Psychological Research, 2,* 187 - 197.

Goldstein, M., Mahanand, P., Lee, J., & Coleman, M. (1976). Dopamine-beta-hydroxylase and endogenous total 5-hydroxyindole levels in autistic patients and controls. In M. Coleman (Ed.), *The autistic syndrome.* Amsterdam: Elsevier/North Holland.

Hanley, H. G., Stahl, S. M., & Freedman, D. X. (1977). Hyperserotoninemia and amine metabolism in autistic and retarded children. *Archives of General Psychiatry, 34,* 521 - 531.

Heh, C. W. C., Smith, R., Wu, J., Hazlett, E., Russel, A., Asarnow, R., Tanguay, P., & Buchsbaum, M. S. (1989). Position emission tomography of the cerebellum in autism. *American Journal of Psychiatry, 146,* 242 - 245.

Hier, D. B., LeMay, M., & Rosenberger, P. B. (1979). Autism and unfavourable left-right asymmetries of the brain. *Journal of Autism and Developmental Disorders, 9,* 153 - 159.

Hutt, C., Forrest, S. J., & Richer, J. (1975). Cardiac arrhythmia and behavior in autistic children. *Acta Psychiatrica Scandinavica, 19,* 361 - 372.

Kalat, J. W. (1978). Speculations on similarities between autism and opiate addiction. *Journal of Autism and Childhood Schizophrenia, 8,* 477 - 479.

Katsui T., Okuda, M., Usuda, S., & Koizumi, T. (1986). Kinetics of -H-serotonin uptake by platelets in infantile autism and developmental language disorder (including five pairs of twins). *Journal of Autism and Developmental Disorders, 16,* 69 - 76.

Kuperman, S., Beeghly, J. H., Burns, T. L., & Tsai, L. (1985). Serotonin relationships of autistic probands and their first-degree relatives. *Journal of the American Academy of Child Psychiatry, 24,* 189 - 190.

Lake, C. R., Ziegler, M. G., & Murphy, D. L. (1977). Increased norepinephrine levels and decreased dopamine-beta-hydroxylase activity in primary autism. *Archives of General Psychiatry, 34,* 553 - 556.

Launay, J. M., Bursztejn, C., Ferrari, P., Dreux, C., Braconnier, A., Zarifian, E., Lancrenon, S., & Fermanian, J. (1987). Catecholamine metabolism in infantile autism: A controlled study of 22 autistic children. *Journal of Autism and Developmental Disorders, 17,* 333 - 347.

Leckman, J. F., Cohen, D. J., Shaywitz, B. A., Caparulo, B. K., Heninger, G. R., & Bowers, M. B., Jr. (1980). CSF monoamine metabolites in child and adult psychiatric patients. *Archives of General Psychiatry, 37,* 677 - 681.

Lelord, G., Callaway, E., Muh, J. P., Arlog, J. C., Sauvage, D., Garreau, B., & Domenchi, J. (1978). Modification in urinary homovanillic acid after ingestion of vitamin B6: Functional study in autistic children. *Revue Neurologique, 134,* 797 - 801.

MacCulloch, M. J., & Williams, C. (1971). On the nature of infantile autism. *Acta Psychiatrica Scandinavica, 47,* 295 - 314.

Mason-Brothers, A., Ritvo, E., Guze, B., Mo, A., Freeman, B. J., Funderburk, S. J., & Schroth, P. C. (1987). Pre-, peri-, and postnatal factors in 181 autistic patients from single and multiple incidence families. *Journal of the American Academy of Child and Adolescent Psychiatry, 26,* 39 - 42.

Minderaa, R. B., Anderson, G. M., Volkmar, F. R., Akkerhuis, G. W., & Cohen, D. J. (1987). Urinary 5-hydroxyindoleacetic acid and whole blood serotonin and tryptophan in autistic and normal subjects. *Biological Psychiatry, 22,* 933 - 940.

Minderaa, R. B., Anderson, G. M., Volkmar, F. R., Akkerhuis, G. W., & Cohen, D. J. (1988). Neurochemical study of dopamine functioning in autistic and normal subjects. *Journal of the American Academy of Child and Adolescent Psychiatry, 28,* 190 - 194.

Minshew, N. J., Payton, J. B., Wolf, G. L., & Latchaw, R. E. (1986). -H NMR imaging of autistics: Implication for neurobiology. *Annals of Neurology, 20,* 417.

Ogawa, T., Suqiyama, A., Ishiwa, M., Ishihara, T., & Sato, K. (1982). Ontogenic development of EEG-asymmetry in early infantile autism. *Brain and Development, 4,* 439 - 449.

Ornitz, E. M., Forsythe, A. B., & de la Pena, A. (1973a). The effect of vestibular and auditory stimulation on the rapid eye movement of REM sleep in normal children. *Electroencephalography and Clinical Neurophysiology, 34,* 379 - 390.

Ornitz, E. M., Forsythe, A. B., & de la Pena, A. (1973b). Effect of vestibular and auditory stimulation on the REMs of REM sleep in autistic children. *Archives of General Psychiatry, 29,* 786 - 791.

Ornitz, E. M. (1974). The modulation of sensory input and motor output in autistic children. *Journal of Autism and Developmental Disorders, 4,* 197 - 215.

Ornitz, E. M. ((1983). The functional neuroanatomy of infantile autism. *International Journal of Neuroscience, 19,* 85 - 124.

Ornitz, E. M. (1985). Neurophysiology of infantile autism. *Journal of the American Academy of Child Psychiatry, 24,* 251 - 262.

Panksepp, J. (1979). A neurochemical theory of autism. *Trends in Neurosciences, 2,* 174 - 177.

Partington, M. W., Tu, J. B., & Wong, C. Y. (1973). Blood serotonin levels in severe mental retardation. *Developmental Medicine and Child Neurology, 15,* 616 - 627.

Prior, M. R. (1979). Cognitive abilities and disabilities in infantile autism: A review. *Journal of Abnormal Child Psychology, 7,* 357 - 380.

Prior, M. R., Tress, B., Hoffman, W. L., & Boldt, D. (1984). Computed tomographic study of children with classic autism. *Archives of Neurology, 41,* 482 - 484.

Reichelt, K. L., Sœlid, G., Lindback, T., & Bøler, J. B. (1986). Childhood autism: A complex disorder. *Biological Psychiatry, 21,* 1279 - 1290.

Ritvo, E., Freeman, B. J., Scheibel, A. B., Duong, T., Robinson, H., Guthrie, D., & Ritvo, A. (1986). Lower Purkinje cell counts in the cerebella of four autistic subjects: Initial findings of the UCLA-NSAC autopsy research report. *American Journal of Psychiatry, 143,* 862 - 866.

Rose, D. L., Klykylo, W. M., & Hitzeman, R. (1985). Cerebrospinal fluid beta endorphin immunoreactivity is elevated in infantile autism and decreased by fenfluramine treatment. *Annals of Neurology, 18,* 418.

Rosenbloom, S., Campbell, M., George, A., Kricheff, I., Taleporos, E., Anderson, L., Reuben, R., & Korein, J. (1984). High resolution CT scanning in infantile autism: A quantitative approach. *Journal of the American Academy of Child Psychiatry, 23,* 72 - 77.

Rosenblum, S. M., Arick, J. R., Krug, D. A., Stubbs, E. G., Young, N. B., & Pelson, R. O. (1980). Auditory brainstem evoked responses in autistic children. *Journal of Autism and Developmental Disorders, 10,* 215 - 225.

Rotman, A., Caplan, R., & Szekeley, G. A. (1980). Platelet uptake of serotonin in psychotic children. *Psychopharmacology, 67,* 245 - 248.

Rumsey, J. M., Creasy, H., Stepanek, J. S., Dorwart, R., Patronas, N., Hamberger, S. D., & Duara, R. (1988). Hemispheric asymmetries, fourth ventricular size, and cerebellar morphology in autism. *Journal of Autism and Developmental Disorders, 18,* 127 - 137.

Rumsey, J. M., Duara, R., Grady, C., Rapoport, J. L., Margolin, R. A., Rapoport, S. I., & Cutler, N. (1985). Brain metabolism in autism: Resting cerebral glucose utilization rates measured with positron emission tomography. *Archives of General Psychiatry, 42,* 448 - 455.

Rumsey, J. M., Grimes, A. M., Pikus, A. M., Duara, R., & Ismond, D. R. (1984). Auditory brainstem responses in pervasive developmental disorders. *Biological Psychiatry, 19,* 1403 - 1418.

Rutter, M. (1978). Language disorder and infantile autism. In M. Rutter & E. Schopler (Eds.), *Autism: A Reappraisal of Concepts and Treatment.* New York: Plenum Press.

Safai-Kutti, S., Kutti, J., & Gillberg, C. (1985). Impaired in vivo platelet reactivity in infantile autism. *Acta Paediatrica Scandinavica, 74,* 799 - 800.

Schain, R. J., & Freedman, D. X. (1961). Studies on 5-hydroxyindole metabolism in autistic and other mentally retarded children. *Journal of Paediatrics, 58,* 315 - 320.

Small, J. G. (1975). EEG and neurophysiological studies of early infantile autism. *Biological Psychiatry, 10,* 385 - 397.

Skoff, B. F., Mirsky, A., & Turner, D. (1980). Prolonged brainstem transmission time in autism. *Psychiatry Research, 2,* 157 - 166.

Stubbs, E. G. (1976). Autistic children exhibit undetectable hemagglutination-inhibition antibody titers despite previous rubella vaccination. *Journal of Autism and Childhood Schizophrenia, 7,* 49 - 55.

Student, M., & Sohmer, H. (1978). Evidence from auditory nerve and brainstem evoked responses for an organic brain lesion in children with autistic traits. *Journal of Autism and Developmental Disorders, 8,* 13 - 20.

Sutton, H. E., Read, J. H., & Arbor, A. (1958). Abnormal amino acid metabolism in a case suggesting autism. *American Journal of Diseases of Children, 96,* 23 - 28.

Tanguay, P. E., Edwards, R. M., Buchwald, J., Schwafel, J., & Allen, W. (1982). Auditory brainstem evoked responses in autistic children. *Archives of General Psychiatry, 39,* 174 - 180.

Taylor, M. J., Rosenblatt, B., & Linschoten, L. (1982). Auditory brainstem response abnormalities in autistic children. *The Canadian Journal of Neurological Sciences, November,* 429 - 433.

Todd, R. D., & Ciaranello, R. D. (1985). Demonstration of inter- and intraspecies differences in serotonin binding sites by antibodies from an autistic child. *Proceedings of the National Academy of Sciences of the United States of America.*

Todd, R. D., Hickok, J. M., Anderson, G. M., & Cohen, D. J. (1988). Antibrain antibodies in infantile autism. *Biological Psychiatry, 23,* 644 - 647.

Trygstad, O. E., Reichelt, K. L., Foss, I., Edminson, P. D., Saelid, G., Bremet, J., Ørbech, H., Johansen, J. H., Bøler, J. B., Titlestad, K., & Opstad, P. K. (1980). Patterns of peptides and proteinassociated peptide complexes in psychiatric disorders. *British Journal of Psychiatry, 136,* 59 - 72.

Tsai, L. (1987a). Pre-, peri-, and neonatal factors in autism. In E. Schopler & G. B. Mesibov (Eds.), *Neurobiological Issues in Autism.* New York and London: Plenum Press.

Tsai, L. (1987b). Neurophysiologic studies of infantile autism. In M. Wolraich (Ed.), *Advances in Developmental and Behavioral Pediatrics.* Greenwich, Connecticut: JAI Press Inc.

Tsai, L., Jacoby, C. G., & Stewart, M. A. (1983). Morphological cerebral asymmetries in autistic children. *Biological Psychiatry, 18,* 317 - 327.

Warren, R. P., Margaretten, N. C., Pace, N. C., & Foster, A. (1986). Immune abnormalities in patients with autism. *Journal of Autism and Developmental Disorders, 16,* 189 - 197.

Warren, R. P., Foster, A., & Margaratten, N. C. (1987). Reduced natural killer cell activity in autism. *Journal of the American Academy of Child and Adolescent Psychiatry, 26,* 333 - 335.

Weizman, A., Weizman, R., Szekely, G. A., Wijsenbeek, H., & Livni, E. (1982). Abnormal immune response to brain tissue antigen in the syndrome of autism. *American Journal of Psychiatry, 139,* 1462 - 1465.

Weizman, R., Weizman, A., Tyano, S., Szekely, G., Weissman, B. A., & Sarne, Y. (1984). Humoral endorphin blood levels in autistic, schizophrenic and healthy subjects. *Psychopharmacology, 82,* 368 - 370.

Weizman, R., Gil-Ad, I., Dick, J., Tyano, S., Szekely, G. A., & Laron, Z. (1988). Low plasma immunoreactive ß-endorphin levels in autism. *Journal of the American Academy of Child and Adolescent Psychiatry, 27,* 430 - 433.

Westall, F. C., & Root-Bernstein, R. S. (1983). Suggested connection between autism serotonin, and myelin basic protein. *American Journal of Psychiatry, 140,* 1260 - 1261.

Williams, R. S., Hauser, S. L., Purpura, D. P., DeLong, G. R., & Swischer, C. N. (1980). Autism and mental reatardation. *Archives of Neurology, 37,* 749 - 753.

Young, J. G., Kyprie, R. M., Ross, N. T., & Cohen, D. J. (1980). Serum dopamine-beta-hydroxylase activity: Clinical applications in child psychiatry. *Journal of Autism and Developmental Disorders, 10,* 1 - 14.

Young, J. G., Kavanagh, M. E., Anderson, G. M., Shaywits, B. A., & Cohen, D. J. (1982). Clinical neurochemistry of autism and associated disorders. *Journal of Autism and Developmental Disorders, 12,* 147 - 165.

Chromosomes, Genes and Autism

RANDI J. HAGERMAN

Advances of the last decade in medical science, particularly in the fields of cytogenetic and metabolic disease, have elucidated specific etiologies for many individuals with autism. Although the largest group still remains idiopatic, detailed studies have demonstrated a documentable organic etiology in over 25 % of children with autism (Gillberg & Wahlström, 1985). The most prevalent single etiology for autism is the fragile X syndrome. Since the association was first identified by Brown and co-workers in 1982, cytogenetic studies have become an integral part of the medical workup of children with autism and pervasive development delays. The search for fragile X has enhanced our appreciation of all types of cytogenetic abnormalities in individuals with developmental disabilites. When fragile X is not found, occasionally other abnormalities, including autosomal or sex chromosomal problems, are present (Gillberg & Wahlström, 1985; Hagerman et al., 1988). This chapter will review the association of autism with cytogenetic abnormalites, including the fragile X syndrome and, to a lesser degree, single gene disorder.

Our understanding of the genetic influences in autism is dependent on accurate subtyping within the overall clinical spectrum. A variety of medical problems can interfere with optimal CNS function and eventually create the constellation of behaviors and responses identified in autism. The genetic etiologies have been the most productive so far in identifying subgroups because most of the known medical causes of autism have a genetic basis. They will also eventually clarify the interaction of genes and brain development, including structure and neurochemistry, which goes awry in autism.

Single gene disorders were first appreciated in the etiology of autism because untreated PKU was prevalent in the past and the majority of individuals who did not receive dietary restrictions manifested a spectrum of autistic features (Friedman, 1969). Chromosomal disorders were considered only rarely associated with autism, as documented by an occasional case report (Wolraich et al., 1970; Coleman, 1976). The advent of fragile X has forced us to reevaluate this association.

Approximately one-half of all fertilized ova have a chromosomal abnormality, but 99% of all fetuses with chromosomal problems die prenatally (Gilbert & Opitz, 1982). Of those that survive to birth, 5.8% of stillborn infants and 5.9 per 1,000 live born infants have a chromosomal defect (not including fragile X) (Jacobs, 1977). One-third of chromosomal problems are sex chromosomal abnormalities, one-fourth are autosomal trisomies and 40% are structural defects, not including fragile X (Jacobs, 1977). The single most common chromosomal abnormality after birth is trisomy 21, Down syndrome. It rarely causes autism and with the advent of prenatal diagnosis its incidence has decreased to appoximately 1 per 1,000 live births. Fragile X syndrome has a very similar incidence and furthermore, it is heritable. Fragile X commonly causes autism, so we will begin our discussion with this disorder.

Fragile X Syndrome

The fragile X syndrome (Figs. 1 and 2) has had a significant impact on the field of autism because it is common and the majority of males affected by fragile X demonstrate a spectrum of autistic features. At the present time, it is the most common identifiable cause of autism that exists.

The fragile X chromosome was first visualized in 1969 by Lubs, after evaluating a family with 4 retarded males. The syndrome was not widely recognized, however, until Sutherland (1977) clarified the tissue culture requirements for eliciting the fragile site in the Xq27.3 region, on the lower end of the long arm of the X chromosome. Expression of the fragile site required that the cells be cultured under conditions of folic acid/thymidine deprivation. Most cytogenetic laboratories did not routinely use folate/thymidylate deficient culture conditions until the 1980's, so that the majority of individuals with this syndrome remain undiagnosed.

The prevalence of this disorder is approximately 0.9 per 1,000 to 1 per 1,360 as measured by a review of mental retardation and birth records (Herbst & Miller, 1980), and by a total screen of retarded individuals in Coventry County, England (Webb et al., 1986). Since nonpenetrant, or unaffected, carrier males and females exist, the rate of individuals who carry the fragile X gene in the general population may be as high as 1 in 750 (Opitz,

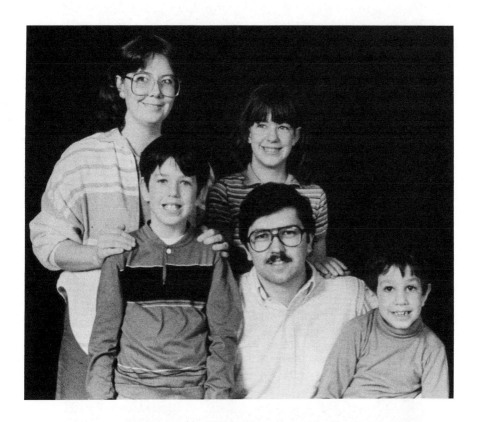

Figure 1. All three children have fragile X syndrome. The boy on the right presented with hyperactivity and a low normal I. Q., the boy on the left is mildly retarded with attention deficits and the daughter is learning disabled with shyness and math problems. All three children demonstrate prominent ears and the mother is a normal, unaffected carrier female.

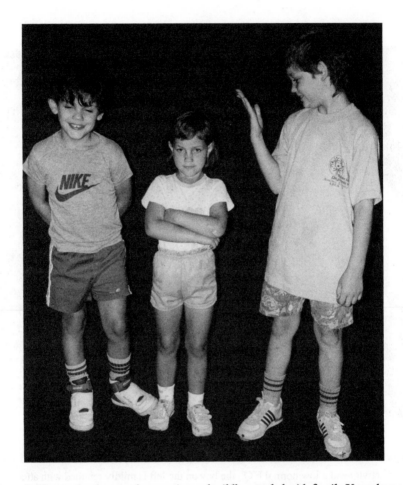

Figure 2. The two brothers are hyperactive and mildly retarded with fragile X syndrome. The sister in the center demonstrates subtle physical features with slightly prominent ears, learning disabilities and shyness.

1986). Approximately one-third of heterozygous females function intellectually in the borderline or retarded range (Sherman et al., 1985). Of heterozygotes with a normal IQ, more than half have significant learning disabilities, particularly in math (Kemper et al., 1986).

Male individuals affected by this syndrome usually demonstrate a long face, large and prominent ears, hyperextensible finger joints, flat feet, and macroorchidism or large testicles (Turner et al., 1986; Opitz & Sutherland, 1984). This last feature is most notable during and after puberty when 80% of fragile X males will have a testicular size $\geq$ 30 ml in volume. Heterozygous females who are cognitively affected by fragile X syndrome also commonly demonstrate large and prominent ears, a long face and hyperextensible finger joints.

In prepubertal males, the classical physical features, particularly macroorchidism, are often not present and therefore the behavioral phenotype can be most helpful in suggesting the diagnosis (Hagerman, 1987a). Young fragile X boys are usually hyperactive with a short attention span and have problems with impulsivity and distractibility (Mattei et al., 1981; Largo & Schinzel, 1985; Fryns et al., 1984). However, they also demonstrate a variety of unusual features such as poor eye contact, hand-biting, hand-flapping, and perseverative speech and mannerisms. These behaviors have stimulated an interest in the association of autism and fragile X syndrome.

In the past, several investigators reported the occasional case of autism in fragile X (Turner et al., 1980; Proops & Webb, 1981; Maryash et al., 1982), but it was Brown et al. (1982) who first reported a close association in that 5 of 27 (18.5%) fragile X males identified at their institute fulfilled Rutter's (1978) criteria for autism. Subsequently, several authors (Levitas et al., 1983; Brøndum-Nielsen, 1983; August & Lockhart, 1984; Kerbeshian et al., 1984; Varley et al., 1985) confirmed this association which occasionally occurred in brothers and even in triplets (Gillberg, 1983).

Levitas et al. (1983) performed a detailed analysis of autism in 10 fragile X males. Six of the 10 patients fulfilled DSM III criteria for autism but the similarities in the behaviors of these patients, including the short, perseverative bursts of speech, hand-biting, and other mannerisms, suggested that they represented a unique subgroup of autism without dramatic savant skills and typically functioning in the moderately retarded range of ability. This study was further expanded to include the first 50 males diagnosed with fragile X syndrome at the Child Development Unit of The Children's Hospital in Denver (Hagerman et al., 1986). None of the fragile X males fulfilled the classical Kanner syndrome as described by the E2 questionnaire developed by Rimland (1971). However, 16% fulfilled the DSM III criteria for Infantile Autism and 31% were autistic by the ABC checklist developed by Krug et al. (1980). The spectrum of autistic features was the most dramatic finding of this study in that all of the 50 fragile X males demonstrated some features. Poor eye contact and eye avoidance were seen in 90% of the subjects, even in those who were described as friendly and interested in social interaction. This finding was also noted by Gillberg et al. (1986) in 7 of 10 autistic fragile X males. Hand-flapping, hand-biting or hand stereotypies were present in 88% and language peculiarities, usually perseverative bursts of speech, were present in 96% of 50 males (Hagerman et al., 1986). The DSM III criteria of a pervasive lack of relatedness was the most difficult criterion to fulfill because the majority of fragile X males demonstrated less severe problems with relatedness. Many were friendly but socially anxious, tactilely defensive and avoidant of eye contact. More recently Wolff et al. (1989) has described the greeting behavior of fragile X males as involving a turning of the whole body away from the person who is greeting them. This avoidant behavior, along with poor eye contact, is often juxtaposed with a desire for social contact and friendliness, basically an approach-withdrawal demeanor, which makes fragile X males somewhat unique among individuals with pervasive developmental delays.

Table 1. Frequency of autism in fragile X males.

Author	No.Autistic Fra(X)/Total No. Fra(X)	%
Jacobs et al., 1983	2/9	22%
Brøndum-Nielsen, 1983	9/27	33%
Fryns et al., 1984	3/21	14%
Partington, 1984	3/61	5%
Benezech et al., 1985	15/28	54%
Hagerman et al., 1985	8/50 DSM III	16%
	15/48 ABC criteria	31%
Brown et al., 1986	24/150 DSM III	17%
Borghgraef et al.,1987	9/23 autistic behavior	39%
Bregman et al., 1988	1/14 DSM III	7%

The combination of friendliness and socially avoidant behavior has also fueled the controversy concerning the association of fragile X and autism. In order to understand this association, one must be aware of the spectrum of autistic behaviors which occur in fragile X males. On one end of the spectrum is a small percentage of fragile X males who fulfill all of the DSM III criteria for autism, including a pervasive lack of relatedness. These individuals tend to be more significantly retarded, as noted by Borghgraef et al. (1987), although higher functioning males often demonstrate an improvement of autistic symptoms as they mature. At the other end of the spectrum are friendly males who have no problems with social interactions. The majority of fragile X males, however, have minor problems with social interactions, including poor eye contact and shyness, along with unusual hand mannerisms and perseverations which are commonly seen in other autistic populations and are important factors for the diagnosis of autism using criteria such as the ABC checklist (Krug et al., 1980; Rutter, 1978). Therefore, the criteria for the diagnosis of autism and the number of males who fulfill this criteria are variable in the reports concerning the frequency of autism in fragile X males (Table 1).

The DSM III-R (APA 1987) has less stringent criteria for the diagnosis of autism or Autistic Disorder. A "pervasive lack of relatedness" has been replaced by a "qualitative impairment in reciprocal social interaction." The majority of fragile X males will fulfill two of the examples under this criterion including gross impairment in ability to make peer friendships and abnormal social play. A second criteria is "qualitative impairment in verbal and nonverbal communication and in imaginative activity." From the subsequent examples, the majority of fragile X males have abnormal nonverbal communication including problems with eye contact and hand mannerisms, marked abnormalities in the production, form and content of speech including cluttering, dysfluencies, perseverations and echolalia (Hanson et al., 1986; Newall et al., 1983; Madison et al., 1986), and an impairment in the ability to initiate and sustain a conversation. Lastly, the third criterion is "markedly restricted repertoire of activities and interests" including stereotyped body movements, persistent preoccupation with parts of objects or attachment to unusual objects, marked distress over changes in trivial aspects of the environment, unreasonable insistence on following routines in precise detail, and markedly restricted range of interests and a preoccupation with one narrow interest. Again, the majority of fragile X males will fulfill one or more of these examples. Therefore, the diagnosis of Autistic Disorder (DSM III-R) will probably be made much more readily in fragile X males than the diagnosis of Infantile Autism.

The question of whether fragile X represents a unique subgroup of autism has been further addressed by comparative studies of behavior and language. Cohen and co-workers (1988) have shown that nonautistic fragile X males show a greater degree of social avoidance than matched retarded children and that autistic fragile X males show a greater degree of social avoidance with strangers, compared to parents, than IQ-matched nonfragile X autistic children. In a further study of gaze patterns, Cohen et al. (1989) have shown that an initial adult look to the child suppressed the child looking to the adult and subsequent mutual gaze more readily in fragile X males than nonfragile X autistic males. This study suggests that fragile X males have an aversion to mutual gaze and a greater sensitivity to their parent's initiation of social gaze than the autistic nonfragile X males who simply had an overall dampening of social gaze, suggesting a lack of interest or an inability to read social cues. In contrast, the fragile X males were very sensitive to the initial parental gaze and their subsequent aversion to mutual gaze is another example of the approach-withdrawal behavior previously described. Clinically, these males appear to be overwhelmed and become anxious from stimuli such as social interactions. This anxiety then leads to avoidance behavior as seen in gaze and greeting behaviors (Wolff et al., 1989; Bregman et al., 1989). On occasion, we have seen anxiety escalate and precipitate aggressive behavior and episodic violent outbursts particularly in fragile X adult males.

Comparative studies in the language area include the report by Wolf-Schein et al. (1987), who studied nonautistic fragile X males and IQ-matched individuals with Down syndrome. A blinded analysis revealed more jargon, perseveration, echolalia and episodes of talking to themselves in fragile X males compared to controls. This language behavior was similar to autistic fragile X males and supports the notion of a fragile X language and behavior style that is unique.

In an analysis of the autistic features in fragile X males, it is important to include the high functioning male with a borderline or normal IQ (Hagerman et al., 1985; Goldfine et al., 1987; Gillberg et al., 1986). These individuals are not nonpenetrant males because they are fragile X positive males with both cognitive and physical features of the syndrome. However, the cognitive deficits are not typical since the IQ is relatively preserved and they are better described as having severe learning disabilities. They still, however, demonstrate similar deficits to those seen in the more affected males including math problems and abstract reasoning problems. Most importantly, behavioral problems also persist and poor eye contact and shyness continue to be problems for many of these males.

We are presently following 3 normal to borderline IQ fragile X males who are adults. Two of these males are best described as having Asperger syndrome (Asperger, 1944; Wing, 1981). The diagnostic features as restated by Gillberg (1985) include: 1) inability to relate normally to other people, social isolation, peculiarities of gaze and naive abnormal behaviour; 2) pedantic and perseverative speech; 3) nonverbal communication is deviant including reduced facial expression, monotonous intonation and limited or inappropriate gestures; 4) repetitive activities and strong attachments to certain possessions; 5) gross motor movements are clumsy and poorly coordinated. These males have encountered significant difficulties in the working situation because excessive stimulation can be overwhelming and confusing and occasionally lead to emotional if not physical outbursts. They do not possess the social skills and flexibility to deal successfully with a variety of personalities in a working situation. They have also had significant problems in establishing intimate relationships and none of these males have married. Asperger (1944) originally described males with superior verbal abilities although Wing (1971) later expanded the description of Asperger syndrome to include individuals with language deficits. Higher functioning fragile X males do not have the severe language deficits typically associated with fragile X syndrome. Their problems, therefore, often fit the diagnostic description of Asperger syndrome (Hagerman, 1987b). In a study of 20 high functioning (IQ >65) children with Kanner type autism or Asperger syndrome, Gillberg et al. (1987) reported that 4 had the fragile X syndrome.

The spectrum of autistic features in individuals with fragile X syndrome is also seen in females who are affected by the syndrome. Although females are usually affected less severely and less frequently, an occasional female will demonstrate autism (Hagerman et al., 1986; Edwards et al., 1988; LeCouteur et al., 1988; Gillberg et al., 1988). In general, approximately one-third of heterozygotes are retarded (Sherman et al., 1985). Of those heterozygotes with a normal IQ, approximately one-half will demonstrate learning disabilities, including math deficits and attentional problems, usually without hyperactivity. Social anxiety, shyness and feelings of isolation are more frequent complaints among heterozygotes than the learning disabilities and are commonly seen in normal and superior IQ heterozygotes (Hagerman & Sobesky, 1989). Tranel et al. (1987) has described a combination of learning and social problems including math difficulties, visual spatial perceptual problems, shyness and social withdrawal as secondary to right hemisphere dysfunction. This description sounds so similar to fragile X females that further neuropsychological testing of heterozygotes is warranted to clarify the neuropathology.

Learning disabilities and social interactional difficulties, combined with the stresses of rasing a fragile X child, often lead to depression in heterozygous mothers (Reiss et al., 1988). Depression, however, is more common in cognitively unaffected heterozygotes than in cognitively impaired heterozygotes, whereas schizotypal features, such as poor relatedness and odd communication patterns, are more common in cognitively impaired heterozygotes (Reiss et al., 1988; Hagerman & Sobesky, 1989). Impaired heterozygotes more frequently demonstrate difficulties in social interaction and poor eye contact than heterozygotes without cognitive deficits (Cronister et al., 1988). These problems appear to be on the same spectrum as the autistic features of the males and directly caused by the fragile X gene, whereas depression may be a secondary environmental effect.

The autistic heterozygous females reported by Hagerman et al. (1986) were both retarded. Two subsequent heterozygous females with autism were reported by Edwards et al. (1988), one with mild mental retardation and the other with a borderline IQ. LeCouteur et al. (1988) has also reported autism in one fragile X retarded female twin, whereas the twin sister, who was higher functioning, demonstrated social withdrawal and shyness without autism. Gillberg et al. (1988) has also reported autism in fragile X female twins but both were affected and mildly retarded, whereas the mother demonstrated constant gaze aversion without autism. Autism in fragile X females appears to be more common significant cognitive impairment also exists. Although heterozygotes do not demonstrate autism and cognitive deficits as frequently as the males, they demonstrate the mildest form of the effects of the fragile X gene on brain development. Since social deficits, specifically shyness, persist in the normal IQ heterozygotes, they perhaps represent a mild form of the autistic spectrum.

To further assess the association of autism and fragile X, autistic males were studied to identify the prevalence of fragile X syndrome in autism (Table 2).

Table 2. Prevalence of fragile X in autistic males.

Author	No. Fra(X)/Total No. Autistic	%
Venter et al., 1984	0/40	0%
Goldfine et al., 1984	0/34	0%
McGillivrary et al., 1984	3/40	7.5%
In Opitz & Sutherland, 1984		
Leckman	0/25	0%
Turner	1/70	1.4%
Mikkelsen	1/20	5%
Chudley	1/16	6.3%
White	0/6	0%
Jørgensen et al ., 1984	1/11	9%
Pueschel et al., 1985	0/18	0%
Jayakar et al., 1986	0/20	0%
Wright et al., 1986	1/31	3%
Watson et al., 1984	4/76	5%
Blomquist et al., 1984	13/83	16%
Brown et al., 1986	24/183	13%
Crowe et al., 1988	2/20	10%
Total	51/693	7.4%

When small numbers were studied, only an occasional fragile X male was found (McGilliviary et al., 1986; Venter et al., 1984: Goldfine et al., 1984; Opitz & Sutherland, 1984). However, the 2 largest screening studies have now reported a significant prevalence of fragile X syndrome. Blomquist et al. (1985) screened 83 autistic males in Sweden and reported 13 (15.7%) positive for the fragile X chromosome. Brown et al. (1986) screened 183 autistic males with 24 (13.1%) positive for the fragile X chromosome. Perhaps the variable frequency represents differences again in the diagnosis of autism and in selection of patients. The larger studies have used DSM III criteria and tend to avoid the bias of screening only a limited number of patients (Fish et al., 1988). The Swedish study represents a total ascertainment of all autistic males in several counties. Brown et al. (1986) pooled the results of 12 studies and found the frequency of fragile X among autistic males to be 7.7% (47/614), which is similar to the total percentage calculated in Table II including studies through 1988. This figure is similar to the updated results reported by Cohen (1989) for screening in New York. They have presently screened 363 autistic males and 8.0% are fragile X positive. Thirty-five males with a diagnosis of Pervasive Developmental Disorder not otherwise specified were also screened and 6 (17%) were fragile X positive. Although previous limited screening of autistic females has not demonstrated fragile X, Cohen et al. (1989) have screened 33 autistic females and 4 (12.1%) were fragile X positive. The overall prevalence of autism in affected fragile X females is similar to the prevalence in males (Table 3).

Table 3. Prevalence of fragile X in autistic females.

Author	No. Fra(X)/Total No. Autistic	%
McGillivary et al., 1984	0/5	0%
Venter et al., 1984	0/17	0%
Jørgensen et al., 1984	0/4	0%
Goldfine et al., 1984	0/3	0%
Blomquist et al., 1985	0/19	0%
Wright et al., 1986	0/9	0%
Cohen et al., 1989	4/33	12.1%
Total	4/90	4.4%

A recent finding of hypoplasia of the posterior cerebellar vermis particularly lobules VI and VII in 18 males with autism is interesting (Courchesne et al., 1988). Reiss et al. (1988a) has reported a similar finding in fragile X males along with a smaller total area of the pons and enlargement of the fourth ventricle compared to normal controls. The cerebellum not only modulates motor function but has significant connections with other areas of the brain, particularly the limbic system and brain stem. Dysfunction in these areas may account for both emotional and cognitive dysfunction or may occur concomitantly with damage to other neural sites. Reiss (1988b) has also found that the degree of autism in fragile X males does not correlate with the degree of cerebellar vermal hypoplasia. This anatomical abnormality, therefore, may be a nonspecific finding or may be a predisposing but independently insufficient factor for producing autism.

Sex Chromosome Abnormalities

Sex chromosome numerical abnormalities are frequent in the general population but usually do not cause mental retardation. Instead, learning disabilities or mild cognitive deficits are seen, particularly in the language and motor areas. Although the frequency of sex chromosome aneuploidy is increased in prison and mental institutions compared to the normal population (Hook, 1973; Polani, 1977), prospective studies of development since birth in unbiased cohorts have shown that institutionalization is rare (Robinson et al., 1982). Instead learning disabilities, with a concomitant psychosocial overlay, are common features (Bender and co-workers, 1987). Crandall and co-workers (1972) evaluated 700 children referred to a child psychiatry clinic and found 1.6% with sex chromosome and behavior problems. Autism has been occasionally reported (Table 4) in each of these

Table 4. Autism associated with sex chromosome aneuploidy.

Author	Karyotype	Case Features
Campbell et al., 1972	47, XXY	Self-mutilation
Wolraich et al., 1970	47, XXX	Identified from screening 25 autistics
Abrams & Pergament, 1971	47, XYY	Hypertelorism, high palate
Mallin & Walker, 1972	47, XYY	Congenital adrenal hyperplasia
Nielsen et al., 1973	47, XYY	IQ 50 at age 7, normal physical phenotype
Gillberg et al., 1984	47, XYY	Aggressive, hyperactive, tantrums, minor motor epilepsy
	47, XYY	Asperger syndrome
Ornitz et al., 1977	48, XXYY	Severe neonatal distress, hypotonia

disorders and the mild language and social-emotional problems which are prevalent may predispose this population to a higher incidence of autism (Gillberg et al., 1984). Each of the aneuploidies will be discussed separately.

Klinefelter syndrome, 47,XXY karyotype, has an incidence of approximately 1:1000. Although these boys usually have a normal IQ, their verbal IQ is often lower than their performance IQ. Moderate problems are typically present in receptive language skills, particularly auditory processing problems (Bender et al., 1983). Mild to moderate problems in sensory motor integration are also frequently seen and their early motor development is described as awkward, slow, poorly organized and uncoordinated (Tennes et al., 1977). The majority of individuals are referred for special education help in school and their psychosocial development is often hampered by a poor self-image and emotional difficulties, particularly if their family is dysfunctional (Bender et al., 1987). Their personality has been described as timid and their self-confidence is often low. They have also been shown to have more problems in relating to their peer group than controls (Bancroft et al., 1982). Perhaps the rare XXY autistic individual represents the worst end of the spectrum of mild social interactional problems based on mild neuropsychological deficits which are secondary to carrying an additional X chromosome. A greater number of X chromosomes in males has been associated with more severe social interactional problems. Borghgraef et al. (1988) reported extremely shy and timid behavior, combined with avoidance of eye contact, in three boys with 49,XXXXY karyotype. There is also an increase of nondysjunction in fragile X, such that 1 in 155 fragile X males also has a 47,XXY karyotype (Fryns & Van den Berghe, 1988).

Girls with 47,XXX (prevalence 1:1000) have more significant language dysfunction than individuals with other types of sex chromosome aneuploidy. Their problems exist in both receptive and expressive language abilities, with auditory comprehension and articulation most deficient (Bender et al., 1983). The full scale IQ is usually lower than other types of sex chromosome abnormality and sibling controls, but it typically remains within the low normal range. A longitudinal study of 11 females with 47 XXX, followed since birth, has shown the need for special education help in 82% although all had speech problems by the first grade, four of whom were nonverbal. Shyness and immaturity were behavior problems seen in the majority and 7 had a psychiatric diagnosis of depression, undersocialization or conduct disorder. They tended to be tall and poorly coordinated compared to controls and their expressive language difficulties appeared to contribute to their shyness (Linden et al., 1988). Only a rare case of autism has been reported (Table IV) but other psychiatric problems are common and their prevalence in institutions is four- to fivefold greater than their birth incidence (Polani et al., 1977). Fragile X has also been reported in a female with XXX and normal cognitive and behavioral features, although her son is retarded with the fragile X syndrome (Fuster et al., 1988).

Turner syndrome (XO) females usually have a lower performance IQ compared to a relatively preserved verbal IQ. In the study by Bender et al. (1983), they did not demonstrate significant receptive or expressive language deficits compared to controls nor significant shyness. Autism has not been reported in this syndrome.

In males with 47,XYY karyotype neuromuscular problems including hypotonia and sensory motor integration problems are usually seen (Salbenblatt et al., 1987) although language deficits are mild (Bender et al., 1983). Impulsivity and aggression are recurrent themes in a review of psychological studies of selected XYY males (Dorus, 1980). In a study of the early childhood of XYY males, Nielsen et al. (1973) reported significant behavior problems including impulsiveness, hyperactivity, difficulties in establishing contact with people, aggression and frequent admission to psychiatric hospitals. This study, similar to others, represented a selected group of 22 XYY patients who were not followed in a prospective fashion from birth and, therefore, would have a higher incidence of behavior problems. The IQ was usually in the normal range although Nielsen et al. (1973) reported that 3 of his 22 patients were below normal and the autistic patient he described was retarded. Poor relatedness was seen in 64% of XYY males in this study although autism was only diagnosed in one. Case histories of autism are most common in sex chromosome aneuploidy with this karyotype (Table IV).

A long Y variant has also been associated with autism and was first reported by Judd and Mandell (1968) in 3 of 8 autistics and subsequently by Hoshino et al. (1979) in 9 of 32 autistics. Later reports have also occasionally noted this finding in autistic males (Gillberg & Wahlström, 1985) but it has also been reported in other types of psychopathology as well, including antisocial behavior, character disorders, alcohol abuse and criminality (Dorus, 1980). Variation of the length of the Y chromosome is seen in 2 to 3% of men in the normal population, and it is particularly common in certain racial groups, i.e. Orientals. This variation usually involves changes in the length of heterochromatic material on the long arm of the Y (Buhler, 1980). This material includes highly repetitive DNA sequences and its presence or absence may not have any consequences for the ultimate phenotype, unless euchromatic Y material is involved. Dorus (1980) has reviewed the studies concerning the length of the Y chromosome in institutionalized males and no consistent relationship between the Y chromosome length and psychiatric diagnosis has been found. Many studies, however, contain case histories that are reminiscent of problems with impulsivity and aggression which have been described in many XYY males.

The findings of a spectrum of behavior difficulties involving social interactional problems with occasional cases of autism in patients with XXY and XXX but not in XO patients suggests that an increased number of X chromosomes predisposes to autistic features. Social interactional problems are also frequently seen in XYY males and part of the Y chromosome contains DNA which is homologous to material on the X chromosome. The homologous regions, however, are on the short arm of the X and not near the Xq27.3 region where dysfunction predisposes to autistic features in the fragile X syndrome. There are probably multiple genes on the X which code for cognitive language, social and behavioral problems and perhaps abnormalities with several loci may cause autistic features.

Autosomal Chromosome Abnormalities

The most common autosomal chromosomal abnormality is trisomy 21 but it has been relatively infrequently associated with autism (Table 5). Social withdrawal or poor relatedness is not typical of children with Down syndrome and the cases reported with autism have been profoundly retarded when cognitive abilities have been documented. Maltz (1979) has pointed out that both his case and Wakabayashi's case (1979) demonstrated global withdrawal and primitive interactions which resulted from general and severe brain damage. Although these children fit behavioral criteria for autism (Rutter, 1978), they were too retarded to see the unique deficits in relatedness which characterize the development of autistic children. An additional case reported by Gillberg and Wahlström (1985) demonstrated spastic diplegia in conjunction with trisomy 21 suggesting additional brain damage.

A theme of severe cognitive deficits tends to characterize almost all of the autosomal chromosomal abnormalities associated with autism (Table 5). Only one individual with a low normal IQ is described who also demonstrates autism. Because of the rarity and frequently sporadic nature of these autosomal chromosome problems, a spectrum of autistic features cannot be traced through those individuals who are less affected, as in the fragile X syndrome and in sex chromosome aneuploidies. The autism caused by autosomal chromosomal abnormalities appears to be related to global cognitive deficits and subsequent severe or profound retardation, whereas disorders associated with the X chromosome often have a very specific impact on socialization skills and other features which are associated with autism. Although the prevalence of autism in fragile X and sex chromosome aneuploidy may be increased in those with a lower IQ, the spectrum of autistic-like features is broad and includes those from borderline to normal IQ also.

A discussion of chromosomal abnormalities is not complete without reporting fragile sites other than Xq27.3 which have been associated with autism. Gillberg and Wahlström (1985) reported the presence of the common fragile site (16) (q23) in 17% of

46 children with autism. However, Jayakar et al. (1986) found this fragile site in equal frequencies in control and autistic children. Wright et al. (1986) have reported that 55% of 22 autistic boys demonstrate a variety of autosomal fragile sites. The heritable fragile site (2) (q13) was reported in 2 of 20 autistic patients and not in controls (Jayakar et al., 1986). However, its significance and the importance of other common and inherited fragile sites will require further population studies (Sutherland & Hecht, 1985).

Single Gene Disorders

A variety of single gene disorders which are not associated with chromosomal abnormalities have been reported in autistic patients. Most disorders which cause metabolic problems are autosomal recessive, and phenylketonuria (PKU) is the most common and best understood single gene disorder associated with autism. PKU is a deficiency of phenylalanine hydroxylase, and the majority of individuals who are untreated with dietary restriction of phenylalanine will manifest a spectrum of autistic features (Friedman, 1969). The incidence of autism in PKU is decreasing dramatically because newborn screening has led to early diagnosis and treatment which can be curative. However, PKU has given us insight into the neuroanatomical changes which can lead to autism since untreated patients have widespread demyelination in the cerebellum and in cerebral white matter (reviewed by Reiss et al., 1986). Neurochemically, phenylalanine hydroxylase is an important step in catecholamine metabolism and its functional inadequacy appears to be associated with a relative dopamine depletion syndrome, even in treated PKU patients (Pennington & Smith, 1988). This finding coincides with the results of metabolic studies in non-PKU autistic patients who show evidence of dopamine depletion (Barthelemy et al., 1988), which may be important in the pathogenesis of autism.

Other autosomal recessive disorders associated with autism are only documented by single case reports for each disorder including neurolipidosis (Creak, 1963), mucopolysaccharidosis (Knobloch & Passamanick, 1975) and histidinemia (Rutter & Bartak, 1971; Kotsopoulous & Kutty, 1979). Autosomal dominant disorders associated with autism include neurofibromatosis (Gillberg & Wahlström, 1985) recently mapped to chromosome 17 (Ledbetter et al., 1989), and tuberous sclerosis (Mansheim, 1979). Multiple case reports for each of these disorders have been reviewed by Reiss et al. (1986). They suggest that the problems with neuroglia differentiation in both of these disorders leads to areas of deficient or disordered myelin formation which would interfere with information transfer in the CNS and may be one neuropathologic mechanism leading to autism. Hunt and Dennis (1987) have evaluated 90 children with tuberous sclerosis, most of whom suffered from infantile spasms or other seizures. Two-thirds had severe behavioral problems which impaired social interaction and 58% were autistic. Hyperactivity was seen in 59% and severely aggressive behavior in 13%. This disorder has a spectrum of behavioral manifestation with a propensity for autistic features. Those patients with more severe cognitive deficits were more frequently described as autistic, that is, over 80% with severe mental retardation were autistic.

The last syndrome which must be addressed is Rett syndrome although the genetic etiology is still unclear. The most likely mechanism is an X-linked dominant mutation with lethality in males. The affected females show deterioration in their cognitive

Table 5. Autism associated with autosomal chromosome abnormalities.

Author	Karyotype	Case Features
Wakabayashi, 1979	Trisomy 21	Profound MR
Maltz, 1979	Trisomy 21	Profound MR, autistic by behavior criteria
Gillberg & Wahlström, 1985	Trisomy 21	Spastic diplegia
Knobloch & Pasamanick, 1985	Trisomy 21	IQ not reported
Mariner et al., 1986	46,XY,inv,dup,del(3) (p21.1;p24.3;p12.3;q21.1)	Prominent ears, pectus excavatum, severe MR
	46,XY,5p+	Increased tone, tremor moderate MR
	46,XX,inv,dup(16) (p13;q22.3)	Short stature, prominent brow ridge, increased tone, mild MR
	46,XY,del(17)(p11.2p11.2)	Hypertelorism, polydactyly, prominent, low-set ears, severe MR
Burd et al., 1988	46,XY,dup(6)(p23-pter) del(2)(q27-qter)	Microcephaly, large low-set ears, epicanthal ears, severe MR
Wenger et al., 1988	46,XY,del(1)(p35)	Unusual facies, epicanthal folds, motor incordination, ataxia
Ritvo et al., 1988	46,XX,del(13)(q12q14)	Retinoblastoma, reduced esterase D activity in rbcs. Developmentally delayed
Turner & Jennings, 1961	Trisomy 22	Low normal intelligence, myopia, small chin

and motor abilities after the first year with a clinical picture involving ataxia, hyperventilation, repetitive hand-clasping and eventual deterioration (Hagberg et al., 1983). Global cognitive and subsequent motor deficits characterize this syndrome so the pathology is not only specific for autistic characteristics, although autism is the typical behavioral picture.

CONCLUSION

The advent of the fragile X syndrome has focused our attention on the association of chromosome abnormalities and autism. Although fragile X is the most common known cause of autism affecting approximately 7% of autistic males and females, there exists a spectrum of problems of social interaction in individuals who are affected by this syndrome. A similar spectrum also exists in some individuals with sex chromosome abnormalities, particularly those with a higher number of X chromosomes such as XXX females or XXXXY males. These problems are not typical of individuals with autosomal chromosomal abnormalities who typically demonstrate more global CNS dysfunction and significant retardation when reported with autism.

When chromosomal disorders are combined with single gene disorders, they represent the majority of known etiologies of autism. Therefore, studies of the genetics of autism (reviewed by Smalley et al., 1988; Folstein & Rutter, 1988) must first identify these known genetic disorders before characterizing the genetic mechanism that may be responsible for those without a known etiology.

REFERENCES

American Psychiatric Assocation. (1980). *Diagnostic and Statistical Manual of Mental Disorders. DSM-III (3rd ed.)* (pp 87-90). Washington, DC: Author.

American Psychiatric Assocation. (1987). *Diagnostic and Statistical Manual of Mental Disorders. DSM III-R (3rd revised ed.)* (pp 38 - 89). Washington, DC: Author.

Asperger, H. (1944). Die autistishen Psychopathen im Kindersalter. *Archiv für Psychiatrie und Nervenkrankheiten, 117,* 6-136.

August, G. J., Lockhart, L. H. (1984). Familial autism and the fragile X chromosome. *Journal of Autism and Developmental Disorders,14,* 197-204.

Bancroft, J., Axworthy, D., & Ratcliffe, S. (1982). The personality and psycho-sexual development of boys with 47XXY chromosome constitution. *Journal of Child Psychology and Psychiatry, 23,* 169-180.

Barthelemy, C., Bruneau, N., Cottet-Emard, J. M., Domenech-Jouve, J., Garreau, B., Lelord, G., Muh, J. P., & Peyrin, L. (1988). Urinary free and conjugated catecholamines and metabolites in autistic children. *Journal of Autism and Developmental Disorders, 18,* 583-591.

Bender, B., Fry, E., Pennington, B., Puck, M., Salbenblatt, J., & Robinson, A. (1983). Speech and language development in 41 children with sex chromosome anomalies. *Pediatrics, 71,* 262-267.

Bender, B. G., Linder, M. G., & Robinson, A. (1987). Environment and developmental risk in children with sex chromosome abnormalities. *Journal of the American Academy of Child and Adolescent Psychiatry, 26,* 499-503.

Benezech, M., & Noel, B. (1985). Fragile X syndrome and autism. *Clinical Genetics, 28,* 93.

Blomquist, M. K., Bohman, M., Edvinsson, S. O., Gillberg, C., Gustavson, K. H., Holmgren, G., & Wahlström, J. (1985). Frequency of the fragile X syndrome in infantile autism. A Swedish multicenter study. *Clinical Genetics, 27,* 113-117.

Borghgraef, M., Fryns, J. P., Dielkens, A., Dyck, K., & Van den Berghe, H. (1987). Fragile (X) syndrome: a study of the psychological profile in 23 prepubertal patients. *Clinical Genetics, 32,* 179-186.

Borghgraef, M., Fryns, J. P., Smeets, E., Marien, J., & Van den Berghe, H. (1988). The 49,XXXXY syndrome. Clinical and psychological followup data. *Clinical Genetics, 33,* 429-434.

Bregman, J. D., Leckman, J. F., & Ort, S. I. (1988). Fragile X syndrome: genetic predisposition to psychopathology. *Journal of Autism and Developmental Disorders, 18,* 343-354.

Brøndum-Nielsen, K. (1983). Diagnosis of the fragile X syndrome (Martin-Bell syndrome), clinical findings in 27 males with the fragile site at Xq28. *Journal of Mental Deficiency Research, 27,* 211-226.

Brown, W. T., Jenkins, E. C., Friedman, E., Brooks, J., Wisnicwski, K., Raguthu, S., & French, J. (1982). Autism is associated with the fragile X syndrome. *Journal of Autism and Developmental Disorders, 12,* 303-308.

Brown, W. T., Jenkins, E. C., Cohen, I. L., Fisch, G. S., Wolf-Schein, E. G., Gross, A., Waterhouse, L., Fein, D., Mason-Brothers, A., Ritvo, E., Rittenberg, B. A., Bentley, W., & Castells, S. (1986). Fragile X and autism: a multicenter survey. *American Journal of Medical Genetics, 23,* 341-352.

Buhler, E. M. (1980). A synopsis of the human Y chromosome. *Human Genetics, 55,* 145-175.

Chudley, A. E., Knoll, J., Gerrard, J. W., Shepel, L., McGahey, E., & Anderson, J. (1983). Fragile (X) X-linked mental retardation. I: relationship between age and intelligence and the frequence of expression of fragile (X) (q28). *American Journal of Medical Genetics, 14,* 669-712.

Chudley, A. E., & Hagerman, R. J. (1987). Fragile X syndrome. *Journal of Pediatrics, 110,* 821-831.

Cohen, I. L., Fisch, G. S., Wolf-Schein, E. G., Sudhalter, V., Hanson, D., Hagerman, R. J., Jenkins, E. C., & Brown, T. W. (1988). Social avoidance and repetitive behavior in fragile X males: a controlled study. *American Journal of Mental Retardation, 92,* 436-446.

Cohen, I. L. (1989). Autism and the fragile X syndrome. Paper presented at the 2nd National Fragile X Conference sponsored by the National Fragile X Foundation, April 5-8, Denver, Colorado.

Cohen, I. L., Vietze, P. M., Sudhalter, V., Jenkins, E. C., & Brown, W. T. (1989). Parent-child dyadic gaze patterns in fragile X males and in nonfragile X males with autistic disorder. *Journal of Child Psychology and Psychiatry* (in press).

Coleman, M. (1976). *The Autistic Syndromes.* Amsterdam: North-Holland Publishing Co.

Courchesne, E., Yeung-Courchesne, R., Press, G. A., Hesselink, J. R., & Jernigan, T. L. (1988). Hypoplasia of cerebellar vermal lobules IV and III in autism. *New England Journal of Medicine, 318,* 1349-1354.

Crandall, B. F., Carrel, R. E., & Sparkes, R. S. (1972). Chromosome findings in 700 children referred to a psychiatric clinic. *Journal of Pediatrics, 80,* 62-68.

Creak, E. M. (1963). Childhood psychosis. *British Journal of Psychiatry, 109,* 84-89.

Cronister, A., Hagerman, R., Schreiner, B., Wittenberger, M., Harris, K., & Shadwell, D. (1988). Physical, historical and cognitive features of heterozygous females (abstract). *American Journal of Human Genetics, 43,* A44 (0176).

Crowe, R. R., Tsai, L. Y., Murray, J. C., Patil, S. R., & Quinn, J. (1988). A study of autism using X chromosome DNA probes. *Biological Psychiatry, 24,* 473-479.

Dorus, E. (1980). Variability in the Y chromosome and variability of human behavior. *Archives of General Psychiatry, 37,* 587-594.

Dykens, E. M., Hodapp, R. M., & Leckman, J. F. (1987). Strengths and weaknesses in the intellectual functioning of males with fragile X syndrome. *American Journal of Mental Deficiency, 92,* 234-236.

Edwards, D. R., Keppen, L. D., Ranells, J. D., & Gollin, S. M. (1988). Autism in association with fragile X syndrome in females: implications for diagnosis and treatment. *Neurotoxicology, 9,* 359-366.

Fisch, G. S., Cohen, I. L., Jenkins, E. C., & Brown, W. T. (1988). Screening developmentally disabled male populations for fragile X: The effect of sample size. *American Journal of Medical Genetics, 30*, 655 - 663.

Folstein, S. E., & Rutter, M. L. (1988). Autism: familial aggregation and genetic implications. *Journal of Autism and Developmental Disorders, 18*, 3-20.

Friedman, E. (1969). The autistic syndrome and phenylketonuria. *Schizophrenia Bulletin, 1*, 249-261.

Fryns, J. P., Jacobs, J., Kleczkowska, A., & Van den Berghe, H. (1984). The psychological profile of the fragile X syndrome. *Clinical Genetics, 25*, 131-134.

Fryns, J. P., & Van den Berghe, H. (1988). The concurrence of Klinefelter syndrome and fragile X syndrome. *American Journal of Medical Genetics, 30*, 109-113.

Fuster, C., Templado, C., Miro, R., Barrios, L., & Egozcue, J. (1988). Concurrence of the triple-X syndrome and expression of the fragile site Xq27.3. *Human Genetics, 78*, 293.

Gilbert, E. F., & Opitz, J. M. (1982). Developmental and other pathologic changes in syndromes caused by chromosome abnormalities. In H. S. Rosenberg & J. Bernstein (Eds.), *Perspectives in Pediatric Pathology*, Vol. 7, New York: Masson Publ.

Gillberg, C. (1983). Identical triplets with infantile autism and the fragile X syndrome. *British Journal of Psychiatry, 143*, 256-260.

Gillberg, C., Winnergård, I., & Wahlström, J. (1984). The sex chromosomes - one key to autism? An XYY case of infantile autism. *Applied research in Mental Retardation, 5*, 353-360.

Gillberg, C., & Wahlström, J. (1985). Chromosome abnormalities in infantile autism and other childhood psychoses: a population study of 66 cases. *Developmental Medicine and Child Neurology, 27*, 293-304.

Gillberg, C. (1985). Asperger's syndrome and recurrent psychosis - a case study. *Journal of Autism and Developmental Disorders, 15*, 389-396.

Gillberg, C., Persson, E., & Wahlström, J. (1986). The autism-fragile X syndrome (AFRAX): a population based study of ten boys. *Journal of Mental Deficiency Research, 30*, 27-39.

Gillberg, C., Steffenburg, S., & Jakobsson, G. (1987). Neurobiological findings in 20 relatively gifted children with Kanner-type autism or Asperger syndrome. *Development Medicine and Child Neurology, 29*, 641-649.

Gillberg, C., Ohlson, V. A., Wahlström, J., Steffenburg, S., & Blix, K. (1988). Monozygotic female twins with autism and the fragile-X syndrome (AFRAX). *Journal of Child Psychology and Psychiatry, 29*, 447-451.

Goldfine, P. E., McPherson, P. M., Heath, G. A., Hardesty, V. A., Beauregard, L. J., & Gordon, B. (1985). Assocation of fragile X syndrome with autism. *American Journal of Psychiatry, 142,* 108-110.

Goldfine, P. E., McPherson, P. M., Hardesty, V. A., Heath, G. A., Beauregard, L. J., & Baker, A. A. (1987). Fragile-X chromosome associated with primary learning disability. *Journal of the American Academy of Child and Adolescent Psychiatry, 26,* 89-592.

Hagberg, B., Aicardi, J., Dias, K., & Ramos, O. (1983). A progressive syndrome of autism, dementia, ataxia, and loss of purposeful hand use in girls: Rett syndrome: report of 35 cases. *Annals of Neurology, 14,* 471-479.

Hagerman, R. J., & Smith, A. C. M. (1983). The heterozygous female. In *The Fragile X Syndrome: Diagnosis, Biochemistry and Intervention.* Dillon, Colorado: Spectra Publishing, Co.

Hagerman, R. J., Kemper, M., & Hudson, M. (1985). Learning disabilities and attentional problems in boys with the fragile X syndrome. *American Journal of Diseases of Children, 139,* 674-678.

Hagerman, R. J., Chudley, A. E., Knoll, J. H., Jackson, A. W., Kemper, M., & Ahmad, R. (1986). Autism in fragile X females. *American Journal of Medical Genetics, 23,* 375-380.

Hagerman, R. J., Jackson, A. W., Levitas, A., Rimland, B., & Braden, M. (1986). An analysis of autism in 50 males with the fragile X syndrome. *American Journal of Medical Genetics, 23,* 359-370.

Hagerman, R. J., Jackson, A. W., Levitas, A., Braden, M., McBogg, P., Kemper, M., McGavran, L., Berry, R., Matus, I., & Hagerman, P. (1986). Oral folic acid versus placebo in the treatment of males with fragile X syndrome. *American Journal of Medical Genetics, 23,* 241-262.

Hagerman, R. J. (1987a). Fragile X syndrome (monograph). *Current Problems in Pediatrics, 17,* 621-674.

Hagerman, R. J. (1987b). Possible similarities between the fragile X and Asperger syndrome (letter). *American Journal of Diseases of Children, 141,* 601-602.

Hagerman, R. J., Berry, R., Jackson, A. W., Campbell, J., Smith, A. C. M., & McGavran, L. (1988). Institutional screening for the fragile X syndrome. *American Journal of Diseases of Children, 142,* 1216-1221.

Hagerman, R. J., & Sobesky, W. E. (1989). Psychopathology in fragile X syndrome. *American Journal of Orthopsychiatry, 59,* 142-152.

Hansen, A., Brask, B. H., Nielson, J., Rasmussen, K., & Silesen, I. (1977). A case report of an autistic girl with an extra bisatellited marker chromosome. *Journal of Autism and Childhood Schizophrenia, 7,* 263-267.

Hanson, D. M., Jackson, A. W., & Hagerman, R. J. (1986). Speech disturbances (Cluttering) in Mildly Impaired Males with the Martin-Bell/Fragile X Syndrome. *American Journal of Medical Genetics, 23*, 195-206.

Hook, E. B. (1973). Behavioral implications of the human XYY genotype. *Science, 179*, 139-150.

Hoshino, Y., Yashima, Y., Tachibana, R., Koneko, M., Watanabe, M., Kumashiro, H. (1979). Sex chromosome abnormalities in autistic children: long Y chromosome. *Fukushima Journal of Medical Science, 26*, 31-42.

Hunt, A., & Dennis J. (1987). Psychiatric disorder among children with tuberous sclerosis. *Developmental Medicine and Child Neurology, 29*, 190-198.

Jacobs, P. A. (1977). Epidemiology of chromosomal abnormalities in man. *American Journal of Epidemiology, 105*, 180.

Jacobs, P. A., Mayer, M., Matsuura, J., Rhoades, F., & Yu, S. C. (1983). Cytogenetic study of a population of mentally retarded males with special reference to the marker X chromosome. *Human Genetics, 63*, 139-148.

Jayakar, P., Chudley, A. E., Ray, M., Evans, J. A., Perlov, J., & Wand, R. (1986). Fra(2) (q13) and Inv(9) (p11p12) in autism: casual relationship. *American Journal of Medical Genetics, 23*, 381-392.

Jørgensen, O. S., Brøndum-Nielsen, K., Isager, T., & Mouridsen, S. E. (1984). Fragile X-chromosome among child psychiatric patients with disturbances of language and social relationships. *Acta Psychiatrica Scandinavica, 70*, 510-514.

Judd, L. L., & Mandell, A. J. (1968). Chromosome studies in early infantile autism. *Archives of General Psychiatry, 18*, 450-457.

Kemper, M., Hagerman, R. J., Ahmad, R. S., & Mariner, R. (1986). Cognitive profiles and the spectrum of clinical manifestations in heterozygous fragile X females. *American Journal of Medical Genetics, 23*, 139-156.

Kerbeshian, J., Burd, L., & Martsolf, J. (1984). A family with fragile X syndrome. *Journal of Nervous and Mental Disease, 172*, 549-551.

Kotsopoulous, S., & Kutty, K. M. (1979). Histidinemia and infantile autism. *Journal of Autism and Developmental Disorders, 9*, 55-60.

Krug, B. A., Arick, J. R., & Almond, P. J. (1980). *Autism Screening Instrument for Educational Planning, revised.* Portland, Oregon: ASIEP Educational Co.

Largo, R. H., & Schinzel, A. (1985). Development and behavioral disturbances in 13 boys with fragile X syndrome. *European Journal of Pediatrics, 143*, 269-275.

LeCouteur, A., Rutter, M., Summers, D., & Butler, L. (1988). Fragile X in female autistic twins. *Journal of Autism and Developmental Disorders, 18*, 458-460.

Ledbetter, D. H., Rich, D. C., O'Connell, P., Leppert, M., & Carey, J. (1989). Precise localization of NFI to 17q11.2 by balanced translocation. *American Journal of Human Genetics, 44*, 20-24.

Levitas, A., Hagerman, R. J., Braden, M., Rimland, B., McBogg, P., & Matus, I. (1983). Autism and the fragile X syndrome. *Journal of Developmental Behavioral Pediatrics, 4,* 151-158.

Linden, M. G., Bender, B. G., Harmon, R. J., Mrazek, D. A., & Robinson, A. (1978). 47XXX: what is the prognosis? *Pediatrics, 82,* 619-630.

Lubs, H. A. (1969). A marker X chromosome. *American Journal of Human Genetics, 21,* 231-244.

Madison, L. S., George, C., & Moeschler, J. B. (1986). Cognitive functioning in the fragile X syndrome: a study of intellectual memory and communication skills. *Journal of Mental Deficiency Research, 30,* 129-148.

Mallin, S. R., & Walker, F. A. (1972). Effects of the XYY karyotype in one of 2 brothers with congenital adrenal hyperplasia. *Clinical Genetics, 3,* 490-494.

Mansheim, P. (1979). Tuberous sclerosis and autistic behaviour. *Journal of Clinical Psychiatry, 40,* 97-98.

Mariner, R., Jackson, A. W., Levitas, A., Hagerman, R. J., Braden, M., McBogg, P. M., Berry, R., & Smith, A. C. M. (1986). Autism, mental retardation and chromosomal abnormalities. *Journal of Autism and Developmental Disorders, 16,* 425-440.

Mattei, J. F., Mattei, M. G., Aumeras, C., Auger, M., & Giraud, F. (1981). X-linked mental retardation with the fragile X, a study of 15 families. *Human Genetics, 59,* 281-289.

McGillivray, B. C., Herbst, D. S., Dill, F. J., Sandercock, H. J., & Tischler, B. (1986). Infantile Autism: an occasional manifestation of fragile X mental retardation. *American Journal of Medical Genetics, 23,* 353-358.

Meryash, D. L., Szymanski, L. S., & Gerald, P. S. (1982). Infantile autism associated with the fragile X syndrome. *Journal of Autism and Developmental Disorders, 12,* 295-301.

Newall, K., Sanborne, B., & Hagerman, R. (1983). Speech and language dysfunction in the fragile X syndrome. In R. J. Hagerman & P. McBogg (Eds.), *The Fragile X Syndrome: Diagnosis, Biochemistry and Intervention.* Dillon, Colorado: Spectra Publishing Co.

Nielsen, J., Christensen, K. R., Friedrich, U., Zeuthen, E., & Ostergaard, O. (1973). Childhood of males with XYY syndrome. *Journal of Autism and Chilhood Schizophrenia, 3,* 5-26.

Opitz, J. M., & Sutherland, G. R. (1984). Conference report: international workshop on the fragile X and X-linked mental retardation. *American Journal of Medical Genetics, 17,* 5-94.

Opitz, J. M. (1986). On the gates of hell and a most unusual gene. *American Journal of Medical Genetics, 23,* 1-10.

Ornitz, E. M., Guthrie, D., & Farley, A. H. (1977). The early development of autistic children. *Journal of Autism and Childhood Schizophrenia, 7,* 207-229.

Pennington, B., & Smith, S. D. (1988). Genetic influences on learning disabilities: an update. *Journal of Consulting and Clinical Psychology, 56,* 817-823.

Polani, P. E. (1977). Abnormal sex chromosomes, behavior and mental disorder. In J. M. Tanner (Ed.), *Developments in Psychiatric Research.* London: Hoddler and Straughton, Ltd.

Proops, R., & Webb, T. (1981). The fragile X chromosome in the Martin-Bell-Renpenning syndrome and in males with other forms of familial mental retardation. *Journal of Medical Genetics, 18,* 366-373.

Pueschel, S. M., Herman, R., Groden, G. (1985). Brief report: Screening children with autism for fragile-X syndrome and phenylketonuria. *Journal of Autism and Developmental Disorders, 15,* 335 - 338.

Reiss, A. L., Feinstein, C., & Rosenbaum, K. N. (1986). Autism and genetic disorders. *Schizophrenia Bulletin, 12,* 724-738.

Reiss, A. L. (1988a). Cerebellar hypoplasia and autism. *New England Journal of Medicine, (letter), 319,* 1152-1153.

Reiss, A. L. (1988b). Neuroanatomical variation in the fragile X syndrome, paper presented to American College of Neuropsychopharmacology, San Juan, Puerto Rico, December 1988.

Reiss, A. L., Hagerman, R. J., Vinogradov, S., Abrams, M., & King, R. J. (1988). Psychiatric disability in female carriers of the fragile X chromosome. *Archives of General Psychiatry, 45,* 25-30.

Rimland, B. (1971). The differentiation of childhoood psychoses: an analysis of checklists for 2,218 psychotic children. *Journal of Autism and Childhood Schizophrenia, 1,* 161-174.

Ritvo, E. R., Mason-Brothers, A., Menkes, J. H., & Sparkes, R. S. (1988). Assocation of autism, retinoblastoma, and reduced esterase D activity. *Archives of General Psychiatry, 45,* 600.

Robinson, A., Bender, B., Borelli, J., Puck, M., Salbenblatt, J., & Webber, M. L. (1982). Sex chromosomal abnormalities (SCA): a prospective and longitudinal study of newborns identified in an unbiased manner. *Birth Defects: Original Article Series, 18,* 7-39.

Rutter, M., & Bartak, L. (1971). Causes of infantile autism, some considerations from recent research. *Journal of Autism and Childhood Schizophrenia, 1,* 20-32.

Rutter, M. (1978). Diagnosis and definition. In M. Rutter & E. Schopler (Eds.), *Autism: a reappraisal of concepts and treatment.* New York: Plenum Press.

Salbenblatt, J. A., Meyers, D. C., Bender, B. G., Linden, M. G., & Robinson, A. (1987). Gross and fine motor development in 47XXY and 47XYY males. *Pediatrics, 80,* 240-244.

Sherman, S. L., Jacobs, P. A., Morton, N. E., Froster-Iskenius, U., Howard-Peebles, T. N., Nielsen, K. B., Partington, M. W., Sutherland, G. R., Turner, G., & Watson, M. (1985). Further segregation analysis of the fragile X syndrome with special reference to transmitting males. *Human Genetics, 69,* 289-299.

Smalley, S. L., Asarnow, R. F., & Spence, A. (1988). Autism and genetics. *Archives of General Psychiatry, 45,* 953-961.

Sutherland, G. R. (1977). Fragile sites on human chromosomes: demonstration of their dependence on the type of tissue culture medium. *Science, 197,* 265-266.

Sutherland, G. R., & Hecht, F. (1985). *Fragile Sites on Human Chromosomes.* New York: Oxford University Press.

Tennes, K., Puck, M., Orfanakis, D., & Robinson, A. (1977). The early child development of 17 boys with sex chromosome anomalies: a prospective study. *Pediatrics, 59,* 574-583.

Tranel, D., Hall, L. E., Olson, S., & Trand, N. N. (1987). Evidence for a right hemisphere developmental learning disability. *Developmental Neuropsychology, 3,* 113-127.

Turner, B., & Jennings, A. N. (1961). Trisomy for chromosome 22. *Lancet, 1,* 49-50.

Turner, G., Daniel, A., & Frost, M. (1980). X-linked mental retardation, macroorchidism and the Xq27 fragile site. *Pediatrics, 96,* 837-841.

Turner, G., Opitz, J. M., Brown, T. W., Davies, K. E., Jacobs, P. A., Jenkins, E. C., Mikkelsen, M., Partington, M. W., & Sutherland, G. R. (1986). Conference report: second international workshop on the fragile X and on X-linked mental retardation. *American Journal of Medical Genetics, 23,* 11-67.

Varley, C. K., Holm, V. A., & Eren, M. O. (1985). Cognitive and psychiatric variability in 3 brothers with fragile X syndrome. *Journal of Developmental and Behavioral Pediatrics, 6,* 87-90.

Venter, P. A., Op't Hof, J., Coetzee, D. J., Van der Walt, C. A., & Retief, A. E. (1984). No marker (X) syndrome in autistic children. *Human Genetics, 67,* 107-111.

Wahlström, J., Gillberg, C., Gustavson, K. H., & Holmgren, G. (1986). Infantile autism and the fragile X, a Swedish multicenter study. *American Journal of Medical Genetics, 23,* 403-408.

Watson, M. S., Leckman, J. F., Annex, B., Breg, W. R., Boles, D., Volkmar, F. R., Dohen, D. J., & Carter, C. (1984). Fragile X in a survey of 75 autistic males (letter to the editor). *New England Journal of Medicine, 310,* 1462.

Webb, T. P., Bundy, S., Thake, A., & Todd, J. (1986). The frequence of the fragile X chromosome among school children in Coventry. *Journal of Medical Genetics, 23,* 396-399.

Wenger, S. L., Steele, M. W., & Becker, D. J. (1988). Clinical consequences of deletion 1p35. *Journal of Medical Genetics, 4,* 263.

Wing, L. (1981). Asperger's syndrome: a clinical account. *Psychological Medicine, 11,* 115-129.

Wolf-Schein, E. G., Sudhalter, V., Cohen, I. L., Fisch, G. S., Hanson, D., Pfadt, A. G., Hagerman, R. J., Jenkins, E. C., & Brown, T. W. (1987). Speech-language and the fragile X syndrome: initial findings. *Journal of the American Speech and Hearing Association, 29,* 35-38.

Wolf-Schein, E. G., Jenkins, E. C., Sklower, S., Cohen, I. L., Wisniewski, K. E., & Brown, W. T. (1988). On the association of fragile X with autism. *Journal of Autism and Developmental Disorders, 18,* 457-458.

Wolff, P. H., Gardner, J., Paccia, J., & Lappen, J. (1989). The greeting behavior of fragile X males. *American Journal of Mental Retardation, 93,* 406-411.

Wolraich, M., Bzostek, B., Neu, R. L., & Gardner, L. I. (1970). Lack of chromosome abervations in autism. *New England Journal of Medicine, (letter), 38,* 1231.

Wright, H. H., Young, S. R., Edwards, J. G., Abramson, R. K., & Duncan, J. (1986). Fragile X syndrome in a population of autistic children. *Journal of the American Academy of Child Psychiatry, 25,* 641-644.

Autism:Immunological Investigations

AUDRIUS V. PLIOPLYS

Blood samples were obtained from a total of 17 patients with autism. There were 16 males and 1 female. The age range was from 8 to 23 years with a mean age of 17. The diagnosis of autism conformed to the DSM-III (APA, 1980) and DSM-III-R (APA, 1987) criteria for autism. There were no identified neurobiologic causes of autism in any of the studied population. Parental signed consent was obtained prior to phlebotomy. This study was approved by ethics review committies. Simultaneously drawn blood samples from healthy young adults served as controls for the lymphocyte stimulation studies and for the pokeweed mitogen stimulations. For comparison of IgG anti-central nervous system (CNS) reactivity the results from a study of 348 children were used (Plioplys, 1989). For the IgM results a comparison group of 101 normal young adults was used. For comparison of neural cell adhesion molecule (NCAM) determinations the results from seven physically and neurologically normal controls (4 male, 3 female) were used with a mean age of 19 years.

The results can be summarized in the following three areas:

LYMPHOCYTE ABNORMALITIES

Peripheral blood lymphocytes were separated on a Ficoll-hypaque density gradient. Autistic patients had normal numbers of T and B cells and T cells subsets.

However, the CD4:CD8 ratios were normal only in 4 individuals (Figure 1) while 6 patients had elevated ratios (>2.2) and 5 patients had decreased ratios (>1.5). Although the mean value of 2.09 ± 0.97 (± one standard deviation, SD) was within normal limits, there was a clustering of the CD4:CD8 ratios into two general groups: those >2 and <2 (Figure 1).

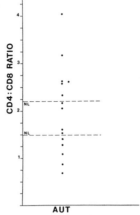

Figure 1. CD4:CD8 ratio in patients with autism. Normative values are indicated. Only 4 values are within normal limits. The CD4:CD8 distributions cluster into those >2 and <2.

There was an increased number of DR+ (activated) T cells in patients with autism (normal <2 %; Figure 2). For the group as a whole, the percentage of DR+ T lymphocytes was 7.73 ± 5.75. Within the DR+ group (11 patients) there was a decrease in percentage of DR+ T cells with increasing age (Figure 2). No patients demonstrated an increased number of interleukin-2 (IL-2) receptor positive cells.

There was an inverse correlation between CD4:CD8 ratios and number of circulating DR+ lymphocytes. In those patients with CD4:CD8<2 there was an increased number of DR+ cells (10.71 ± 2.87%) as compared to the patients with CD4:CD8>2 (5.12 ± 6.5 %; p<0.05).

Mitogen-induced proliferation of both concanavallin-A (5 µg/ml and 50 µg/ml) and phytametagglutinin (1 µg/ml and 10 µg/ml) in patients with autism did not differ from controls. The autologous mixed lymphocyte reaction (AMLR) was within normal limits when the group was examined as a whole. However, there was a significantly decreased AMLR (8630 ± 3045; counts per minute ± one SD) for the 5 patients with CD4:CD8<1.5 as compared to the 9 patients with a normal or elevated CD4:CD8 (15213 ± 7700; p<0.05). In contrast when patients were divided by numbers of DR+ (activated) T cells into normal numbers of DR+ T cells and increased number of DR+ T cells, there was no difference in AMLR (12887 ± 4351 vs 12863 ± 8181).

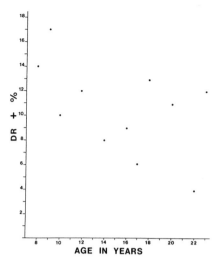

Figure 2. DR+ percentage as plotted against age for those patients with autism who had DR+ T lymphocytes. The DR+ percentages are all elevated (normal <2 %). There is a decrease in DR+ percentage with age.

Autistic patients have an abnormally increased percentage of DR+ but not IL-2 receptor ± lymphocytes suggesting "incomplete" activation, a finding which is seen in autoimmune diseases. The decrease in activated cells with increasing age suggests that there may be an autoimmune process which is more active earlier in life. Further details concerning this line of investigation may be found elsewhere (Plioplys et al., 1989).

ANTI-CENTRAL NERVOUS SYSTEM IMMUNOREACTIVITY

B cell function (proliferation and in vitro IgG and IgM synthesis in response to two different concentrations of pokeweed mitogen) was normal. Quantitative serum immunoglobulins (IgG, IgA and IgM) were normal. When tested against Western blots prepared from normal, human cerebellar tissue, there was an increased incidence of IgG anti-210K neurofilament subunit reactivity (41 % vs 7 % in 348 controls; p<0.001). IgM anti-210-K reactivity occurred in 53 % of the patients (25 % in 101 controls; p<0.05) with an overall incidence of IgM anti-cerebellar Western blot banding of 88 % (26 % in controls; p<0.001). IgG or IgM reactivity against frontal cortex Western blots was not observed.

There was no correlation between the anti-CNS results and abnormalities in CD4:CD8 lymphocyte ratios, AMLRs and the expression of DR surface antigen. There was no correlation between any of these results and medication intake (one patient was taking each of the following medications: carbamazepine, haloperidol, methylphenidate and pimozide; two were taking thioridazine).

Reported cerebellar magnetic resonance imaging abnormalities in autism (Courchesne et al., 1983) may be related to this demonstrated anti-cerebellar immunoreactivity. Further details concerning this line of research may be found elsewhere (Plioplys et al., 1989).

NCAM LEVELS

The biochemical structure of neural cell adhesion molecule (NCAM) is homologous to immunoglobulins in that five extracellular NCAM domains share structural homology with members of the immunoglobulin superfamily (Berthels et al., 1987; Cunningham et al., 1987). The homophilic binding of NCAM molecules may be on the basis of complementary interactions between the immunoglobulin domains (Cunningham et al., 1987). If immunoglobulins are abnormally regulated in autism (as the above data suggests), then possibly other molecular members of the immunoglobulin superfamily, such as NCAM, may also be abnormally regulated.

The level of a NCAM serum fragment in autistic patients was determined by using an antiserum prepared with immunoaffinity purified mouse NCAM. There was a significant decrease in serum NCAM concentration in autistics as compared to controls. In autism, the mean level was 42.34 ± 8.85 optical density units per ml of serum, whereas in the controls it was 98.84 ± 16.91 (p<0.0005; Figure 3).

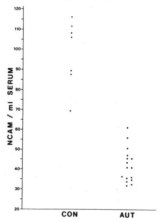

Figure 3. NCAM serum concentration expressed in optical density units per ml of serum in controls (CON) and autistics (AUT). There was a significant decrease in the mean value of NCAM levels in autistics when compared to controls (42.34 ± 8.85 vs 98.84 ± 16.91; p<0.0005).

When calculated as optical density units of NCAM per mg of serum protein, again there was a highly significant decrease in autistics as compared to controls. In autism the results was 0.63 ± 0.13 and in the controls 1.27 ± 0.19 (p<0.0005; Figure 4).

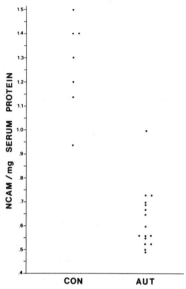

Figure 4. NCAM serum concentration expressed in optical density units per mg of serum protein in controls (CON) and autistics (AUT). There was a significant decrease in the mean value of NCAM levels in autistics when compared to controls (0.63 ± 0.13 vs 1.27 ± 0.19; p<0.0005).

The difference between autistics and controls could not be attributed to a medication induced effect in the autistic serum samples. Approximately one third of the autistic population were receiving medications at the time of phlebotomy. When the patients taking medications are grouped and compared to the control population the significant difference in NCAM serum levels remained when expressed as either NCAM/ml serum of NCAM/mg protein (in both cases p<0.0005). There was no statistically significant difference between NCAM serum levels, either as NCAM/ml or NCAM/mg protein, in autistics taking medications when compared to autistics not taking medications.

Depressed serum NCAM levels in autism are distinct from schizophrenia where the levels are elevated (Lyons et al., 1988). It is possible that the elevated serum NCAM levels in schizophrenia reflect an increase in natural central nervous system synaptic turnover rate, as has been suggested (Lyons et al., 1988), whereas its depression in autism may reflect a decreased turnover rate. Furthermore, these results demonstrate that autism and schizophrenia are biologically distinct entities and suggest that circulating

NCAM levels may be useful in distinguishing autism from childhood schizophrenia within the diagnostic grouping of pervasive developmental disorders (APA, 1980; APA, 1987). Further details concerning this line of investigation may be found elsewhere (Plioplys et al., 1989).

REFERENCES

American Psychiatric Assocation. (1980). *Diagnostic and statistical manual of mental disorders. (3rd ed.).* Washington DC: Author.

American Psychiatric Assocation. (1987). *Diagnostic and statistical manual of mental disorders. (3rd rev ed.).* Washington DC: Author.

Barthels, D., Santoni, M-J., Wille, W., Ruppert, C., Chaix, J-C., Hirsch, M-R., Fontecilla-Camps, J. C., & Goridis, D. (1987). Isolation and nucleotide sequence of mouse NCAM cDNA that codes for a Mr 79,000 polypeptide without a membrane-spanning region. *EMBO Journal 6,* 907 - 914.

Courchesne, E., Yeung-Courchesne, R., Press, G. A., Hesselink, J. R., & Jernigan, T. L. (1988). Hypoplasia of cerebellar vermal lobules VI and VII in autism. *New England Journal of Medicine, 318,* 1349 - 1354.

Cunningham, B. A., Hemperly, J. J., Murray, B. A., Prediger, E. A., Brackenbury, R., Edelman, G. M. (1987). Neural cell adhesion molecule; structure, immunoglobulin-like domains, cell surface modulation, and alternative RNA splicing. *Science, 236,* 799 - 806.

Lyons, F., Martin, M. L., Maguire, C., Jackson, A., Regan, C. M., & Shelley, R. K. (1988). The expression of an N-CAM serum fragment is positively correlated with severity of negative features in type II schizophrenia. *Biological Psychiatry, 23,* 769 -775.

Plioplys, A. V., Greaves, A., & Yoshida, W. (1989). Anti-CNS antibodies in childhood neurologic diseases. *Neuropediatrics* (in press).

Plioplys, A. V., Greaves, A., Kazemi, K., & Silverman, E. (1989). Lymphocyte function in autism. *Canadian Journal of Neurological Sciensies* (abstract in print); manuscript submitted for publication.

Plioplys, A. V., Greaves, A., Kazemi, K., & Silverman, A. (1989). Autism: anti-210K neurofilament immunoglobulin reactivity. *Neurology* (abstract in print); manuscript submitted for publication.

Plioplys, A. V., Hemmens, S. E., & Regan, C. M. (1989). Expression of a NCAM serum fragment is depressed in autism. *Annals of Neurology* (abstract in print); manuscript submitted for publication.

The First Evaluation: Treatment Begins Here

CHRISTOPHER GILLBERG

INTRODUCTION

In autism literature it is exceptional to see a declaration of what should and what should not be included in the diagnostic evaluation of the individual child and rarer still to find even a paragraph commenting on the fundamental importance of this evaluation both in terms of crisis intervention and as a basis for any treatment plan. The present chapter represents an attempt to fill some of this gap.

THE THERAPEUTICAL IMPACT OF DIAGNOSIS IN AUTISM

Families with a child who suffers from autism often say, several years after the first evaluation which led to a correct diagnosis of "autistic disorder" or "autism" that the day on which they received that information has remained in their minds not as a day of doom but rather as the point of departure for realistic hope. Before that day they have often felt themselves to be "left in the dark" or vaccillating in a destructive manner between fear and hope. I now have very considerable experience (several hundred families) of diagnostic evaluations and long-term follow-up of families with children with autism and I think I am not overstating the case if I say that early and correct diagnosis makes a positive difference. We have not yet compiled the systematic data, but parents of children with autism who received a correct diagnosis after the child's sixth birthday (which was common in the seventies when I started out in the field) report more negative things about society, themselves and the child than parents who had a full expert assessment before the child's fourth birthday. The first evaluation is the corner-stone of all treatment in autism.

DECIDING ON LABELS

The family should be thoroughly informed about the nature of the child's handicap and the precise name of the diagnosis the doctor has made as soon as possible. Psychiatrists and psychologists inexperienced in the field sometimes refrain from this procedure and may tell the parents that the child "will grow out of it", "is delayed", "has something not clearly classifiable" or suffers from "(mild) autistic traits" or even "a touch of autism". Information of this kind usually does more harm than good. The child should be examined by someone very knowledgeable in the field who dares decide on an appropriate label, be it "autistic disorder", "Asperger syndrome", "Rett syndrome" or "still unclassifiable" for that matter. This is not to say that diagnoses along the "autism spectrum" should be made hastily, but rather that they should be established with as much certainty as possible so that the family has a name for the child's disorder.

In the case of more intelligent children with autism - those currently often given the clinical diagnosis of Asperger syndrome - the "name" of the disorder should, sooner or later, be told to the child itself. When to do this depends on the child's developmental level and age and the family's wishes. The 8 - 12-year age period has often been the most appropriate period to do this in my experience.

THE HISTORY TAKING

A careful history taking provides the backbone of any diagnosis. Autism spectrum disorders are no exception to this rule. In optimal circumstances both mother and father should be carefully interviewed. Other important care-givers such as grandparents, siblings, day-nursery personell, school-teachers etc usually provide important information too provided that somebody asks them. Unstructured interviews are sometimes unhelpful, whereas semi-structured and even highly structured systematic questioning often inspire a sense of relief in the parents who feel that they can give even very "difficult" information to somebody who obviously knows something about the child's handicap. "How can you know so well which questions to ask?" "You are describing my child!" "I feel you know him without having seen him more than a couple of minutes". Of course, one has to caution against the risk of jumping to hasty conclusions if questions are too directive and answers are not allowed to be elaborated. Always ask the informant to exemplify!

There are often great differences in the quality of histories obtained depending on the child's position in the sibship and parental "maturity" (but not necessarily education). Young parents of first-born children usually are less likely to have observed some of the more subtle signs of deviance in young children with autism than are, for instance, mothers of number three of three brothers. Parents who have heard about autism often give a very adequate description of the child's development and symptoms. Those, on the other hand, who have already studied books on autism may or may not provide a realistic picture of the child. Some, after having recognized certain traits, actually want to make the whole picture fit and "overdo things" in an effort to comply with what they believe to be the doctor's wishes in respect of diagnosis. Sure enough, the doctor's education, temperamental style and way of interviewing also have some part to play in this connection.

Areas which must be covered in the interview comprise hereditary factors (in minute detail, going through one relative after another and inquiring about developmental delays, mental retardation, autism, Asperger-type problems, speech-problems, dyslexia, other learning disorders, epilepsy and known neurological or psychiatric disorder - this part often has to be repeatedly analysed on different occasions), pregnancy and perinatal periods (and medical records should always be analysed: there is relatively poor agreement between mother's and medical report in this respect [Bax et al., 1978]), associated medical conditions (including seizures), social factors, a developmental history, a description of the child's symptoms (the latter often best achieved in connection with specific questionnaire interview - see below) and last - but not least - the parents' expectations, hopes and reasons for consulting you.

The use of highly structured questionnaires

There is now a variety of more or less well examined questionnaires which can be used in connection with autism diagnostics. Three of the most well-established rating scales instruments are the CARS (Childhood Autism Rating Scale) (Schopler et al., 1980, Morgan, 1988) the PEP (Psychoeducational Profile) (Schopler & Reichler, 1979) and its counterpart for adolescents and adults (AAPEP) (Mesibov et al., 1989) and the ABC (Autism Behavior Checklist) Krug et al., 1980; Brand Teal & Wicbe, 1986; Volkmar et al., 1988).

In clinical practice I have found the ABC to be useful in that it highlights most of the symptom areas which are relevant in the field of autism and that it requires relatively little time to complete (c 30 minutes). The ABC consists of a number of statements (e g "walks on tiptoe" and "has no friends") and the informant (usually the mother in my experience, even though the instrument was not originally developed for use with parents) is required, very simply, to say whether that statement applies or not. I have found the ABC to be a good help, particularly with children 3 - 10 years of age and especially with those who have some speech. For a good critical review of the ABC (and other autism rating scales) see Morgan (1988) The ABC should not be regarded as "a test of whether or not the child has autism" but rather as a helpful tool in eliciting pertinent information.

For detailed clinical examination and research, the CARS, the PEP, the HBS (Handicaps, Behaviours and Skills schedule) (Wing, 1971) and the BSE (Behaviour Summarized Evaluation Scale) (Barthelemy et al., 1989) in my opinion provide some of the best published assessment tools currently available, and there is burgeoning work on their validity, reliability and applicability. The CARS in particular now has a considerable literature to support its reliability and validity (Morgan, 1988).

I think it can also be of help to use a short screening chart covering the sixteen "symptoms" outlined in the DSM-III-R (APA 1987).

The highly structured questionnaire interview, if performed in a sensitive way by someone knowledgeable in the field of autism, often provides a good opportunity for the parents to "come forward" with a number of problems in the child which they have never before had the opportunity to talk to anyone about. The simple reasons for this could be that they may not have had words to describe the "symptom" or they have had a diffuse feeling that something was wrong but they didn't realize that this particular phenomenon (e g the interest in casette tapes) could be regarded as a problem characteristic of the underlying handicap.

PSYCHOMETRY

A cognitive test is essential in any first work-up of a child who presents with autistic features. This is for several reasons, perhaps the most important being that an overall estimate of cognitive functions is necessary when planning a treatment programme (Howlin & Rutter, 1987) and that IQ at diagnosis has high predictive power as regards outcome in the long-term perspective (e g Gillberg & Steffenburg, 1987). A psychologist well acquainted with "testing in autism" should always perform the test in order to avoid the child being diagnosed (which is done all too frequently) as being "untestable". Verbal and non - verbal tests should be used. In Sweden, the Griffiths developmental scale is often used but it yields relatively little information apart from that apparent at the clinical examination. The Leiter performance scale, the new Vineland scale covering social and adaptive skills and the Reynell test of language are often useful in the pre-school period. For school-age children with high-level autism or Asperger syndrome, the WISC is usually informative (with characteristic low results in the fields of word comprehension and picture arrangement) (Lockyer & Rutter, 1979: Freeman et al., 1988; Lincoln, et al., 1988). For speaking children with autism, a careful evaluation by a speech pathology therapist is usually required.

In our centre, we have recently included a battery of tests suggested by the Frith group (Baron-Cohen, 1989), in the basic "psychometrics" used with all but the youngest and most severely retarded groups of children and adolescents with autism and Asperger syndrome. These are tests which are thought to reflect the child's capacity to conceive of other people as having minds. The tests clinically provide a very useful point of departure for discussing with the parents the basic nature of their child's "mystical" handicap. In many cases such a discussion makes the child much less mystical (mystical that is in a negative way) in the minds of the parents.

So called "projective tests" are rarely useful in the evaluation of the child's "inner world".

NEUROPSYCHIATRIC WORK-UP

A thorough neuropsychiatric work-up in the field of autism <u>must always</u> include a meticulous physical and neurological examination, a psychiatric state examination and an appropriate set of laboratory investigations. I shall summarize the most important issues in this field and would like to underline that this part of the investigation in a case of autism remains the most essential basis for any treatment programme. In my opinion there can be no good treatment for children, youngsters and adults with autism without a comprehensive neuropsychiatric work-up.

Physical examination

Table 1 outlines what needs to be looked for in the physical examination of every case with suspected autism. Apart from the necessity to try and fit obvious physical anomalies into the picture of a known specific syndrome (e g Williams syndrome, Rett syndrome, Martin - Bell syndrome etc), there is always a special need to look for diagnostic skin changes (e g tuberous sclerosis, neurofibromatosis, hypomelanosis of

Ito). This means that the child's skin (and hair) and sometimes that of the parents as well - has to be meticulously examined with the clothes removed. Height, weight, head circumference and curvature of spinal column are also features which must be systematically recorded.

TABLE 1. Physical examination of child with suspected or clear autism.

Always note/score/examine

Height
Weight
Head circumference
Minor physical anomalies (e g according to method described by Waldrop and
   Halvorsen 1971)
Skin and hair changes (dry, cold skin and coarse , dry hair; café-au-lait spots;
   depigmented spots; fibromas; adenoma sebaceum; cheek rash; polyosis; hypopigmented
   areas; freckles in armpits; peau de chagrin etc)
Eyes and eye-movements including squint
Spinal column
Heart rate and variability
Abdomen (enlarged spleen, liver etc)
External genitals (large testicles, abundant prepuce)
Neuromotor performance (e g walks, crawls, walks on tip-toe, uses pens or crayons
   (in)appropriately, handedness in 5 different settings, hypo- or hypertonus, ataxia,
   balance, routine reflexes)

The psychiatric state examination

The present psychiatric state examination must include a "broad" description of the child with regard to overall functioning (e g "7-year old mute child who looks younger than chronological age, avoids eye-contact with parents and examiner, has little facial mimicry, flaps his hands and walks high on tip-toe. Appears to pay no attention to surroundings and does not react to strong noise, hand-claps etc. Clearly hyperactive in that he moves incessantly from one thing to another. No signs of hallucinations". Psychomotor activity, ability to relate to examiner and other people present, presence of hallucinations, irrelevant speech, other speech-language abnormalities, stereotypies and presence of special skills should be particularly noted and described.

Laboratory investigations

Table 2 details the essential and laboratory investigations that should always be made. It is necessary to take the child's age into account since certain diagnoses are more likely in younger and others more likely in older children (see below). All children with autism, regardless of age, must have at least a chromosomal culture, a neuroimaging test (CT or MRI) of the brain, an EEG and tests of hearing and vision. In a young child (under school-age) all the "essential investigations" of Table 2 have to be performed, whereas in an older child the extent of the investigation could vary somewhat from case to case.

TABLE 2. Essential and optimal laboratory investigations in autism and autistic-like conditions.

Essential (unless clinical examination has already revealed etiology)
    Blood
    Phenylalanine
    Serotonin and platelet count
    Uric acid
    Calcium
    Phosphorus
    Magnesium
    Lactic acid
    Pyruvic acid
    Herpes titer
    Cytomegalovirus titer
    Mumps titer
    Chromosomal culture - folate deficient media (all males and females)
    BUN
    24-hour Urine
    Uric acid
    Magnesium
    Calcium
    Phosphorus
    Metabolic screen (including test for mucopolysaccharides)
    Creatinine
    HVA
    Other laboratory tests
    EEG
    CT or NMR
    Ophtalmological
    Auditory evaluation (including brainstem auditory evoked potential if the
      child is mute)
    Otological examination, including test of vestibular function such as
      Barany's rotation test for elicitation of nystagmus
Optional
    72-hour stool for lipid and occult blood
    24-hour urine for amino acids, organic acids, urinary peptide excretion,
      succinyl purines, niacin metabolites and zinc
    Cerebrospinal fluid-protein, cell count, glucose, monoamine and
      endorphin and amino-acid content
    Brainstem and cortical auditory evoked potential

DEVELOPMENTAL AND AGE ASPECTS

Developmental aspects and the child's age need to be taken into account when planning the laboratory investigation programme. A two-year old girl with autism should have the whole "essential" programme. The same girl, presenting for diagnostic evaluation three years later might then well turn out to have all the characteristic symptoms of the Rett syndrome and should then, of course, receive the laboratory work-up warranted in that syndrome rather than the "essential" battery in autism. A nine-year old boy with autism, epilepsy and an adenoma sebaceum-like rash in all probability suffers from tuberous sclerosis and the laboratory investigation should be tailored to that diagnosis rather than to "unspecific autism".

DIAGNOSIS: STATIC AND DYNAMIC ASPECTS

Autism is a behavioural syndrome and a developmental disorder. This - among other things - means that symptoms vary according to age and overall developmental level. The symptoms considered typical of autism have usually been extracted from the clinical stereotype once provided by Leo Kanner's original descriptions (Kanner, 1943). These generally referred to preschool and young school-age children, usually with mild degrees of mental retardation. Autism in many respects has a different face in infancy (Dahlgren & Gillberg, 1989) and in older children, adolescents and adults (Wing 1980, Gillberg & Schaumann, 1981; Wing, 1983). Suggestions have been made for changing the diagnostic labels accordingly. For instance "infantile autism residual state" appeared in the DSM-III (APA, 1980) to cover cases who had once fulfilled criteria for infantile autism but no longer did so. In the DSM-III-R (APA, 1987) there is only "autistic disorder", probably indicating the increasingly felt need to have some stability with regard to "basic diagnoses" in the indivudual case. Nevertheless, diagnostic reformulations need to be made continuously both from the behavioural, educational and medical points of view. It is not possible to provide a general recommendation as to the frequency of such reevaluations. However, it is clear that behaviour sometimes changes dramatically over time (e g pubertal changes, the very few who develop hallucinations etc), educational needs can vary enormously from one period to another and underlying medical conditions may not with our current methods of investigation be "diagnoseable" until, for instance, pre-puberty (as is somtimes the case in tuberous sclerosis). Therefore, diagnostic evaluations cannot generally be regarded as a once-and-for-all business.

CONCLUDING REMARKS

It should be self-evident that there can be no treatment in autism without a proper diagnosis and an appropriate work-up. Treatment approaches in many respects must be different depending on the underlying cause (compare for instance PKU, the Rett syndrome, the fragile X syndrome and tuberous sclerosis: diet prescription in one, scoliosis and wheel-chair prognosis in the second, genetic counselling in the third and fourth instances and great differences between the two with regard to behavioural phenotype and associated handicaps). The diagnosis in itself means a word for parents, siblings - and indeed sometimes the patient - to use in communication with others. Uncovering causes and clues with respect to underlying pathophysiology is almost always helpful, both for purely psychological reasons and for better treatment approaches (Barthelemy et al., 1989). It can no longer be acceptable to work for years with children with autism without having a sound neuropsychiatric and medical evaluation as a basis for all further work. We who work in the field must confront those colleagues who still say that: "why do this or that laboratory test when the outcome will not alter the child's prognosis?" Knowing as much as possible about all aspects of the child's handicap is the aim of diagnosis and work-up. Treatment and habilitation begin there!

REFERENCES

American Psychiatric Association. (1980). *Diagnostic and Statistical Manual of Mental Disorders. DSM-III. (3rd ed.).* Washington, DC: Author.

American Psychiatric Association. (1987). *Diagnostic and Statistical Manual of Mental Disorders. DSM-III-R. (3rd rev ed.).* Washington DC: Author.

Baron-Cohen, S. (1989). The autistic child's theory of mind. A case of specific developmental delay. *Journal of Child Psychology and Psychiatry, 30,* 285 - 297.

Barthelemy, C., Adrien, J. L., Tanguay, P., Garreau, B., Fermanian, J., Roux, S., Sauvage, D., & Lelord, G. (1989). The behavioural summarized evaluation (B.S.E.). Development and validation of a clinical assessment scale for autistic children (submitted).

Brand-Teal, M., & Wiebe, J. (1986). A Validity Analysis of Selected Instruments used to Assess Autism. *Journal of Autism and Developmental Disorders, 4,* 485 - 494.

Dahlgren, S-O., & Gillberg, C. (1989). Symptoms in the First Two Years of Life. A preliminary Population Study of Infantile Autism. *European Archives of Psychiatric and Neurological Science, 386,* 1 - 6.

Dahlgren, S-O., & Gillberg, C. (1989). Symptoms in the First Two Years of Life. A preliminary Population Study of Infantile Autism. *European Archives of Psychiatric and Neurological Science, 386,* 1 - 6.

Freeman, B. J., Ritvo, M. D., Mason-Brothers, A., Pingree, C., Yokota, A., Jenson, W., McMahon, W., Petersen, B., Mo, A., & Schroth, P. (1988). Psychometric Assessment of First-Degree Relatives of 62 Autistic probands in Utah. *American Journal of Psychiatry, 146,* 361 - 364.

Gillberg, C., & Schaumann, H. (1981). Infantile autism and puberty. *Journal of Autism and Developmental Disorders, 11,* 365 - 371.

Gillberg, C., & Steffenburg, S. (1987). Outcome and prognostic factors in infantile autism and similar conditions. A population based study of 46 cases followed through puberty. *Journal of Autism and Developmental Disorders, 17,* 271 - 285.

Hart, H., Bax, M., & Jenkins, S. (1978). The value of a developmental history. *Developmental Medicine and Child Neurology 20,* 442 - 452.

Howlin, P., & Rutter, M. (1987). *Treatment of Autistic Children.* Chichester: John Wiley & Sons.

Kanner, L. (1943). Autistic disturbances of affective contact. *Nervous Child 2,* 217 - 250.

Krug, D. A., Arick, J., & Almond, P. (1980). Behaviour checklist for identifying severely handicapped individuals with high levels of autistic behaviour. *Journal of Child Psychology and Psychiatry, 21,* 221 - 229.

Lincoln, E. J., Courchesne, E., Kilman, B. A., Elamsian, R., Allen, M. (1988). A Study of Intellectual Abilities in High-Functioning People with Autism. *Journal of Autism and Developmental Disorders, 18,* 505 - 524.

Lockyer, L., Rutter, M. (1970). A five to fifteen year follow-up study of infantile autism: Patterns of cognitive ability. *British Journal of Social and Clinical Neuropsychology, 4,* 27 - 41.

Mesibov, G. B., Schopler, E., & Caison, W. (1989). The Adolescent and Adult Psychoeducational Profile: Assessment of Adolescents and Adults with Severe Developmental Handicaps. *Journal of Autism and Developmental Disorder, 19,* 33 - 40.

Morgan, S. (1988). Diagnostic Assessment of Autism: a review of objective scales. *Journal of Psychoeducational Assessment, 6,* 139 - 151.

Rumsey, J. M., Hamburger, S. D. (1988). Neuropsychological Findings in High-Functioning Men with Infantile autism, Residual State. *Journal of Clinical Experimental Neuropsychology, 2,* 201 - 221.

Schopler, E., Reichler, R. J., DeVellis, R. F., & Daly, K. (1980). Toward objective classification of childhood autism: Childhood Autism Rating Scale (CARS). *Journal of Autism and Developmental Disorders, 10,* 91 - 103.

Schopler, E., Reichler R. J., & Renner B. R. (1985). *Childhood Autism Rating Scale (CARS).* New York: Irving.

Waldrop, M., & Halvorsen, C. (1971). Minor physical anomalies and hyperactive behaviour in young children. In J. Hellmuth (Ed.), *Exceptional Infant. Vol 2. Studies in Abnormalities* (pp 343 - 380). New York: Brunner/Mazel,

Wing, L. (1971). Schedule of Children's Handicaps, Behaviour and Skills. London: Medical Research Council.

Wing, L. (1980). Childhood autism and social class: a question of selection. *British Journal of Psychiatry, 137,* 410 - 417.

Wing, L. (1983). Social and interpersonal needs. In E. Schopler & G. B. Mesibov (Eds.), *Autism in Adolescents and Adults* (pp 337 - 354). New York: Plenum Press.

Volkmar, F. R., Sparrow S. S., Godreau D., Cicchetti D. V., Paul, R., & Cohen D. J. (1987). Social deficits in autism: an operational approach using the Vineland adaptive behaviour scales. *Journal of the American Academy of Child and Adolescent Psychiatry 26,* 156 - 161.

Educational Evaluation

MARGARET D. LANSING

INTRODUCTION

Educational evaluation is an essential step in planning optimal treatment for the autistic child. It has been frequently stated (Rutter, 1978, Lansing & Schopler, 1978; Wing, 1976) that education is the treatment of choice for this population. Due to the idiosyncratic needs of an autistic child, an appropriate educational plan must be based on a broad evaluation that includes three essential areas: 1. CONTENT; An assessment of the skills and concepts already acquired and those the child shows a readiness to learn; 2. BEHAVIOR; The autistic behaviors and deficits that must be understood; 3. TECHNIQUES; The teaching techniques that will improve attention, motivation, and learning. The assessment of these three areas will form the basis for specific individualized recommendations that result from this educational evaluation. In order to illustrate the value of this type of broad evaluation, I will be describing it in the context of our TEACCH evaluation using the Psychoeducational Profile (PEP-R) (Schopler et al., in press).

     The unusual and uneven development across various function areas, or domains, in children with autism has been widely recognized (Johnson-Martin, 1988). Likewise, variations in behavioral response and self-control occur all too frequently in children with autism. The evaluator must therefore be alert to the wide variations in skill level, be familiar with the attentional and motivational deficits, and be able to adapt the test environment in order to reduce the stress experienced by the child. Through this process she can help the child demonstrate his best skills and intrinsic interests. (For the purpose of clarity, the child will be referred to as, "he", and the examiner as, "she".) The test results and clinical observations obtained during the evaluation are translated into recommendations used by teachers and parents at home. (Schopler et al., 1980, 1983).

The educational evaluation at TEACCH uses the Psychoeducational Profile (PEP) (Schopler & Reichler, 1979). This test has been used in our program for over 15 years and more recently translated into five languages. Due to an increasing number of referrals for evaluation of younger or more retarded children, we have revised the PEP (Schopler et al., in press) and added several new items at the lower developmental age ranges. In this way we are able to provide more specific educational recommendations for this very young or developmentally delayed population. These new items will be described in the text that follows.

CONTENT

Developmental Function Areas

The test consists of 131 developmental items arranged in seven function areas. Each function area measures skills ranging from ages 6 to 80 months. The seven areas are: Imitation, Perception, Fine Motor, Gross Motor, Eye-Hand Integration, Cognitive Performance, and Cognitive Verbal (Figure 1). The separation of each test item into the various function areas makes it possible to see clearly the uneven development that is so characteristic of autism. The pattern of this uneven development is illustrated by the profile below, showing a 3 yr old child with strengths in gross motor and eye-hand integration skills and marked deficits in language and imitation. The total developmental age score shows functioning overall at the 18 month level. This pattern is quite common in the young population seen in our clinic.

Since our recommendations for educational content and teaching strategies has always been to use the child's strengths to build up the deficit areas (Schopler et al., 1980), it is vitally important to understand each child's individual pattern.

To more fully illustrate the content and range of our educational evaluation, the chart below lists items at the lowest and highest developmental level in each of the seven function areas.

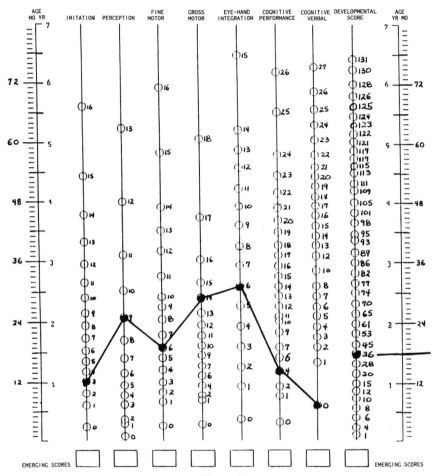

Figure 1

Range of Development Test Items

FUNCTION AREA	LOW	HIGH
Imitation	Responds to baby games Repeats own action after being imitated	Copies rhythmic pattern Repeats 4-5 digits
Perception	Tracks movement Hears and orients to noise makers	Matches colors Matches shapes

Fine Motor	Releases object into
	  container
	Flips light switch
		Touches thumb to each
		  finger
		Uses pencil for drawing

Gross Motor	Drinks from a cup Transfers objects	Swings beads in pendulum motion Climbs, alternating feet
Eye-Hand Integration	Scribbles Fits shape to hole	Copies diamond Copies letters
Cognitive Performance	Finds hidden object Anticipates routines	Follows written directions Solves simple math problem

Cognitive
  Verbal
	Gestures for help
	Names common object
		Repeats complex sentences
		Reads orally and answers
		  questions

In addition to the seven function areas described above, the PEP also scores the child's behavior in four main areas of behavior relevant to the diagnosis of autism. These are: Relating: Play and Interest in Materials: Sensory Modalities: and Language. Each behavioral item is scored in one of three ways: Absent, Mild, or Severe. The criteria for each score refers to the frequency and intensity of the behavior, a score of Severe indicating the behavior is frequent and intense, and Absent indicating the lack of the autistic behavior. The value of combining behavior observations with the assessment of skills is reported by Powers (1988), who notes that simultaneous observation of skills and behaviors allows the examiner to see the relationship between these two facets.

Scoring the Test

We use three different scores: 1) Pass: This indicates that the child clearly understands and performs the task to the criteria stated in the manual. 2) Emerge: This score indicates that the child has some understanding but cannot yet complete the task. 3) Fail: This indicates that the task is clearly above the child's level of understanding or ability to perform. As soon as the examiner sees that the child is not going to be able to receive a passing score, she is then permitted to give help in any way that will further evaluate just where the difficulty lies. One can experiment with different teaching techniques and the successful ones are then incorporated into recommendations that follow each evaluation. From the child's point of view, the evaluation consists of a series of different activities, some of which he can do by himself, some he can do with help, and some he can watch the examiner complete. Each activity is completed in one of these three ways and put away as "finished". The child is not aware of failing and not left to struggle for long. Young children who come to us as formerly labelled "untestable" can work in this situation and are testable.

In the past the autistic child's low tolerance for frustration or confusion often produced many behavioral problems that led an examiner to the conclusion that the child is untestable. Oppositional behavior or tantrums occurred when a task was difficult or when the directions were confusing. Both the use of the Emerge score, and the sequential arrangement of tasks in the PEP minimizes this stress. The test does not sequence the tasks according to developmental levels, making each successive task harder than the one before. It is arranged to provide variety in type of activity and degree of difficulty. However, the examiner may perform this sequence according to clinical judgement. When a child has difficulty with one task, the next one presented is at a simpler level, or in a different function area that may be easier. For example, we might move from a language task, commonly difficult and stressful to the child, to a gross motor task, usually a strength and therefore pleasurable. We may move from a fine motor task, often a weak area, to a task involving work with puzzles.

Test Administration

Autistic children may have difficulty demonstrating their skills in one area due to deficits in another function area. For example: If they do not understand language, they will not be able to perform tasks only presented by verbal directions: If they do not understand WH questions, (What, Who, Where, etc.) they cannot respond. However, when the same question is presented in a sentence completion format, e.g. "This is a __ - (pause)", or "They are ___ (pause)", the child may be able to finish the phrase. The administration of test items is quite flexible allowing the examiner to adjust to the child's uneven development. We make a careful effort to be sure that we are in fact assessing the function area we think we are measuring. For example; if we are testing imitation skills we do not give verbal directions. We may say, "Do this" (as we raise our hand up), but not say, "raise your hand". But if we are testing motor abilities we can give any type of direction that will help the child understand what he is to do. Some children may understand verbal directions, but more commonly receptive language is also a deficit area. In this case the examiner will give demonstrations, may give gestural prompts, and in some cases give manual assistance. For example: when asked to "kick the ball" the child is confused. When this is demonstrated and he does not understand imitation, this is also confusing. But when he is given physical guidance, he then can understand what is wanted and subsequently continue to kick the ball without help. It is important to make the directive understood before judging that the child does not have the ability that is being measured on each test item.

The examiner needs to be familiar with the uneven development commonly seen in autism in order to avoid erroneous assumptions about either basal or ceiling levels. Quite frequently we hear children using single words, short phrases, or even complete sentences that are echolalic in nature. They may occur immediately after hearing a word or phrase, or they may come from television, songs or repetitive phrases heard at home. Upon hearing this language it is natural for us to expect this child to label pictures or objects, to ask for help, or use simple social language. When this does not happen we might assume the child is shy or oppositional. In fact we need to back down and assess skills in expressive communication at a lower level. On the PEP this involves tasks that require gestural communication such as waving "bye-bye" or handing an object to ask for help.

Unusual and very important peak skills are also discovered when the examiner does not assume ceiling levels. We have been surprised at the number of autistic pre-school children who either are already reading single words, or who have the potential for becoming hyperlexic. The hermetic reading ability has been noted by others (Goldberg, 1987), but how the child learns to decode is not fully understood. Sight recognition and oral reading ability can exist without comprehension. However, it can be used to teach both receptive and expressive language and therefore needs to be assessed during an evaluation. Just in the past year in our clinic we have evaluated and subsequently worked with five pre-school children who were non-verbal and had extremely limited receptive language. Their intrinsic interest in letters of the alphabet, observed during the PEP, combined with excellent visual perception and visual memory enabled them quickly to learn to match words, to match words to objects and pictures, and then to begin to verbalize (orally read), these words. Once learned in this fashion, their verbal vocabulary has become fluent and is used independently. New words and concepts can then be introduced in written form first and later incorporated into natural receptive and expressive language. Perhaps the most extreme example of this unexpected peak skill is a profoundly retarded and severely autistic boy who showed visual interest in letters and logos in the telephone book during the educational evaluation. Four years later he remains non-verbal and without receptive understanding of verbal language, but is following written directions and pointing to written words to communicate his needs. When a child experiences the power of communication we often see a marked increase in social interest and interactions.

BEHAVIOR (Common reasons for behavior problems)

During the evaluation most autistic children present behaviors that interfere with optimal assessment of the child's level of ability. Rather than focusing directly on the behavior we try to understand the motivation or autistic deficits that underlie the child's actions. We do this by adjusting the test environment, by changing the sequence of tasks presented, by providing concrete rewards, and by teaching more appropriate ways for the child to express his needs. The information gained in this way is incorporated into the recommendations stated in the written report (Schopler, Reicher & Lansing, 1980). We are told by both parents and teachers that the recommended techniques for minimizing problem behaviors combined with a fuller understanding of the child's autistic deficits and uneven development of skills, is more valuable than knowing test scores or just being given specific educational goals. To illustrate the variety of behaviors the examiner will need to understand I have grouped them into seven general areas.

Problems with Motivation

When children lack intrinsic interest in the test materials and do not understand the need to complete any activity the tester must find ways to increase motivation and thus cooperation. We start the evaluation with information from home and classroom concerning what the child likes, what he does in his free time, and what rewards have been used in the past. We closely observe him during free play time during the test to gain further insights into possible motivators. With the young child or developmentally delayed child, we commonly see intrinsic interests in body movements, such as rocking, hand flapping or other self-stimulatory behaviors. We often see high interest in visual or auditory elements such as music, rattles, shiny objects or string. Often a child will bring with him a favored object that provides security. The test administration includes interactions involving physical play and tickling. This is often the first time we see a smile or hear a laugh. The test also includes the use of a drink and a candy edible. In addition we can use other edible rewards if needed. Although we combine concrete rewards with social praise, the latter is not always a high motivator.

Problems in Understanding the Contingencies

Many young or very delayed autistic children do not understand that something they see and want is contingent on behavior. The child becomes frustrated by any postponed gratification and his anger leads to oppositional behavior and the term "untestable". He will attempt to get what he wants for himself by reaching and grabbing, leaving the table, or expressing anger by throwing materials or beginning self-abusive behaviors. To reduce this frustration we adapt the environment to make it clearer to the child just when he can have what he wants. This is achieved in three ways. 1.) We keep rewards and distractors out of sight until it is time to give them. 2.) We structure the test materials in a way that visually clarifies just when he can have what he wants. (This will be described further when I discuss Testing Techniques.) 3.) We decrease the frequency with which we give these rewards. Over a period of several repetitions; e.g. task, then reward, the child begins to understand this sequence and can accept it without anger. Although he may not develop a true understanding of contingencies, he is able to recognize the sequence of events, recognize that he will be given what he wants, and can predict when this will happen.

Problems with Organization

Due to the autistic child's confusion, distractibility and disorganization when too many materials are presented at one time, the examiner needs to be prepared to reorganize, limit and control the test materials. Common deficits in organization include: 1.) inability to think ahead and appropriately sequence the steps within one given task, such as threading and puzzle assembly; 2.) inability to plan ahead and pick up just one item at a time instead of quickly grabbing a handful; 3.) inability to perceive the whole set of items to be used, becoming distracted by small details or perseverating on just one part of the whole. For example: One test item asks the child to select one common object from a group when it is named, (cup, spoon, shoe, toothbrush, etc). One child immediately took the toothbrush and mouthed it. As long as this object was in reach, he could not listen and select a different one. The toothbrush was therefore put away because it was too distracting. Now the child could listen and did demonstrate a simple receptive vocabulary for the other objects. Observations of these organizational deficits and the trial of techniques to provide help in organization lead to important goals and techniques for teaching. The flexible administration of the PEP combined with the use of the Emerge score permits the examiner to assist in helping the disorganized child perform tasks without hindering the validity of the test score.

Problems in Processing Sensory Modalities

Observations of sensory responses include the type of stimuli that is attended to most easily, the child's ability to integrate two sensory modalities at the same time, and the time needed for processing information and organizing a response. The PEP assesses a variety of auditory, visual and tactile perceptions which are scored in the Perception function scale. However, the child's ability to perceive may not necessarily indicate his ability to process these perceptions and use them to learn new information. Frequently we notice that the child does not attend to auditory stimuli when he is involved with visual items. The same child may not attend to visual stimuli when he is involved with auditory stimuli, such as music or sounds coming from outside the testing room. When language is involved, the integration of both modalities becomes even harder. For example: one child may be able to look at a picture, hear a word, and then select the matching picture. Another child may not hear the word if he is looking at pictures and will need the stimulus word given first, and then be shown the pictures. In addition to the problems with integration of two perceptions, there is a wide variation in the processing time needed by each child. The examiner must be sensitive to this variation and give the child enough time before assuming he does not understand or know the appropriate response.

Problems with Attention Span and Activity Level

The duration of organized attention given to an activity varies according to the child's developmental age and to the type of activity. The child may attend for long periods to his own free-play activity or to easy and familiar tasks, but have a much shorter attention span to new tasks or harder ones. We see children who do concentrate on puzzles or a drawing task, for example, who give much shorter attention to language tasks or ones involving pretend play. The ability to maintain organized attention also influences the child's activity level. Frequently we are evaluating children who are reported to be hyperactive, with requests coming from teachers for medication to control this. If a child can remain calm and physically inactive for relatively long periods when he is organized and attentive to tasks that are easy or ones he has chosen himself, then medication is not the solution. On the other hand, if we observe the child's excessive activity interrupts his clear efforts to maintain organized attention at all times, then this might be a medical issue.

Problems with Preoccupations, Rituals and Stereotypies

Observations pertaining to the child's preoccupations, rituals, and stereotypic physical behaviors are a necessary part of any evaluation of autistic children. Preoccupations may take the form of repetitive questions or, at a younger level, repetitive sounds. Obsessive rituals are often observed in the way a child handles and arranges concrete materials. Stereotypies occur more frequently during unstructured free play time, but can also be observed during the directed tasks. Most frequently seen are behaviors of rocking, spinning, hand flapping and posturing. The PEP materials include items that elicit these behaviors such as a large mirror, a long string, shiny objects and ones that can spin. The content of the preoccupations and rituals as well as the situations that elicit the stereotypies are recorded and incorporated into the report and recommendations.

Problems with Acceptance of Change

One of the major characteristics of autism is a resistance to change. The evaluation procedures involve many changes, some of which are visually structured and therefore predictable and some are not. This characteristic is observed as the child perseverated on one behavior, refuses to give up one material, or dislikes moving from one area to another. The discomfort from the transition may not be related to a preference for what he is doing or a dislike of what will happen next, but simply to the process of change. The most dramatic illustration of this difficulty is seen in the young child who has a tantrum on leaving his parents and moving to the testing room. Quite naturally one assumes this is separation anxiety. However, when testing is completed and it is time to return to his parents, the same tantrum occurs. Moreover, upon meeting his parents he seems uninterested in approaching them. The child's inability to predict or accept change is a major cause of tantrums or self-abusive behaviors. Parents and teacher, faced with these disturbing behaviors, need help in understanding the cause and in finding ways to adjust the environment to minimize the child's stress. The examiner should not only observe but experiment with various techniques that will minimize the problem. Some suggested techniques we have found helpful for all the behaviors discussed in this section will be described below.

TESTING TECHNIQUES

The fullest educational evaluation is obtained when the examiner is able to experiment with various techniques that may assist the child to attend, understand directions, and respond appropriately. Through experimentation the tester can discover techniques that are effective and can be incorporated into the recommendations. The use of the Emerge score gives freedom to the examiner for this purpose that is not usually possible with standardized tests which permit only a Pass or Fail rating. This flexible administration also encourages the tester to observe and think more closely about how and why the child responds as he does to each situation. Inferences and assumptions can be immediately tested through these variations in testing techniques. Following are examples of these techniques.

Visual Structure

The autistic child is more comfortable when he can see where he should be, what material he should attend to, and what will happen next. We use visual cues to indicate where different types of activities will take place, and this, in turn, suggests the behavioral expectations for each area. His coat or favored object may be placed on his chair for seated work. The table may be moved to a position that blocks him from running off, one that visually indicates he is expected to stay seated. Free play is indicated by a mat or rug on which are placed age appropriate toys. Gross motor equipment in another area suggests that physical activity is appropriate in this place.

Testing Structure

Distractibility is reduced by removing distractors from sight, by placing only one activity on the table, and by having a bin at the far right of the table into which all tasks are placed when finished. Children who tend to become confused by tasks requiring organized placement of many materials may be helped by being given only one item at a time. Some children have difficulty initiating placement of materials until they understand exactly where to put them. For example, when asked to sort colored shapes into categories, a child may just stack them or line the cards up in a row. But when given three trays and cued to place each card into one of the three trays he can often demonstrate the ability to categorize even though he cannot organize the task without this help. The examiner can then pin-point the real area of difficulty. The score, in this case, would be Emerge because help was given,but the informaion discovered is immediately useful to his teacher.

Attention span is lengthened when the child knows how long an activity will last. If he cannot see the end in sight he may assume it will be endless and refuse to continue. For example, one task assesses the child's ability to stack eight blocks. Children who tend to grab, sift or throw blocks must be given them one at a time. We may even need to have a colored paper on the table to indicate just where he should place them. The tester will have all eight blocks clearly visible to the child, but out of reach. As she hands each block the child can see how he is progressing and how much more is expected. We are often surprised to observe the child's concentration and effort increase as he nears the end of such a task. This type of help does not interfere with the test score since we are not judging task organization, but only the ability to stack. If, on the other hand, we have a child who cannot stack all the blocks, obvious because the stack topples after the first three, the tester can then remove several of her blocks from sight. Now the child sees that only one or two more remain and is often willing to try once more. In this case the score will be lowered, but the information obtained gives appropriate expectations to the teacher.

Sequence of Tasks

During the evaluation the examiner is permitted to be quite flexible in her choice of tasks presented. The manual and score form of the PEP suggests a sequence that works well for most children, but due to individual variations it is helpful to vary this in response to the child's observed responses. We begin with short and visually clear tasks that do not involve verbal directions. The behavioral responses noted during the first few tasks indicate to the tester how it may help to choose subsequent tasks. We avoid presenting a harder task after observing a failure. This fluctuation between difficult and easier tasks helps the child to maintain attention and cooperative behavior. We may also offer a second try later in the testing session if the child seemed anxious or confused initially but relaxed later on once he became familiar with the routines and expectations. This often occurs with young children who settle down to the repetitive structure and sequence of each task.

Each task, or group of tasks is presented in a visually clear way. Some children may be able to complete three or four tasks before leaving the table for a play break. Others may need a play time more frequently. Each task, or group of tasks, is placed on the table to the left of the child. It is then administered, help given if necessary, and once completed is put in a box labeled "finished" on the far right of the child. In this way he can see how much is to be done, and can observe his own progress.

Communication

Many autistic children, and especially young ones, find verbal language somewhat aversive. They may be comfortable, even reassured, with familiar voice intonations but stressed when they are expected to process and respond to verbal language. Anyone who has been asked to respond appropriately to a foreign language they do not understand will recognize this stressful situation. It is important, therefore, for the examiner to obtain as much information as possible before the evaluation starts concerning the probable level of receptive language that can be expected from the child. Teacher and parent reports are useful for this purpose. Test rapport is established through the visual structure already described, through gestural communication, and through voice intonation. Long verbal explanations of where their mother is, why they will have a good time, etc. are seldom helpful. In addition, the first few test items do not require verbal directions and for some children they are administered silently.

Communication throughout the test is given at a level the child can understand. This may involve combining words with gestures or even physical assistance, when gestures are not noticed or understood. When a test item is measuring the child's receptive language no gestures are permitted, but the examiner should speak slowly and clearly. When a test item is not measuring receptive language but rather assessing the child's information and expressive abilities, then the examiner can vary the form of her questions. The most common example of this occurs when asking for information in the form of the question, "What is this?" (color, shape, number, letter). Many children do not understand WH questions yet do have the labels asked for. The examiner can then change her question into an unfinished sentence; e.g. "This is a (pause)?" The child can score Pass if he responds to this technique since the test item is not judging his understanding of questions, but his information and expressive ability. Throughout the test we are attentive to the exact functions that are being scored and adjust our communicative techniques accordingly.

Prompts

The Emerge score allows the examiner to give various prompts to help the child get started on a task, or to give help when he has difficulty. As mentioned previously, this increases cooperation and attention and provides useful information to be incorporated into the recommendations for beginning teaching goals. Prompts that prove helpful are discovered through experimentation. A hierarchy of possible prompts, from the advanced to simplest level is: 1.) Verbal prompts; "go ahead...look...that is good... try again..." etc; 2.) Gestural prompts; pointing, clapping, smiling, and common graphic signs; 3.) Demonstrations; doing part of the task while the child watches; 4.) Physical prompts; touching the child's hands, moving the child's hands or body for him. We frequently try all four types of prompts before we learn which will be most helpful to the child. Individual variations include children who find physical contact aversive; children who do not understand imitation so cannot learn from a demonstration; children who seldom look so cannot observe a gesture; children who find verbal language confusing and thus unpleasant.

CONCLUSION

The purpose of an educational evaluation is to obtain information that will be useful to those responsible for the child's education, both at home and in school. This assessment may be the first step in planning an optimal program, or it may be used to measure progress and adjust an existing program. Assessment techniques for autistic children need to be flexible and adjusted to their individual strengths, deficits and general learning style. Flexible test administration is possible when children are scored in three ways: Pass, Emerge, Fail. The intermediate score provides important information for education without interfering with standard developmental age equivalents. Adapting the environment to the autistic deficits helps the child maintain appropriate behaviors and eliminates the label, "untestable".

REFERENCES

Goldberg, T. (1987). On Hermetic Reading Abilities. *Journal of Autism and Developmental Disorders, 17,* 29 - 44.

Johnson-Martin, N. (1988). Assessment of Low-Functioning Children. In E. Schopler & G. Mesibov (Eds.), *Diagnosis and Assessment in Autism.* New York: Plenum Press.

Lansing, M., & Schopler, E. (1978). Individualized Education: A Public School Model. In M. Rutter & E. Schopler (Eds.), *Autism. A Reappraisal of Concepts and Treatment.* New York: Plenum Press.

McKinney, B., & Peterson, R. A. (1987). Predictors of stress in parents of developmentally disabled children. *Journal of Pediatric Psychology, 12,* 133 - 150.

Parks, S. (1988). Psychometric Instruments for Assessment. In E. Schopler & G. Mesibov (Eds.), *Diagnosis and Assessment in Autism.* New York: Plenum Press.

Powers, M. (1988). Behavioral Assessment of Autism. In E. Schopler & G. Mesibov (Eds.), *Diagnosis and Assessment in Autism.* New York: Plenum Press.

Rutter, M. (1978). Developmental Issues and Prognosis. In M. Rutter & E. Schopler (Eds.), *Autism. A reappraisal of Concepts and Treatment.* New York: Plenum Press.

Schopler, E., & Reichler, R. (1979). *Individual Assessment and Treatment for Autistic and Developmentally Disabled Children,* Vol I, Psychoeducational Profile. Austin, Texas: Pro-Ed.

Schopler, E., Reichler, R., & Lansing, M. (1980). Assessment and Evaluation. In *Individualized Assessment and Treatment of Autistic and Developmentally Disabled Children,* Vol III. Baltimore: University Park Press.

Schopler, E., Lansing, M., & Waters, L. (1983). Teaching Activities for Autistic Children. In *Individual Assessment and Treatment of Autistic and Developmentally Disabled Children,* Vol III. Baltimore: University Park Press.

Wing, L. (1976). Provision of Services. In L. Wing (Ed.), *Early Childhood Autism.* Oxford: Pergamon Press.

Principles for Directing Both Educational Treatment and Research

ERIC SCHOPLER

This chapter is based on 25 years' involvement with children diagnosed with autism or related developmental disorders. During this period of time, my colleagues and I have developed a statewide, community-based system located in our Psychiatry Department at the University of North Carolina School of Medicine: The Division for the Treatment and Education of Autistic and Communications Handicapped Children (TEACCH). Described in detail elsewhere (Reichler & Schopler, 1976; Schopler & Olley, 1982; and Schopler, Mesibov, Shigley, & Bashford, 1984), TEACCH is North Carolina's statewide system for providing children and adults with autism and related developmental disorders with comprehensive service, relevant research, and training of professionals. Home and family adjustment is facilitated through six regional TEACCH Centers. Individualized educational programming is developed through 92 TEACCH-affiliated public school classrooms under our program direction. Community integration is facilitated through parent groups attached to Centers and classrooms and affiliated with state and national parent organizations. Parental perspective is implemented at each program level.

In this discussion, I will review both the primary obstacles to the development of our community-based system, and also the most useful and important concepts and principles that have made it viable for this relatively extended period. By now, it is quite widely recognized that following Kanner's (1943) publication of autism, psychoanalytic theory was the primary and mistaken basis for explaining and treating that condition. The children were said to be withdrawn from pathological parents - "refrigerator mothers" -

whose unconscious attitudes and wishes produced the autistic symptoms. Treatment was primarily a parentectomy, or placement away from parents in a residential institution (Bettelheim, 1967).

Our own research (Schopler, 1971; Schopler & Loftin, 1969, a & b) and that of others (Cantwell & Baker, 1984) produced a consensus of empirical data showing that parents were not the primary cause, but victims of autism much like their children. On the strength of these data, we began helping these children through their parents as co-therapists (Schopler, 1971). We evolved a parent-professional collaborative relationship in which we developed an optimum individualized teaching and behavior management program for each child.

We found that we could accept parents' statements of concerns, without reinterpreting them according to theoretical assumptions about their unconscious motives and attitudes. In those cases where parents misunderstood their children or how to manage them, we made it the staff's burden to show evidence for such misunderstanding or mismanagement, rather than the parents'. We incorporated parental experience into our diagnostic formulations, and incorporated parental perspectives into our individualized educational programming, research, and professional training. The resulting TEACCH system for the study and treatment of autistic children has been used as a model in many states and countries, and has been shown effective in several outcome studies (Marcus et al., 1978; Short, 1984; and Schopler et al., 1982). Figure 1 shows long-range outcome (Schopler et al., 1982) for our children compared with six other studies. In these six studies, between 38% and 76% of the autistic children were institutionalized in mental hospitals after they reached adulthood (Creak, 1963; DeMyer et al., 1973; Lotter, 1974; Mittler et al., 1966; and Rutter, 1970). In the TEACCH sample, on the other hand, only 7% of the sample was institutionalized, including 4% placed in group homes. The remainder stayed in the community. This study confirmed what we believed clinically: that autistic and similar children can remain with their families, function better, and at a lower cost to the community when there is a viable community support system.

BACKGROUND APPRAISAL

Looking back over the past 25 years, it is intriguing to identify some of the factors contributing both obstacles and progress to the understanding and treatment of autistic children. In the field of mental health and education, Freudian theory and psychodynamic variations had achieved pre-eminence during the post World War II period. Both specific etiologial explanation and specific treatment techniques were frequently overused or misapplied. Theoretical justification, rather than empirical evidence,

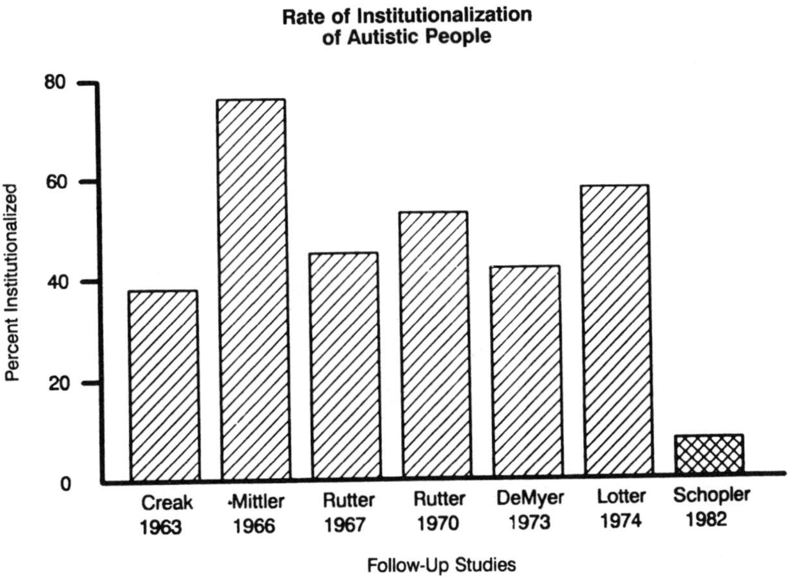
Rate of Institutionalization
of Autistic People
Percent Institutionalized
80
60
40
20
0
Creak 1963
Mittler 1966
Rutter 1967
Rutter 1970
DeMyer 1973
Lotter 1974
Schopler 1982
Follow-Up Studies

Figure 1

was considered sufficient for guiding intervention. Empirical research was of interest to only a few scientists, and they were not primarily involved in education or treatment. During this same period from 1940 to 1960, there appeared an increasing proliferation of specific therapies or educational techniques. These were sometimes introduced by untrained people, or representing special interests. No doubt the professional establishment's preoccupation with treatment based on theory rather than empirical evidence contributed to the proliferation of specific techniques.

From the field of autism alone, I have compiled a list of specific treatment techniques that have appeared in the literature during the past 20 years. This list is intended to be suggestive rather than all inclusive:

TABLE 1   Specific Treatment Techniques for Autism

Aversive therapy	Goldfine treatment	Patterning therapy
Behavior therapy	Holding therapy	Psychical therapy
Dance therapy	Interactive therapy	Speech therapy
Deinstitutionalization	Logo therapy	Pony therapy
Developmental therapy	Megavitamin therapy	Play therapy
Fenfluramine treatment	Mainstreaming	Music therapy
Electroconvulsive shock therapy	Phenothiazine treatment	Sensory integration

Extensive comparisons between these specific techniques or concepts could be made. But for the purpose of this discussion, it is sufficient to identify some of the features they all seem to share in common with each other:

(1) Each seemed like a reasonably good idea to the initiator. Sometimes it had been known to correct a similar problem or to add a corrective element. Sometimes it was based on a coincidental observation or intuition. But regardless of source, the initiator was convinced it was reasonable to try this technique with someone in this clinical population.

(2) By the time a particular treatment technique or concept has appeared in print, it has invariably appeared effective for one or more cases. The resulting improvement was convincing to one or two observers. But because it was a single case observation, the reason for the observed improvement could not be demonstrated. It may have been caused by any number of other related factors, including spontaneous fluctuation of behavior. Nevertheless, even single case improvement claims attract attention, inspire hope, and are considered worthy of media coverage. This increased interest sometimes promotes further trials or even controlled study.

(3) The third aspect shared by these specific techniques is that they are studied with additional cases in controlled studies. These replications are sometimes based on low probability hypotheses without adequate theoretical justification, but born from desperate clinical frustration. Regardless of the replication method, none of the specific techniques listed has been effective with all children.

(4) Moreover, continued use also shows that each technique has costs or negative side effects not predicted in the flush of pilot study drama. The specific treatment concept or technique in question becomes a short-lived fad which often produces unnecessary disappointment and unintended harm.

The above limits to the use of specific techniques and concepts appear to warrant pessimism or hopelessness. This is not the case. Compelling evidence has been presented (Frank, 1961) that non-specific treatment factors have precedence over specific techniques. These are based on the faith found in the relationship between doctor-patient, parent-child, or teacher-student. It is such a relationship that allows access to the best understanding of the more dependent individual's problems or learning difficulties, along with the best knowledge of the currently available techniques. It is the therapeutic aspirations of this non-specific relationship that permits determining the most favourable technique, evaluated from a cost-benefit ratio for the individual involved. This determination is finally less a scientific decision than one based on the art of treatment or education; that is, knowing the individual with his complex history, and matching it with the best available treatment.

From my perspective as an educator, it appears that any of us can become unwittingly involved in extending a treatment technique or concept beyond the limits of supporting evidence. In so doing, we may caricature that reasonable idea and turn it into a short-lived fad, which can do harm or cost more than it is worth.

In our experience with developing the TEACCH system, we are often pressed to over-extend one of the relevant treatment concepts. For example, we had spent a good deal of research effort on the hypothesis that parents of autistic children can function as co-therapists with professionals (Schopler & Reichler, 1971; Short, 1984). Both clinical experience and empirical data supported a positive answer to this question. However, some tried to interpret these findings to mean that parents' educational priorities should always be given priority, or that the same type of co-therapy relationship should be implemented without modification to parents of psychopaths, suicidal depressives, or schizophrenics.

I am pleased to report that with the TEACCH system so far we have avoided - better, resisted - this fad development, by adhering to certain administrative priorities. These enabled us to develop some viable and lasting guiding principles of treatment and education. Our first administrative priority grew out of our commitment to parent collaboration. It required providing the best treatment and education permitted by the state of the art. Concurrently, we made a commitment to study and support research into problems that were obstacles to understanding the disorder of improving the child's adaptation. In case of conflict between these two priorities, we would be inclined to resist having research interfere with treatment. Our next priority was to develop training and development of staff to implement both service and clinically relevant research.

Given the above priorities, it is not surprising that the most enduring principles and concepts that we have identified are seven capable of generating *both* clinical and empirical research data. These principles evolved at a time when an accumulation of research indicated that autism was not a single-cause emotional illness induced by parental pathology. Instead, it was a multiply-caused chronic developmental disorder. And although biologically based, the adaptation of individuals with autism could be greatly enhanced through special education.

PRINCIPLES AND CONCEPTS GUIDING TEACCH SYSTEM

Improved Adaptation

The first principle is that the child's adaptation can be improved in *two* ways. One is to improve the child's skills, especially for communication and social interaction. Second, when the child's deficit prevents the acquisition of a new skill, then the environment can be modified to accommodate the deficit. Either of these two ways will improve the child's adaptation.

Clinically, this principle is important because it acknowledges that both skill enhancement and environmental modifications are needed for children with developmental disorders like autism. It recognizes that even in the absence of specific cures, optimism can be maintained because two intervention approaches are available that will improve adaptation, rather than only one.

From the perspective of empirical research, this principle was consistent with some of our outcome studies. For example, we studied the effects of parent training on their own children (Marcus et al., 1978) and found that the children showed significant improvement in attention to task and cooperation with adults. In another outcome study, we measured the effects of structured teaching versus unstructured teaching (Schopler et al., 1971), and under structured conditions we found significantly better social relatedness and attentiveness, and also a significant decrease in bizarre behavior, over the unstructured conditions.

Parent Collaboration

Our second principle is that children are best helped through and with their parents as co-therapists or collaborators with professionals. At the clinical level, this principle has had too many applications to summarize easily. However, implications can readily be found in our organizational structures, clinical procedures, and parent-professional relationships (Schopler et al., 1984).

Central to our clinic operation is the one-way observation room. After completing the evaluation, the therapist demonstrates certain teaching or behavior management techniques. These are written out in a home teaching program, and implemented by parents and/or siblings at home. Parents frequently introduce new procedures from their own observation and experience, which become a meaningful component of their child's optimum individualized educational program. Such programs were compiled in Schopler, Lansing & Waters (1983). The parent-as-co-therapist model was extended into collaboration with the child's teachers. Parent-teacher collaboration occurred along a continuum of intensity, ranging from parent functioning regularly as an assistant teacher in the classroom, to monthly telephone contacts. This relationship played a central part in mediating the children's central difficulty in generalizing learned skills from one place to another.

Parent-professional collaboration involves four types of relationship (Schopler, 1987): (1) When professionals are the trainers, and parents are trainees. This approximates the traditional authority dependent interaction. (2) In the next interaction, the traditional roles are reversed: Parents are the trainers, and professionals are trainees. This comes from more recent recognition that parents usually have both the capacity and the motivation to understand their own children. Their experience, observation, and educational priorities are incorporated into the treatment plan. (3) Mutual emotional support from professionals to parents and vice versa. This important interaction comes from the recognition that children with developmental disorders are often slow to learn and can be more frustrating to parents and teachers than other children. (4) The fourth relationship involves social advocacy, in which parents and professionals collaborate to develop community understanding of their children's special needs, and cost effective services not currently available.

Relevant empirical research regarding parent collaboration in our system has included disproving the notion that parents produce their children's autistic symptoms with their own disordered thinking. Our studies showed that parents of autistic children show no more thought disorder than other kinds of parents, and that thought disordered behavior can be induced by test anxiety from professionals' psychodynamic judgments (Schopler & Loftin, 1969, a & b). In a related study, we questioned the conventional professional wisdom of the time that parents misunderstood their severely disturbed children. We compared parental estimates of their children's developmental levels before diagnostic evaluation, with test results of the same functions after formal testing. We found that parents' estimates correlated significantly with test-based estimates, and that parents with mildly disturbed children were relatively poorer estimators than parents with more disturbed children (Schopler & Reichler, 1972). Not only could parents usually estimate their children's level of function reasonably well, they also were effective as trainers and co-therapists (Marcus et al., 1978).

Assessment for Individualized Treatment

The third enduring principle is that individualized educational program and treatment are based on developmental diagnostic evaluation and assessment. The importance of this concept comes from the frequently systematic professional misunderstanding of autistic children. During the early history of the autism syndrome, professionals frequently considered these children untestable (Alpern, 1967). Moreover, some behaviorists have de-emphasized or ignored assessment or testing of autistic children for the purpose of distinguishing the differences between behaviors that can be shaped and modified, versus those whose rigidity was linked to a developmental deficit. More recently, a new treatment ideology has emerged under the banner of "mainstreaming". Some of the fervent mainstream enthusiasts advocate that all handicapped individuals are habilitated by placement in a "normal" environment without appropriate education and assessment.

In the TEACCH system, we have found that both formal and informal diagnosis and assessment are needed in order to determine an individual's educational program, implemented in the least restrictive environment, and safeguarding each individual's right to optimum treatment. At the clinical level, this has meant training staff and students in naturalistic observation and how to make informal assessments of each client in different life contexts (Mesibov, Troxler, & Boswell, 1988).

Empirical research involved the development of a number of assessment instruments. These have included the Childhood Autism Rating Scale (CARS) (Schopler et al., 1980; Schopler et al., 1988). This instrument is used for making the diagnosis of autism from systematic observation. This diagnosis, however, is not sufficient for the individual assessment needed for defining an optimum treatment program. To accomplish this, we developed the Psychoeducational Profile (PEP) (Schopler & Reichler, 1979), currently revised for a more thorough inclusion of the preschool population (Schopler, Reichler, Bashford, Lansing, & Marcus, in press). This assessment instrument was extended to the adolescent and adult population with the Adolescent and Adult Psychoeducational Profile (AAPEP) by Mesibov, Schopler, Schaffer, & Landrus (1988) for the purpose of evaluating the client with autism for the best vocational and living arrangement possible.

Teaching Structures

Our fourth principle is that education is based on structured teaching. Clinically, the importance of this concept was repeatedly observed and reported during the 1960s and 70s when autistic children were primarily treated in non-directive (Axline, 1947) and psychodynamic (Ekstein, 1954) play therapy. These frequently seemed to result in lack of progress and the need for residential treatment, thus giving impetus to the more structured treatment of operant conditioning, and the educational program developed in our system (Lansing & Schopler, 1978).

At the level of empirical research, we were able to demonstrate that autistic children functioned better under structured conditions than they did under unstructured conditions, and that individual variations in response to structure correlated with developmental levels. Children of lower levels of developmental function benefitted more from structure than did children at higher levels (Schopler et al., 1971). This study demonstrated a finding that has become more viable with subsequent experience. Since then, we have evolved more sophisticated teaching structures for different levels of function (Schopler, Lansing, & Waters, 1983). These have been applied to public school classrooms throughout our TEACCH system in North Carolina. This system has been taught in a finely-tuned training program under the leadership of Dr. Mesibov (Schopler & Mesibov, 1988) and has been applied in different cultures, including Japan, Belgium and France. The importance of structured teaching is now widely recognized and implemented.

Skill Enhancement

Our fifth principle underscores that the most effective approach is to enhance skills of children and parents, and to recognize and accept their shortcomings. This concept follows along with our assessment emphasis. One of the primary purposes of the assessment instruments reviewed under the assessment principle is to distinguish between emerging skills which can be enhanced immediately, and deficit areas for which training is better delayed or treated with environment structures. The emphasis on working with existing and emerging skills has been reaffirmed by clinical experience for the past 20

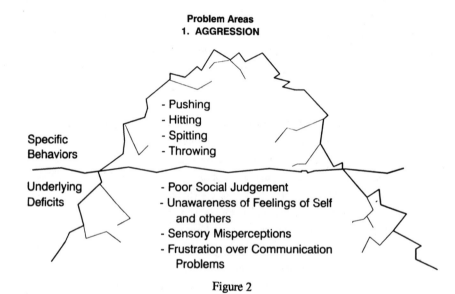

Problem Areas
1. AGGRESSION

Specific
Behaviors

- Pushing
- Hitting
- Spitting
- Throwing

Underlying
Deficits

- Poor Social Judgement
- Unawareness of Feelings of Self
  and others
- Sensory Misperceptions
- Frustration over Communication
  Problems

Figure 2

years. In fact, it is fair to say that this emphasis has been effective not only with children and parents, but also with staff and trainees.

The suggestion is sometimes made that such skill development emphasis is most effective with more able children and parents. Our experience has been to the contrary. For example, recently a schizophrenic mother of an autistic child was referred to us after being released from six months of in-patient treatment. She had improved during hospitalization but felt unable to resume caring for her family and household. After assessment, it was found that she had some recollection of making Jello, a favorite family dessert. After a week of intensive training in Jello making, she was able to prepare it on her own. This gave her the necessary impetus to begin cooking and preparing other meals in the past. Skill emphasis did not cure her schizophrenia, but enhanced her adaptation.

At the empirical research level, we completed a study of parents' perception of program helpfulness (Schopler, Mesibov, DeVellis, & Short, 1981). Parents reported most program helpfulness with problems in their child's social relationships, motor skills, self-help skills, and communication. Children with higher IQs improved more in language and self-help skills than did children with lower IQs. In a pre-and post-treatment study based on observations of children in their own homes, Short (1984) found significant improvement in both parent involvement and in appropriate child behavior.

Cognitive and Behavior Therapy

Our sixth principle refers to the enduring usefulness of cognitive and behavior theory for guiding both special education and research, theoretical systems eloquently reviewed by Gardner (1985). At the clinical level, the application of these two theoretical systems can be illustrated with the management of difficult behavior. Figure 2 outlines an iceberg to represent problems of aggression. The smaller portion of this entity shows above the water line, or is visible in the form of specific behaviors like pushing, hitting, biting, or kicking. Below the water line are possible explanations for the cause of particular aggressive behaviors. It could be frustration over communications deficit; therefore, hitting at the teacher rather than signalling for her attention. It could be a child's misperception of pain or inability to understand behavior rules. Through careful observation and assessment, the best explanatory cause is identified, and used as the basis for intervention. If it is frustration over communication, we can teach a word, a sign, or a signal. If the aggressive hitting behavior decreases, our explanatory theory is supported. If, on the other hand, hitting continues, a different explanatory mechanism is involved.

At the level of empirical research, we have developed a communications curriculum (Watson et al., 1989). It includes data collection in four different semantics categories, especially important in the communication problems of autism. See Table 2. Context in column one refers to the place in which the communication unit was learned or practiced. Column 2 refers to what student said, using word, sign, picture, or body language. The third column represents the student's communicative intent, and the fourth column is for grouping the semantic category used in the student's communication. The assessment of these four communication dimensions offers both a data base for research and a basis for teaching strategies with individual children.

The Generalist Training Model

The seventh principle refers to intervention and training in the TEACCH system. That is, professionals concerned with autism are trained as generalists who are expected to know the entire range of problems raised by this disorder. Traditionally in the United States, the field of mental health has emphasized specialization. Psychologists conducted evaluations, speech pathologists provided speech therapy, social workers specialized in family work, psychiatrists preferred psychotherapy, and so on. This is an understandable phenomenon considering the long training required of professionals in various disciplines. Unfortunately for families seeking help for their handicapped children, specialization structures professionals to be interested in, or accountable for, primarily their own area of specialization. This increases the likelihood that parents receive inconsistent or contradictory opinions on diagnosis and treatment. Moreover, it makes it difficult for anyone to take professional responsibility for the entire child. The generalist model reduces these undesirable consequences of specialization. It enables staff to see the child from the parents' perspective and to work collaboratively with them. It increases staff responsibility, makes the job more interesting, and improves staff ability to use consultation from specialists more effectively.

From the perspective of training, we have developed an intensive multi-disciplinary training model. It incorporates didactic sessions on the eight topics we have found basic to the study and treatment of autism and related developmental disorders. These eight topics, summarized in Table 3, are presented in didactic format during half the training sessions, and illustrated directly with a group of autistic children during the other half session. This training program was filmed by a Japanese documentary film group in 1986, and has been effectively applied in Belgium, France, Japan, and the United States.

TABLE 2 Communication Sample

Student: Ralph. Observer: Warren. Date: 1/17. Time began: 9:30. Time ended: 11.30.

CONTEXT	WHAT STUDENT SAID OR DID	FUNCTIONS							SEMANTIC CATEGORIES				
		Request	Getting attention	Reject	Comment	Give info	Seek info	Other	Object	Action	Person	Location	Other
1. Makes mess while making breakfast	towel (signs)	X							object wanted				
2. Work-folding	finish (signs)				X					own action			
3. Free time - R walks into kitchenette	touches teacher's arm		X										
4. " -	hands t. a cup	X											
5. T: "What?"	drink (signs)	X							object wanted				
6. T. hands R. orange juice	pushes jar away			X									
7. R. opens refrigerator	drink (signs)	X											
8. T: "Drink what?"	R. picks up cola bottle + signs drink	X							object wanted				
9. R. stands up	bathroom (signs)	X										own location	
10. R's shoe untied; to T.	shoe (signs)	X							object acted on				
11. " -	shoe (signs) + holds up untied shoe	X							object acted on				
12. Finishes playing with cards	finish (signs)				X					own action			

179

TABLE 3 Topics for Generalist Training

1. Characteristics of autism
2. Diagnostic assessment, formal and informal
3. Structured teaching and reducing behavior problems
4. Collaboration with parents to expedite client adaptation
5. Communication issues
6. Independence and vocational training
7. Social and leisure skills training
8. Behavior management

CONCLUSION

In this presentation, I have reviewed some of the specific therapy techniques and research concepts that have sprung up in the field during the past four decades. Many of these specific technologies and concepts were used beyond the limits of their supporting data and have become short-lived fads. They do offer brief periods of hope to parents and others, frequently with silence about limits, costs, and side effects. In the evolution of the TEACCH system, we have attempted to reduce overuse of theories and treatment techniques by adhering to the use of empirical research and the rules of evidence. Towards this end, we have identified seven principles or concepts found most viable in our TEACCH system over the past 25 years. These seven principles have remained viable because they apply both to clinical practice and research, fostering the use of empirical evidence in both of these areas.

REFERENCES

Alpern, G. D. (1967). Measurement of "untestable" autistic children. *Journal of Abnormal Psychology, 72,* 478-496.

Axline, V. M. (1947). *Play therapy.* Boston: Hougton Miffin Co.

Bettelheim, B. (1967). *The empty fortress. Infantile autism and the birth of the self.* New York: Free Press.

Cantwell, D. P., & Baker, L. (1984). Research concerning families of children with autism. In E. Schopler & G. B. Mesibov (Eds.), *The effects of autism on the family.* New York: Plenum Press.

Creak, M. (1963). Childhood psychosis: Review of 100 cases. *British Journal of Psychiatry, 109,* 84.

Ekstein, R. (1954). The space child's time machine: a "reconstruction" in the psychotherapeutic treatment of a schizophrenic child. *American Journal of Orthopsychiatry, 24,* 492-506.

DeMyer, M. K., Barton, S., DeMyer, W. E., Norton, J. A., Allen, J., & Steele, R. (1973). Prognosis in autism: a follow-up study. *Journal of Autism and Childhood Schizophrenia, 3,* 199-246.

Gardner, H. (1985). *The mind's new science: A history of the cognitive revolution.* New York: Basic Books, Inc.

Kanner, L. (1943). Autistic disturbance of affect contact. *Nervous Child, 2,* 217-230.

Lansing, M., & Schopler, E. (1978). Individualized education: A public school model. In M. Rutter & E. Schopler (Eds.), *Autism: A reappraisal of concepts and treatment* (pp 439-452). New York: Plenum Press.

Lotter, V. (1974). Factors related to outcome in autistic children. *Journal of Autism and Childhood Schizophrenia, 4,* 263-277.

Marcus, L., Lansing, M., Andrews, C., & Schopler, E. (1978). Improvement of teaching effectiveness in parents of autistic children. *Journal of the American Academy of Child Psychiatry, 17,* 625-639.

Mesibov, G. B., Schopler, E., Schaffer, B., & Landrus, R. (1988). *Individualized assessment and treatment for autistic and developmentally disabled children. Vol. 4 Adolescent and adult psychoeducational profile (AAPEP).* Austin, TX: Pro-Ed.

Mesibov, G. B., Troxler, M., & Boswell, S. (1988). Assessment in the classroom. In E. Schopler & G. B. Mesibov (Eds.), *Diagnosis and Assessment in Autism.* New York: Plenum Press.

Mittler, P., Gilles, S., & Jukes, E. (1966). Prognosis in psychotic children: Report of a follow-up study. *Journal of Mental Deficiency Research, 10,* 73-83.

Reichler, R. J., & Schopler, E. (1976). Developmental therapy: A program model for providing individual services in the community. In E. Schopler & R. J. Reichler (Eds.), *Psychopathology and child development: Research and treatment* (pp 347-372).

Rutter, M. (1970). Autistic children: Infancy to adulthood. *Seminars in Psychiatry, 2,* 435-450.

Schopler, E. (1971). Parents of psychotic children as scapegoats. *Journal of Contemporary Psychology, 4,* 17-22.

Schopler, E. (1987). Specific and nonspecific factors in the effectiveness of a treatment system. *American Psychologist, 42,* 376-383.

Schopler, E., Brehm, S. S., Kinsbourne, M., & Reichler, R. J. (1971). Effect of treatment structure of development in autistic children. *Archives of General Psychiatry, 24,* 415-421.

Schopler, E., Lansing, M., & Waters, L. V. (1983). *Individualized assessment and treatment for autistic and developmentally disabled children. Vol. III: Teaching activities for autistic children.* Austin, TX: Pro-Ed. Translated into German, 1984. Translated into Japanese, 1985.

Schopler, E., & Loftin, J. (1969a). Thinking disorders in parents of psychotic children. *Journal of Abnormal Psychology, 74,* 281-287.

Schopler, E., & Loftin, J. (1969b). Thought disorders in parents of psychotic children: A function of test anxiety. *Archives of General Psychiatry, 20,* 174-181. Also in S. Chess & A. Thomas (Eds.), *Annual progress in child psychiatry and child development* (1970), (pp. 472-486). New York: Bruner/Mazel.

Schopler, E., & Mesibov, G. (1989). Training professionals and parents for teaching autistic children. *Postgraduate advances in autism* (in press).

Schopler, E., Mesibov, G., & Baker, A. (1982). Evaluation of treatment for autistic children and their parents. *Journal of the American Academy of Child Psychiatry, 21,* 262-267.

Schopler, E., Mesibov, G., DeVellis, R., & Short, A. (1981). Treatment outcome for autistic children and their families. In P. Mittler (Ed.), *Frontiers of knowledge in mental retardation. Vol. 1. Special educational and behavioral aspects* (pp. 293-301). Baltimore: University Park Press.

Schopler, E., Mesibov, G. B., Shigley, R. H., & Bashford, A. (1984). Helping autistic children through their parents: The TEACCH model. In E. Schopler & G. B. Mesibov (Eds.), *The effects of autism on the family* (pp 65-81). New York: Plenum Press.

Schopler, E., & Olley, J. G. (1982). Comprehensive educational services for autistic children: The TEACCH model. In C. R. Reynolds & T. R. Gutkin (Eds.), *The handbook of school psychology* (pp. 629-643). New York: Wiley.

Schopler, E., & Reichler, R. J. (1971). Developmental therapy by parents with their own autistic child. In M. Rutter (Ed.), *Infantile autism: Concepts, characteristics, and treatment* (pp. 206-227). London: Churchill-Livingstone.

Schopler, E., & Reichler, R. J. (1972). How well do parents understand their own psychotic child? *Journal of Autism and Childhood Schizophrenia, 2,* 387-400.

Schopler, E., & Reichler, R. J. (1979). *Individualized assessment and treatment for autistic and developmentally disabled children. Vol. 1: Psychoeducational profile.* Austin, TX: Pro-Ed. Translated into German, 1981. Translated into Dutch, 1982.

Schopler, E., Reichler, R., Bashford, A., Lansing, M., & Marcus, L. (1989). *Individualized assessment and treatment for autistic and developmentally disabled children: Vol. 1. Psychoeducational profile revised (PEP-R).* Austin: TX: Pro-Ed. (in press).

Schopler, E., Reichler, R., DeVellis, R., & Daly, K. (1980). Toward objective classification of childhood autism: Childhood autism rating scale (CARS). *Journal of Autism and Developmental Disorders, 10,* 91-103. Translated into Swedish, 1984. Translated into French, 1986. Translated into Japanese, 1985.

Schopler, E., Reichler, R. J., & Renner, B. R. (1988). *The childhood autism rating scale (CARS).* Revised, Western Psychological Services, Inc.

Short, A. B. (1984). Short-term treatment outcome using parents as co-therapists for their own autistic children. *Journal of Child Psychology and Psychiatry and Allied Disciplines, 25,* 443-458.

Watson, L., Lord, C., Schaffer, B., & Schopler, E. (1989). *Teaching spontaneous communication to autistic and developmentally handicapped children.* New York: Irvington.

Help for the Family

PATRICIA HOWLIN

INTRODUCTION

The involvement of parents in therapy and the use of the home as a therapeutic base is important for many reasons.

Clearly, parents are in a unique position when it comes to identifying their child's particular problems and the events that tend to exacerbate or to reduce these. They will also have extensive experience of the best ways to encourage desirable behaviours. Morever, since it is parents who have to cope directly with the child's problems it is they who are most likely to profit from any improvements in behaviour. Thus, their motivation to work for the good of the child is likely to be greater than that of any professional, no matter how caring. Many experimental studies now indicate, too, that working with parents at home is by far the best way of reducing problems of maintenance or generalization, as well as being a relatively economical form of intervention (Howlin & Rutter, 1987; Lovaas, 1987; Short, 1984).

Perhaps most importantly, however, working at home ensures that treatment can take place within a family context. In this way, therapeutic procedures can balance the needs of the child with those of other family members, so that outcome is optimally beneficial for all.

THE GOALS OF INTERVENTION

Although the benefits of home based intervention are considerable, there are, nonetheless, problems associated with this type of approach. The principal of these is that the reliance on parents or siblings as co-therapists, may, if not carefully organized, result in increased strains on families who are already under great pressure. Carr (1984), cites the example of one family, who, having moved from a well resourced area to one where there were relatively few facilities, expressed only relief "at being free of all the professionals who had been overwhelming them". In our own work we have held very strongly to the view that home based interventions must beware of imposing greater burdens on families either in terms of expenditure of time, energy or finances. Instead our aim has always been primarily to reduce the stress that a handicapped child can impose on family life. This can be done in a number of different ways.

Firstly, it is important to ensure that the problems worked on are ones that are relevant for that particular child and his family. They should not be selected according to the preconceived views of the therapist involved.

Secondly, whenever possible, treatment programmes should incorporate management techniques or reward systems that are already part of the family's coping repertoire. It has been our experience that attempts to introduce entirely novel strategies are rarely as effective as the appropriate modification of existing ones.

Thirdly, the types of treatment techniques advised should be ones that, wherever possible, reduce the anxiety levels of both the child and his parents. Methods that result in an increase in distress are unlikely to be carried out with any degree of consistency. Again, we have found that it is generally more successful to compromise and use techniques with which parents feel comfortable (even if they do take longer to have an effect) than to attempt to introduce procedures which, although in principle may be more rapid or effective, will only be carried out half-heartedly or intermittently.

Fourthly, intervention should not seek to increase the amount of time parents spend with their child but should aim to enable them to use this time more effectively. Life should not revolve entirely around the demands of the autistic child. Instead families need help to accommodate to these demands whilst at the same time allowing them to attend to their own needs and those of their other children.

Finally, help also needs to be provided in a variety of different ways, which may not be directly related to the child's problems. Counselling help may be required to deal with emotional or marital or other family problems. Advice about social benefits can sometimes help to reduce the economic burdens suffered by many families. The organization of baby-sitting facilities or respite care may be crucial to the well-being of the rest of the family. Appropriate medical help may be valuable for certain sorts of problems (depression in parents or specific problems such as epilepsy in the child). Other children in the family may need help and advice on their own behalf, for living with impairment is not always easy. And last,but in many ways most importantly, help must be given to ensure that the educational provison offered is appropriate. Schooling will take up the greater part of the child's day for many years; if it is not adequately meeting his needs there will be little that families can do to counteract this. On the other hand, if schooling is appropriate and if there is close liaison between home and school the chances of the child reaching his maximum potential are likely to be enhanced.

CHOOSING THE BEHAVIOURS TO BE TREATED

As noted above, our general procedure, when becoming involved with a family for the first time, has been to allow them to decide on the behaviours to be modified. This obviously has the advantage of increasing parental motivation to take part in therapy. It can also encourage parents to carry out some of the more tedious tasks related to treatment evaluation, such as the collection of base-line data or recordings of progress. However, it must be accepted that parents' selection of problem behaviours does not always accord with that of the therapist. Families may become so resigned to long term difficulties that their concerns centre instead around much more trivial and often more recent problems. A typical example is of one mother who said that her main worry about her hyper-active, incontinent, echolalic child was that he did not recognise colour names. In terms of the child's functioning it seemed to us that not knowing his colours was the least of his problems. Fortunately, it is much easier to work successfully on increasing simple skills than decreasing long standing behavioural difficulties. By using such opportunities to teach basic techniques and to give parents a feeling of control over their child's problems (sometimes for the first time in years) the family's subsequent ability to deal with much more fundamental problems may be greatly enhanced. The therapist can then begin to advise the family about the best order in which to tackle other problems and of ways in which these can be broken down into separate components so that intervention takes place in a progressive, step by step fashion.

THE CHOICE OF TREATMENT TECHNIQUES

Most parents demonstrate successful management strategies at least some of the time in coping with their autistic child. However, they may use these only intermittently or non-contingently so that effectiveness is greatly reduced. With the exception of physical punishment, which we tend strongly to discourage, our general aim has been to utilise strategies already in use by parents, helping them to make more effective use of these. Consistency of approach may well be more important than the specific type of programme used and encouraging cohesion amongst family members is vital. One can than build upon existing strategies, employing these with a wider range of problems or in an increasing number of situations and enhancing their effectiveness by the addition of other techniques relevant to specific problems. For example, a "Time-Out" programme for disruptive behaviour may be made more effective, not only by increasing the consistency with which it is used but by using it in conjunction with other procedures, such as relaxation or desensitization, which may reduce other, related problems. Similarly, when developing self help or constructional skills, although the use of contingent reinforcement is crucial for success, it is not in itself sufficient to teach new behaviours and modelling, shaping and prompting procedures will also be required.

Once new behaviours and skills have been acquired it is also likely that some degree of environmental restructuring will be required in order to ensure that children are encouraged to make the best use of their newly acquired abilities. Indeed the deliberate elicitation of these skills within the child's regular environment seems to be one of the essential ingredients of treatment success. Setting parents specific goals, without necessarily attempting to increase their use of reinforcement or other behavioural techniques, has been found to be highly effective in some studies (Cheseldine & McConkey, 1979). Short (1984) suggests that the amount of physical and verbal guidance provided by parents may actually be more important than rates of reinforcement. Many other intervention studies have also indicated that simple restructuring of the environment can have significant effects on language, social and constructional behaviours (see Howlin & Rutter, 1987).

A further aim of therapy has been to focus as much on positive treatment strategies as possible. Hence, if disruptive or undesirable behaviours result from a lack of appropriate skills (communication, self help, constructional etc.) or from other difficulties, such as obsessional, ritualistic or phobic tendencies, our basic approach has been to increase relevant skills or to develop control over fears or obsessional behaviours rather than to work directly on the elimination of what, in fact, may be secondary problems.

This approach to therapy may not, of course, always prove to be the most rapid way of dealing with difficulties but working together with parents at home frequently demands compromises on both sides. In principle, for example, it may be much more effective in the short term to deal with disruptive behaviours by extinction or "time out" techniques. However, in practice, parents may well have many difficulties in implementing such programmes consistently (especially if feeding or sleeping difficulties are involved) so that alternative strategies, although less rapid, may prove to be much more effective in the long term. Table 1 indicates the type of programme that was found to be most useful with a 12 year old boy who refused to let his mother stop for any reason whilst they were out in the car, until they reached their stated destination. Extinction programmes had worked successfully with him in the past, notably in reducing his tendency to climb in and out ot windows rather than using more conventional means of leaving or entering the house. However, his mother, who was a nervous driver at the best of times, felt unable to ignore his disruptive behaviours in the car. The adoption of a "graded change" approach to this problem proved much more acceptable.

Table 1. Reduction of obsessional behaviour

PROBLEM - Child's refusal to allow the car to stop on journeys

STAGES OF INTERVENTION

1	Predicted stop of 30 seconds close to home. Return to home if child disruptive.
2	Predicted stop of one minute. Journey continues if no resistance, otherwise return home.
3.	Unpredicted stop of one minute.
4	Several stops on journey.
5	Journey length extended.
6	Trips to shops resumed.

The progressively graded introduction of change has also proved to be a very effective method of dealing with a wide range of other problems. Object attachements have been successfully reduced by gradually decreasing the amount of time each day spent with the object; the number of places in which the child has access to the object, or even the size of the object itself.

Figure 1, for example, illustrates how a five year old's attachment to his blanket, which he refused to let out of his sight at any time, was reduced, literally, by his mother cutting a small piece off it each night when he was asleep. He seemed quite undistressed by this shrinkage and eventually the blanket was reduced to a few threads which no longer maintained his interest. Simultaneously, too, the postcards that he carried in his other hand also seemed to lose their attraction, although this obsession was not worked on independently.

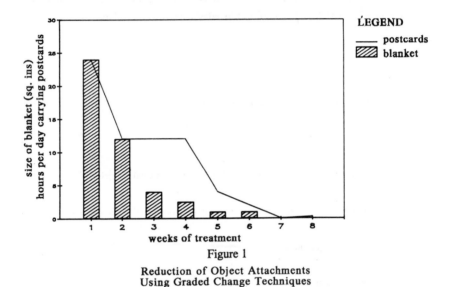

Figure 1

Reduction of Object Attachments
Using Graded Change Techniques

Irrational fears and phobias may also be dealt with effectively using this type of approach (see Table 2).

Table 2. Reduction of phobic behaviour

PROBLEMS - 5 year old boy's fear of baths.

STAGES OF TREATMENT (OVER 2 MONTHS)

1 New bath being installed in house.

  Child allowed to store toys in it.

2 Bath moved into bathroom. Continues as toy store.

3 Child washed fully clothed standing in bath.

4 Washed in bath with clothes removed.

5 Plug placed in bath.

6 Water level gradually raised.

7 Child spending prolonged periods in bath.

Other examples of a graded change approach are illustrated in chapter by Howlin, 1990. Amongst the behaviours for which these techniques have proved valuable are stereotypies and mannerisms, obsessional collecting, ritualistic lining up of toys, repetitive questioning, resistance to change and feeding and sleeping problems. Table 3 provides a summary of the variety of difficulties treated successfully in this way. One of the major advantages of this type of approach is that it tends to avoid any increases in anxiety in either parents or children, even when long standing behavioural problems are involved. As such, these methods generally prove highly acceptable to the great majority of families, who are then more likely to use the recommended strategies consistently. Once problem behaviours are reduced to an acceptable level, that is they no longer disrupt family functioning or interfere with the child's other activities, they may be used as a basis for building up other more acceptable behaviours (see Howlin, 1990) or as highly effective rewards.

Table 3. Reduction of obsessional activities.

PROBLEM	STAGES OF INTERVENTION
Collecting coins	1 Reduction in no. of rooms where coins allowed 2 Access to other enjoyed actitives e. g. T. V., eating, getting into parents' bed made contingent on coins being removed from room 3 Reduction in numbers of coins allowed in any one place 4 Coins allowed only in bedroom
Lining up toy cars	1 Gradual reduction in no. of cars from 50 to 20 2 Further reduction in length of lines to 5 cars only 3 Pairs of cars only allowed in house, though these scattered in various rooms 4 Cars used in imaginative play
Motor mannerisms	1 "Flapping" restricted at certain times of day (e. g. meal or T. V. times) 2 Increase in areas where flapping restricted 3 Further restrictions to certain times only 4 Flapping allowed only in own room
Verbal routines	1 Routines allowed only after period of non-stereotyped conversation 2 No. of repetitive sessions per day gradually reduced 3 No. of repetitive questions per session reduced 4 Routines allowed briefly at bedtimes only
Resistance to change in household	1 Minor change in angle of single chair 2 Chair gradually moved away from usual position 3 Others chairs moved to different angles 4 Gradual changes in other household items (angles of doors, curtains etc.)

MINIMISING DEMANDS ON PARENTS

A further, very deliberate aspect of our intervention programmes has been to ensure that treatment does not result in greater demands on families but that it enables them to organise their time more effectively to meet their own needs as well as those of their autistic and other children. No demands are made on families to change their existing life styles nor to spend more time with the autistic child. Indeed, in many cases, it is recommended that the amount of time devoted exclusively to the handicapped child might be reduced and more time given over to other family activities.

In the early stages of therapy parents will be observed in their interaction with the child at home and their methods of dealing with difficulties recorded, along with details of their child's behaviour. Parents may also be asked to fill out daily diary sheets to establish how they allot time to various activities both with and apart from the child. This allows assessment of how time is spent and how, perhaps, it might be more effectively employed. Some brief sessions of intensive work together may be recommended when trying to establish new skills but, on the whole, emphasis has been placed on the elicitation of skills or the modification of problems within the child's regular daily programme. In this way not only are demands on parents kept to a minimum, but new behaviours become part of an established "habit chain", leading to better generalization and more effective maintenance. Moreover, if parents appear to have difficulty in implementing techniques or keeping necessary records etc., then the demands made on them will be modified until they are able to cope. Very rarely will we ever consider terminating involvement with a family on the grounds that they are not following a programme satisfactorily. Instead we will modify the programme until they can do so.

The general effectiveness of this type of approach was demonstrated in a controlled study of home based therapy with families of autistic children (Howlin & Rutter, 1987). The amount of time mothers spent with their autistic child was assessed using daily time budgets. Few differences were found between treated or control groups in the amount or intensity of interaction, either before or after intervention. However, time sampling analyses of interactional styles indicated that, over time, parents in the treatment group evolved much more directive and informative ways of interacting with their children (see Figure 2). These changes, in turn, were parallelled by improvements in children's behaviour and language. It is clear that it is possible to effect significant changes in behaviour by modifying interactional styles but without necessarily increasing the amount of time spent in therapy.

Subsequent assessments of parents' views of therapy also indicated that improvements could be achieved without undue demands or intrusion. Significantly more

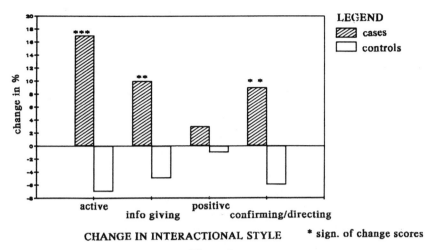

CHANGE IN INTERACTIONAL STYLE   * sign. of change scores

Figure 2

Change in Interactional Style Over 6
Months

parents in the treatment group than amongst the controls reported satisfaction with the help they had received; they felt more problems had been dealt with; the methods advised had been appropriate and successful; relations with their therapist were very positive and treatment had also enabled them to deal with a much wider range of issues and problems (see Figure 3). They felt that some effort had been required in putting the suggested procedures into practice but almost all parents had managed to do so and few reported any difficulties in finding the time necessary for carrying out programmes. On the other hand, they did not particularly enjoy keeping charts or diaries of their child's progress and several felt that therapists' expectations of their child were too high. Despite these last two caveats, however, home intervention was generally welcomed by parents and they did not view it as overintrusive or overdemanding.

THE ALLEVIATION OF OTHER FAMILY PROBLEMS

Dealing with Emotional Problems

Helping parents to develop effective management strategies and providing them with practical means of coping with their children's problems is, of course, central to treatment. Moreover, the acquisition of effective coping strategies plays an important role in helping to reduce worries, anxieties and general feelings of inadequacy. Nevertheless,

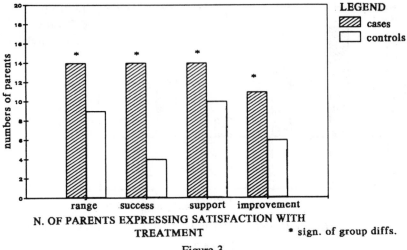

N. OF PARENTS EXPRESSING SATISFACTION WITH
TREATMENT   * sign. of group diffs.

Figure 3

Parental Satisfaction With Treatment

for optimum effect, therapy also needs to be sensitive to parents' needs as individuals. Irrational guilt, overwhelming exhaustion and feelings of anger, frustration, disappointment and hostility are all normal and understandable reactions experienced at some time by most parents of handicapped children. Counselling work is important in helping parents realize that they are not alone in these feelings, that love and anger can co-exist, and that there are ways of coming to terms with these troubling emotions and of channeling them in positive ways.

As well as providing specific help related to the child's problems our work has focused on the provision of guidance and support over the more general issues associated with having a handicapped child. Marital and emotional problems are encountered fairly frequently, with our approach to these issues depending on a careful analysis of the issues involved, for example, the treatment of depressive symptoms might involve medical or cognitive forms of intervention. Marital problems may require referral to other professional agencies or be dealt with by cognitive and/or behavioural techniques. Sleeping difficulties, for example, are a common problem with many autistic children and a programme to remove the child from the parents' bed may be an important step in reviving an ailing relationship. Help in restructuring daily activities may also be essential in encouraging parents to find more time for themselves and for each other. They may also require support to deal with the feelings of guilt that stem from reducing their interaction with the autistic child or leaving him to his own devices for short periods each day.

Providing Information and Advice

A central goal of our intervention with families has been to try to provide them with as much information as possible about the nature of autism and to help them form realistic notions of how far intervention can help and what the long term prognosis is likely to be. Obviously, one can never predict with absolute accuracy what will happen and one is always dealing with probabilities not certainties. Nevertheless, follow up studies of autism do provide some information regarding outcome which can usefully be shared with parents (Kanner, 1973; Rutter et al; 1967). For the severely handicapped it will be important to help parents, from the very early stages, to accept that their child is always likely to need some degree of specialist care. When dealing with older, non-communicating children, for whom the chances of acquiring useful speech are small (Howlin, 1989), encouragement to move to augmentative systems of communication may be important. With more able individuals, it is evident that the existence of specific skills can be crucial for good outcome (Kanner, 1973) and the value of encouraging such abilities (even if they have their basis in obsessional interests) is considerable.

Information of this nature is also important when it comes to setting treatment goals and influencing parents' expectations of these. The child's own deficits and abilities will, ultimately, be the most important factors in determining how much treatment can achieve. It is important that parents are given encouragement to develop their child's capabilities as far as possible, but equally, they should not be given false hopes nor made to feel that if outcome is not as positive as they had once hoped they are somehow at fault.

Choice of schooling will also depend on a careful analysis of the child's strengths and weakness. Whereas integration in mainstream school may be the best placement for some children, there are others who are likely to be greatly disadvantaged in such an environment and who could profit much more in a school for autistic children or perhaps one for the severely learning disabled (Howlin, 1985).

Specific information about what is known about the causes of autism is another crucial aspect of working with parents. Many families still harbour fears that the autism is somehow their fault and attributable to something that they did (or did not do) in pregnancy or early infancy. Factual information about known causes, though still somewhat limited can help to relieve some of these anxieties.

Genetic information may also be important for many families, not only for explaining possible causes of the disorder but in order to clarify the possible risks involved in having more children. For most families these will be small but are obviously important factors to consider (Folstein & Rutter, 1987). Counselling may be required, too, for older siblings worrying about their chances of having a handicapped child and although our knowledge in this area is far from complete it is important to share as much of this as possible. Similarly, if tests are available that might be able to provide further information (Fragile X analyses, for example), families should have right of access to these.

General information about normal development may be needed by many parents. There is often a tendency to assume that all the child's problems are related to his autism whereas, in fact, they may be part and parcel of normal developmental processes. Assertiveness or lack of cooperation in a previously docile child may well be related to advances in linguistic skill or to increased mental age. Similarly, the rejection, by older individuals, of restrictions which they had accepted when younger may be an important part of the process of growing up. Helping parents to accept what is and what is not acceptable at certain stages is important for them and for their child's development. Help with dressing, feeding and toiletting; limited expectations of the child's abilities to take part in normal family life, or close monitoring of his activities, especially away from home, may be appropriate at a certain age but quite inappropriate at another. Increased self reliance and independence, and some cooperation in household chores, should be developed steadily as children grow more capable. The need for greater freedom of choice and a reduction in parental supervision will also be required with time. Support for parents to continually develop the child's potential abilities whilst gradually relinquishing their control is something that needs to be offered on a long term basis. Parents' and children's needs will change over the years and short term programmes, no matter how effective, are unlikely entirely to meet these. Autism is a life long disorder and access to skilled therapeutic help should be available whenever required.

Effects on Siblings

Many parents express considerable anxiety about the extent to which their normal children may be adversely affected by the autistic child. There are suprisingly few good studies of the effects of having an handicapped sibling (Howlin, 1988). Overall, the effects do not seem to be necessarily deleterious and there is some suggestion that children may even profit from the experience, becoming more altruistic, tolerant, considerate and responsible than their peers. Nevertheless, some do show greater signs of disturbance and resentment (McHale et al., 1984). Research and clinical experience suggests that these effects can be minimised in a number of ways.

A positive attitude to the child by the parents is one of the most important factors influencing siblings' responses. If parents are accepting and loving the other children are likely to be so too (Grossman, 1972).

Information about the causes of autism and about practical ways of dealing with problems are viewed by siblings as important in minimising their anxieties and maximising their coping strategies (Fromberg, 1984). Siblings may prove to be extremely efficient therapists and, as long as involvement in treatment does not increase demands on them in any way, this role may be very valuable in increasing their feelings of control and self esteem. Research indicates that feelings of resentment are more likely to occur if the presence of the handicapped child increases the burden of care on siblings; if it reduces the time parents are able to give them, or if it affects their privacy or social lives (Simeonsson & McHale, 1981). These problems can be minimised by helping parents organise their time effectively, so that the autistic child does not require exclusive attention; by ensuring that other children are treated as fairly as possible (for example, by insisting that the autistic child take some part in household activities, no matter how limited) and by making sure they have some degree of privacy so that they can see friends or do homework in peace or keep precious belongings safe.

Help with Practical Issues

In addition to direct intervention at home most families will require help from outside resources. Appropriate schooling is crucial for optimal development but, as noted above, this will differ from child to child. Moreover, as needs change with time, so too may the type of schooling required. We have attempted to maintain links with schools and educational authorities to ensure that educational provision is available as early as possible and that this continues to keep pace with the child's needs. The majority of schools deliberately foster close links between parents and teachers but occasionally problems arise and again we will try to help forge (or repair) such links if necessary.

Cooperation with Social Services is also required if children are to receive all the financial and other support to which they may be entitled. Social Services involvement is necessary when dealing with post school provision and it is always preferable that links are made when the child is younger, rather than waiting until they are about to leave school. Similarly, rather than seeking respite care only in emergencies our aim has been to encourage families to make use of such help on a regular basis. This enables them to take periodic breaks and ensures that the child can experience separations from home under planned and non-stressful circumstances. Some families may decline such help, or Social Services may resist providing it, but if accepted it can prove of great benefit to parents and children alike. In particular, getting used to early, brief separations, makes it easier to cope if residential care is required at some later stage. It also helps the autistic child to develop relationships with adults other than those familiar to him at home or school. Holiday breaks can offer similar benefits and helping parents to make use of specialist holiday provision has often been important. Other aspects of our involvement with families have involved the provision of baby sitters or organising skilled medical or dental help. Conventional medical or para medical provision is often quite inadequate to meet the needs of a sick autistic child and direct intervention in hospitals or surgeries has been required on a number of occasions. We have also encouraged parents to make use of the very valuable services provided by the National or local Autistic Societies.

THE EFFECTIVENESS OF A HOME BASED APPROACH TO TREATMENT

As will be apparent from the foregoing description, our approach towards working with parents at home is an eclectic one. Although behavioural strategies play an essential role, they are but part of the total armamentarium, with the overall focus being on family wellbeing. This approach is one that families have found comfortable and relatively unstressful, and one with which they have been able to cooperate well. It has clearly resulted, too, in many improvements in children's behaviour as the results from individual case studies indicate (Howlin & Rutter, 1987). However, it is also evident that outcome is not always as favourable as might be hoped.

In our comparative study of treated and control children it was apparent that certain behaviours changed much more than others as a result of treatment. After 6 months of intensive work at home there remained few differences between children in IQ or in the quality of their social relationships. In contrast, ritualistic, disruptive and non-cooperative behaviours declined amongst the treated whilst they actually increased amongst the controls. Lingustic skills showed a similar pattern of change in both groups. The extent of improvement was significantly greater in the treatment group but both groups made steady gains in language usage and language level over the first 6 months of therapy (see Figure 4).

A longer term follow-up at 18 months, indicated that, rather than extended treatment increasing language skills, significant treatment effects appeared to be reduced over time. However, although treated children did not necessarily reach higher levels of language complexity than controls they were able to use their language skills in a more communicative fashion.

Follow-up assessments also revealed differential responses to treatment, with those children who were mute when treatment began making least progress. Initially echolalic children, on the other hand, tended to have a good outcome whether or not they were involved in therapy (see Table 4).

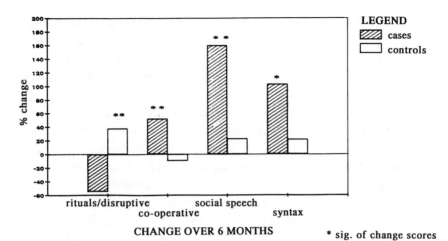

CHANGE OVER 6 MONTHS   * sig. of change scores

Figure 4

Changes in Language and Behaviour
Over the First 6 Months of Treatment

Table 4. Outcome for cases and controls according to initial levels

| INITIAL LEVELS | OUTCOME (%) | | | | | | E=cases | C=control |
| | No speech | | Poor | | Fair | | Good | |
	E	C	E	C	E	C	E	C
No speech	19	13	6	25	6	-	6	-
Single words			-	12	6	-	6	-
Echolalia			6	13	-	6	33	19
Phrase speech							13	13

KEY

Poor = Words only

Fair = Some phrases speech

Good = Conversational speech

Thus, outcome appeared to be dependant not only on the type of skill or behaviour involved but also on individual child characteristics. It might be argued that 18 months was too brief an intervention period to expect dramatic change but in fact the results indicated that the greatest gains all occured within the first 6 months of treatment, with change thereafter being maintained but not greatly increased.

There were other findings too, that gave rise to concern. For example, although direct observations showed rapid improvements in children's behaviour, parents were much slower to report positive change. Moreover, parental ratings made some time after the cessation of treatment indicated that they still had difficulties coping with new behaviour problems and there were few difference between experimental and control parents in their perception of improvement after therapy had ended. Thus, in terms of generalization and parental views of progress, outcome was less than totally satisfactory.

Although comparable with findings from similar studies, notably those carried out by Schopler and his co-workers (Short, 1984), these results clearly fall short of those reported recently by Lovaas (1987). In our own intervention studies attempts to modify behavioural difficulties were, on the whole, highly effective but no changes in I. Q. were found whereas Lovaas recorded significant improvements in this area. Changes in language were very much dependant on the child's initial level and treatment appeared to affect language usage rather than language level. Moreover, although several of our children have been admitted to mainstream schooling, and some of our older clients have done well at college or work (some are even married and have children), they can in no way be considered to show normal social functioning and are easily identifiable as "unusual" by all those with whom they come into contact. Lovaas' findings, in contrast, suggest that intensive therapy resulted in many children being indistinguishable from their normal peers. Obviously, the style of our family intervention has been much less intensive and probably much less demanding on parents than that offered by Lovaas. Indeed, working within the N.H.S system, it would be difficult to envisage setting up a comparative programme. A number of questions remain, therefore, concerning both the short and long term effects of therapy. Would highly intensive behavioural treatments (of 40 hours per week or more) at an early age have resulted in much more impressive results, such as those reported by Lovaas?

Would greater demands on parents have resulted in a reduction in the numbers or types of families able to take part?

Would more detailed assessments of social competence than those applied in the Lovaas' work have revealed the existence of many more social difficulties?

And, finally, how much more effective in the longer term, that is through adolescence and early adulthood, are the results of intensive, early interventions?

It is evident that a fully controlled and long term replication of Lovaas' work is required; unfortunately it is likely to be extremely difficult to obtain funding for such a project.

SUMMARY

Intervention with the families of autistic children requires a long term, multi-faceted approach. Helping parents to develop effective management strategies for coping with behaviour problems is an essential part of therapy. However, if this is to be optimally successful it is important to set the needs of the child within the context of general family requirements. It is the long term improvement in family functioning that is the ultimate goal, not simply the short term alleviation of specific behavioural difficulties. Such an approach requires much longer term support than is usually available and demands resources that can span the whole age range, from infancy to adulthood.

Evaluation is also needed to establish how effective, again in the longer term, is this type of family oriented approach when compared with the much more intensive programmes utilised in some other studies. It is most likely that both types of approach have their advantages and their drawbacks. How to help families achieve the greatest benefits from both should now be our common aim.

REFERENCES

Carr, J. (1984). Family Processes and Parent Involvement. In J. Dobbing (Ed.), *Scientific Studies in Mental Retardation:* Proceedings of First European Symposium. London: MacMillan.

Cheseldine, S., & McConkey, R. (1979). Parental Speech to Young Down's Syndrome Children: An Intervention Study. *American Journal of Mental Deficiency, 83,* 612 - 620.

Folstein, S., & Rutter, M. (1987). Autism: Familial Aggregation and Genetic Implications: In E. Schopler & G. Mesibov (Eds.), *Neurobiological Issues in Autism.* New York: Plenum.

Fromberg, R. (1984). The Sibling's Changing Roles. In E. Schopler & G. Mesibov (Eds.), *The Effects of Autism on the Family.* New York: Plenum Press.

Grossman, F. (1972). *Brothers and Sisters of Retarded Children.* Syracuse: Syracuse University Press.

Howlin, P. (1985). Special Educational Treatment. In M. Rutter & L. Hersov (Eds.), *Child and Adolescent Psychiatry: Modern Approaches.* (2nd edition). Oxford: Blackwell.

Howlin, P. (1988). Living with Impairment: The Effects on Children of Having an Autistic Sibling. *Child Care, Health and Development, 14,* 395 - 408.

Howlin, P. (1989). Changing approaches to language training with autistic children. *British Journal of Communication Disorders, 24,* 151 - 168.

Howlin, P. (1990). Traeting Autistic Children at Home. A London Based Programme. In C Gillberg (Ed.), *Diagnosis and Treatment of Autism.* New York: Plenum Press.

Howlin, P., & Rutter, M. (1987). (with Berger, M., Hemsley, R., Hersov, L., & Yule, W.). *Treatment of Autistic Children.* Chichester: Wiley.

Kanner, L. (1973). *Chilhood Psychosis: Initial Studies and New Insights.* New York: Wiley.

Lovaas, O. I. (1987). Behavioral Treatment and Normal Educational and Intellectual Functioning in Young Autistic Children. *Journal of Consulting and Clinical Psychology, 55,* 3 - 9.

McHale, S., Simeonsson, R., & Sloan, J. (1984). Children with Handicapped Brothers and Sisters. In E. Schopler & G. Mesibov (Eds.), *The Effects of Autism on the Family.* New York: Plenum.

Rutter, M., Greenfield, D., & Lockyer, L. (1967). A Five to Fifteen Year Follow Up Study of Infantile Psychosis. II. Social and Behavioural Outcome. *British Journal of Psychiatry, 113,* 1183 - 1199.

Short, A. B. (1984). Short Term Treatment Outcome Using Parents as Co-therapists for Their Own Autistic Children. *Journal of Child Psychology and Psychiatry, 25,* 443 - 458.

Simeonsson, R., & McHale, S. (1981). Review: Research on Handicapped Children: Sibling Relationships. *Child Care, Health and Development, 7,* 153 - 171.

Pharmacotherapy in Autism: An Overview

MAGDA CAMPBELL

INTRODUCTION

"The promotion of maturation and development constitutes the essence of treatment of young, including psychotic children. Ideally, an effective drug should enhance this process" (Campbell, 1975, p. 399). It has been stated repeatedly, that the role of psychoactive agents in the treatment of autistic children is two-fold: to decrease behavioral symptoms and to promote development (Campbell, 1975). Pharmacotherapy should never be viewed as a sole treatment in autism; it is viewed only as part, however, sometimes an important part, of a comprehensive treatment program. Though there is some information about the type of symptoms which may respond to pharmacotherapy (Perry et al., 1989a) clinical experience shows that the individual child with those very target symptoms may not respond to drug.

Systematic assessment of the efficacy and safety of psychoactive agents in autistic children began by Barbara Fish in the early sixties, and it was Fish who established both the groundwork in this area of research, and clinical practice (Fish, 1968). Since then, progress has been made, particularly in the area of methodology and assessment (Campbell, 1987; Campbell & Palij, 1985; Campbell & Spencer, 1988). In addition, efforts were made to develop a more rational pharmacotherapy. In the past decade or so, it was attempted to relate behavioral and cognitive deviancies and deficits in autism to biochemical alterations, and to correct both the symptoms and intellectual subnormality with an appropriate (corresponding) psychoactive agent (Ritvo et al., 1970, 1984; Campbell and co-workers, 1976, 1988, 1989; Herman et al., 1986). This type of research effort was not always met with therapeutic success. The effectiveness of haloperidol on the other hand, has been demonstrated both in short-term (Anderson et al., 1984, 1989; Campbell et al., 1978; Cohen et al., 1980) and in long-term studies (Perry et al., 1989a). However, the association of tardive and withdrawal dyskinesia with haloperidol limits its use (Campbell et al., 1988a; Perry et al., 1989b).

Attempts were also made to predict response to drug and to define responders (Fish, 1970; Fish et al., 1966; Perry et al., 1989a).

At the present time there is no psychoactive drug which will eliminate the behavioral symptoms in autism and normalize the intellectual deficits. Nevertheless, the effectiveness of certain drugs in subgroups and in individual autistic children has been demonstrated. Concerning side effects, clearly, among the currently available psychoactive drugs, a therapeutically powerful drug has side effects, while a psychoactive drug with minimal or no side effects may be of lower potency or may have only minimal therapeutic activity.

NEUROLEPTICS

It has been demonstrated in carefully designed and double-blind controlled studies, that the high-potency neuroleptics like trifluoperazine (Fish et al., 1966) and haloperidol (Campbell et al., 1978; Anderson et al., 1984, 1989) are not only statistically but also clinically superior to placebo in the treatment of young autistic children. On the other hand, the administration of low-potency neuroleptics, including chlorpromazine, is associated with sedation even at low doses, without significant decrease of such target symptoms as hyperactivity, temper tantrums and aggressiveness (for review, see Campbell, 1975). Furthermore, the administration of chlorpromazine is associated with decrease of seizure threshold and increase of frequency of seizures (Tarjan et al., 1957) and therefore may be contraindicated in many autistic children who require pharmacotherapy. Autism is associated with a relatively high incidence of seizure disorders (Deykin & MacMahon, 1979).

There is some supportive evidence (Cohen et al., 1977; Gillberg et al., 1983) that subgroups of autistic children have increased dopaminergic function though a recent study is in disagreement (Minderaa et al., 1989). Certain symptoms autistic children display, including stereotypies, hyperactivity, attentional and cognitive problems support the notion that a dysfunction of the dopaminergic system exists in this disorder (for review, see Young et al., 1982). This would support the rationale of using a potent antidopaminergic agent, such as trifluoperazine or haloperidol in the treatment of autistic children who display these target symptoms.

Fish et al. (1966) have shown, in a carefully designed and controlled study, that trifluoperazine, at doses 2 to 20 mgs, is an effective drug in children ages 2 to 6 years, and particularly in those who are of low intellectual functioning.

Systematic studies of haloperidol under double-blind conditions have demonstrated the effectiveness of this psychoactive agent in young autistic children as a group, and its superiority over placebo (Anderson et al., 1984, 1989; Campbell et al., 1978; Cohen et al., 1980). All but one (Cohen et al., 1980) of these trials employed large samples of patients; exclusively hypoactive children and those with seizure disorder were excluded. Haloperidol dosage was individually regulated under careful clinical monitoring; optimal doses, ranged 0.25 to 4.0 mg/day or from 0.016 to 0.217 mg/kg/day. Under these conditions, haloperidol was not only statistically but also clinically superior to placebo, in the absence of side effects when given over a period of 1 to 2 months. Furthermore, it was shown that at these therapeutically effective doses the administration of haloperidol facilitates learning in the laboratory (Campbell et al., 1978; Anderson et al., 1984), or at least, it does not interfere with learning (Anderson et al., 1989). Therapeutic changes on haloperidol included decreases of hyperactivity, temper tantrums, irritability, stereotypies and withdrawal. Ratings were carried out by multiple raters, independently, in a variety of situations (playroom, classroom and inpatient ward) on a variety of rating scales. All children were inpatients and compliance was 100%. Side effects occurred only above therapeutic doses; most frequent were excessive sedation and acute dystonic reaction (Anderson et al., 1984). Acute dystonic reaction was treated with and responded to diphenhydramine (25 mg orally or intramuscularly); it could have been avoided in most if not in all cases if the increments were done more gradually and slowly. Parkinsonian side effects were extremely rare in this age group. Other side effects included behavioral toxicity which was also rated in children during treatment with placebo.

The rating scales employed in these studies (Campbell & Palij, 1985a), the computerized laboratories for discrimination learning (Campbell, 1987; Campbell & Palij, 1985a) and the designs (Campbell, 1987) were described elsewhere. Rating conditions and ecological observations are of great importance in evaluating treatment effects and were previously discussed (Campbell, 1978).

Not only the short-term, but also the long-term effectiveness of haloperidol was demonstrated. Some autistic children require pharmacotherapy over a prolonged period of time, mainly because of certain severe behavioral symptoms which include temper tantrums, aggressive and self-mutilating behaviors. A study was designed to evaluate the ability of haloperidol to maintain improvement over time (Perry et al., 1989a). Additional aims of the study were to determine the comparative efficacy of continuous versus discontinuous administration of haloperidol, and whether discontinuous drug administration with a reduced amount of drug intake will also reduce the development of neuroleptic-related dyskinesias. Children, ages 2.3 to 7.9 years who required haloperidol treatment and who responded to a short-term administration of this drug were enrolled in this clinical trial. The duration of treatment was 6 months, followed by a 4-week placebo period. Children were randomly assigned to two groups; group I received haloperidol every day of the week, for 6 months. Children who were in group II received haloperidol only for 5-days a week, and placebo for 2 days, also over a period of 6 months. The 2-day placebo periods were randomly assigned and varied. All medication was dispensed blindly in envelopes, each dose in a separate envelope. The design, assessment and procedures are detailed elsewhere (Perry et al., 1989a). In the 60 children who completed the study, haloperidol was particularly effective in those who had severe symptoms of anger, irritability and labile affect (Perry et al., 1989a). Haloperidol remained effective over the 6-month period irrespective of being administered on a continuous or discontinuous basis. Daily doses of haloperidol ranged from 0.5 to 4.0 mg/day (mean, 1.23 mg/day), or 0.016-0.209 mg/kg/day (mean, 0.059). Except for haloperidol-related dyskinesias, no other side effects were rated at these doses. Of the 12 children who developed dyskinesias, 9 children had withdrawal dyskinesias during the 4-week placebo period, and 3 had dyskinesias during the haloperidol treatment period (Perry et al., 1989a).

It should be noted that administration of haloperidol over a one-year period of time did not have adverse effects on the intellectual functioning of 33 autistic children; at baseline testing their ages ranged from 2 1/2 to 7 8/12 years and at follow-up testing 3 1/2 to 8 8/12 years (Shell et al., 1987).

Dyskinesias represent a serious drawback of treatment with haloperidol, and, with all neuroleptics, in spite of their clinical efficacy. Molindone is not an exception (Greenhill, 1987).

Neuroleptic-related dyskinesias were systematically studied in autistic children, employing a prospective design (Campbell, 1985; Campbell et al., 1983a, 1983b, 1988a; Golden et al., 1987; Meiselas et al., 1989; Perry et al., 1985, 1989b; for review, see Campbell et al., 1983a).

Earlier studies were retrospective and employed relatively high doses of neuroleptics (Engelhardt & Polizos, 1978; Polizos & Engelhardt, 1980; Polizos et al., 1973). These reports suggested that dyskinesias in autistic children differ from those reported in adult psychiatric patients. The topography of movements was found to be different, seen mainly in lower, and in upper extremities in the form of ataxia. Furthermore, in these children only withdrawal dyskinesias were observed and they were reversible in all cases. In a sample of 53 children, 51% developed withdrawal dyskinesias within one to 2 weeks following discontinuation of neuroleptics (Engelhardt & Polizos, 1978).

Subsequent studies were in disagreement as to the topography and type of dyskinesias. A carefully designed prospective study involved 82 autistic children, whose ages, at the time of entry into the study, ranged from 2.3 to 8.2 years. They received relatively conservative doses of haloperidol (0.25-10.5 mg/day, or 0.016 to 0.217 mg/kg/day (median, 0.054). The length of exposure of these children to haloperidol was from 0.84 to 78.48 months (mean 18.1 months). The results showed that 29.27% of the children, or 24 of the 82 children developed dyskinesias (Campbell et al., 1988a). During haloperidol administration only 20.8% of the 24 developed dyskinesias while 79.2% developed dyskinesias after drug withdrawal, while receiving placebo. Most commonly involved were oro-facial muscles, muscles of the tongue, and of upper extremities. In all children the dyskinesias were reversible: they lasted from 7 days to 7.5 months. Several variables were studied in order to define those children who developed dyskinesias from those who did not; females showed a trend toward a greater risk (Campbell et al., 1988a). The demography of the sample, the methods including the rating scales, and the videotaping procedures, are detailed elsewhere (Campbell et al., 1988a; Campbell & Palij, 1985b). A 5 1/2 year old boy, developed Tourette-like symptoms after haloperidol withdrawal (Perry et al., 1989b).

Because stereotypies can occur in the same areas, of the face and body, and because they are difficult to differentiate sometimes from dyskinesias (Campbell et al., 1983a; Meiselas et al., 1989), it is strongly recommended that each child should be carefully examined for abnormal movements prior to pharmacotherapy.

STIMULANTS

The existence of an increased dopaminergic function in at least a subgroup of autistic children (Cohen et al., 1977; Gillberg et al., 1983) would be supported by the negative reports on the use of stimulant drugs in this population. Both dextroamphetamine (Campbell et al., 1972) and levoamphetamine (Campbell et al., 1976), drugs which can be described as dopamine agonists, were explored in this population. All studies have methodological flaws, and one is a single-case report (Strayhorn et al., 1988). Even though administration of dextroamphetamine was associated with decrease of hyperactivity, and increases of attention span and verbal production, these therapeutic effects were frequently accompanied by loss of appetite, worsening of withdrawal, severe behavioral toxicity, and worsening of pre-existing stereotypies and stereotypies *de novo* (Campbell et al., 1972). Levoamphetamine was more toxic and side effects included worsening of pre-existing stereotypies and stereotypies *de novo* (Campbell et al., 1976). Behavioral toxicity with methylphenidate (20 mg/day) included fearfulness, and exacerbation of hyperactivity in a 9 1/2 year old autistic boy, (Realmuto et al., 1989).

Methylphenidate was reported to decrease hyperactivity in a sample of 9 children, without significant side effects (Birmaher et al., 1988). Clearly, this class of drug requires a critical evaluation in autism.

FENFLURAMINE

No other psychoactive agent generated such interest in recent years as fenfluramine, resulting in a multicenter study under the leadership of Ritvo (Ritvo et al, 1986) and several independent studies (for review, see Campbell, 1988). After an initial enthusiasm (Geller et al, 1982) the efficacy and safety of this drug is now being questioned by some investigators and clinicians. Each study consisted of a small, or, at best, a modest sample size; in several, the patients' age range was very wide. Several studies lacked random assignment to treatment conditions in addition to other methodological weaknesses (for review, see Campbell, 1988). Early reports were promising and suggested that administration of fenfluramine, at daily dosis of 1.5 mg/kg is associated with behavioral improvement and increases in intellectual functioning without side effects (Ritvo et al., 1983). Subsequent reports were less positive (August et al., 1985; Ritvo et al., 1986) and even negative (Campbell et al., 1988b; Ekman et al., 1989 in press; Leventhal et al., 1985).

Fenfluramine is a potent antiserotonergic and a mild antidopaminergic drug (for review, Campbell, 1988). Fenfluramine was explored because about one-third of autistic children have hyperserotonemia (Campbell et al., 1975; Ritvo et al., 1970) and there is a supportive evidence that abnormalities of the serotonergic system are underlying certain behavioral symptoms and cognitive problems in autism (Campbell et al., 1975; Ritvo et al., 1983; for review, see Young et al., 1982). Furthermore, it was very important to explore a drug whose administration is not associated with tardive dyskinesia. It should be noted though that dystonic reaction on following a single dose of fenfluramine was reported: it involved the muscles of neck, tongue and throat (Sananman, 1974).

All studies used a fixed dose of fenfluramine (1.5 mg/kg/day) and a crossover design, with the exception of Campbell et al. (1988b). Campbell et al. (1988b) employed a parallel groups design with random assignment of patients to treatment conditions, and a flexible dose schedule; optimal daily doses of fenfluramine ranged from 1.250 to 2.068 mg/kg (mean, 1.747). This study differed from others in terms of patient population: the 28 children were all inpatients and had a narrow age range (2.56 to 6.66 years; mean, 4.57;

median, 4.41). Instead of repeated monthly administration of IQ tests (Ritvo et al., 1983, 1986), the effect of fenfluramine on cognition was assessed in a computerized laboratory, using a discrimination learning paradigm (Campbell et al., 1988b). The study of Campbell et al. (1988b) employing multiple raters and multiple rating scales, failed to show the superiority of fenfluramine over placebo in reducing maladaptive behaviors. There was only a trend favoring fenfluramine in decreasing hyperactivity and stereotypies in the automated laboratory. However, fenfluramine had a retarding effect on discrimination learning as compared to placebo. Most frequent side effects, associated with fenfluramine administration were excessive sedation, irritability, loss of weight and loose bowel movements. Thirteen of the 14 children who received fenfluramine had side effects; 11 of the 14 children who received placebo had similar side effects.

At our present state of knowledge it seems that fenfluramine may be helpful for the individual autistic child, but it cannot be recommended for autistic children as a group. Furthermore, concerns were expressed that fenfluramine administration may result in serotonin depletion (Schuster et al., 1986) though a thorough review of clinical reports in children does not support this (for review, see Campbell, 1988).

NALTREXONE

The rationale for exploring naltrexone, a potent opiate antagonist was three-fold. First, there was supportive, though inconclusive evidence, that abnormalities of endogenous opioids exist in subgroups of autistic children (Gillberg et al, 1985; Weizman et al, 1984). Second, it was hypothesized, that a variety of abnormalities displayed by autistic children are analogous to those seen in opiate addicts, to those in laboratory animals who were administered opiates, and in infants born to mothers who were taking opiates during pregnancy (Kalat, 1978; Panksepp, 1979; Panksepp & Sahley, 1987). Finally, naltrexone is not associated with tardive dyskinesia.

Two acute dose range-tolerance trials of naltrexone were suggestive of its therapeutic efficacy and safety. Reduction of stereotypies, withdrawal and hyperactivity, and increase in verbal production were reported. Herman et al. (1986) administered naltrexone to 5 autistic children, ages 4 to 12 years, all outpatients; Campbell et al. (1989) studied naltrexone in 10 boys, all inpatients, whose ages ranged from 3.42 to 6.5 years (mean 5.04). In both studies, naltrexone was administered in a single dose, ranging from 0.5 to 2.0 mg/kg. At these doses slight sedation was the only side effect. Electrocardiogram, liver function tests and other laboratory tests remained within normal limits (Campbell et al., 1989). Five children lost, and 4 gained weight. Behavioral response was not related to naltrexone levels.

Leboyer et al. (1988) explored naltrexone in a 6-day experiment with a 2-day placebo baseline. The patients, 2 autistic girls with self-injurious behavior continued to receive neuroleptics throughout the experiment. Naltrexone was administered in single dose starting with 1.0 mg/kg followed by 1.5 and finally by 2.0 mg/kg with 2-day intervals between each dose. Marked reduction in hyperactivity, increase in social behavior and decrease in self-injurious behavior were rated. It is of interest that naloxone, also an opiate antagonist, was reported to enhance the effectiveness of neuroleptics in adult schizophrenic but not in manic patients (Pickar et al., 1982). Walters et al. (1989) presented a single-case, a 14-year-old autistic boy, with severe self-injurious behavior, who participated in a double-blind placebo controlled study of naltrexone, employing an intensive B-A-B-A design. The study was designed to assess the effects of naltrexone specifically on self-injurious behavior and on social relatedness. Each treatment condition lasted 21 days, and naltrexone was given daily, 1.0 mg/kg. Increased social relatedness and complete cessation of self-injurious behavior were rated on naltrexone.

In an ongoing study, naltrexone is given on daily basis, over a period of 3 weeks, in an inpatient setting to children of preschool age. Daily doses range from 0.5 to 1.0 mg/kg. The study is double-blind and placebo controlled; following a 2-week baseline placebo period patients are randomly assigned to treatment conditions. Preliminary results are based on clinical consensus ratings of 17 children; they suggest that more children improved on naltrexone, than on placebo as shown in Table 1. All laboratory studies, including liver function tests and electrocardiogram, remained within normal limits, under careful monitoring (Campbell et al., 1990).

TABLE 1. Naltrexone vs placebo. Clinical Global Consensus Ratings.

	Improvement				
	Marked	Moderate	Slight	No Change	Worse
Naltrexone (N=9)	1	5	3	0	0
Placebo (N=9)	0	1	4	4	0

BUSPIRONE

Buspirone is a new antianxiety drug with antiserotonergic properties; it was explored in autistic children because of its antiserotonergic properties. About one-third of autistic children have elevated serotonin levels in plasma (Campbell et al., 1975; Ritvo et al., 1970) or in platelets (Anderson et al., 1989) though not all reports are in agreement (Anderson et al., 1989). Realmuto et al. (1989) administered buspirone to 4 autistic children, ages 9 1/12 to 10 5/12 years in an open fashion. Following a 2-week baseline period, children were administered buspirone for 4 weeks (5 mg TID); after a one-week washout they were given either methylphenidate or fenfluramine for 4 weeks. A variety of rating scales were used. Three of the 4 children showed some improvement on buspirone: decreases in hyperactivity in 2, of aggressiveness in 2, and of stereotypies in 2 were rated, on several rating scales. No side effects were observed. A critical assessment of buspirone is warranted in a larger sample of children.

COMBINATION OF PSYCHOACTIVE DRUG AND PSYCHOSOCIAL TREATMENT

Autism is a pervasive, and in many young children a severe condition. Even though a variety of treatment modalities were developed in the past 4 decades (for review, see Campbell and Schopler, 1989), no currently available method of treatment produces dramatic results. It is important then to determine, which single treatment is better, and whether the effectiveness of one treatment can be enhanced by another treatment modality.

The effectiveness of haloperidol was compared to behavior therapy focusing on language, and the combination of both were assessed under double-blind and placebo-controlled conditions. Forty children, ages 2.6 to 7.2 years completed the study; the children were randomly assigned to 4 treatment conditions, employing a factorial design (Campbell et al., 1978). While haloperidol alone was responsible in decreasing certain behavioral symptoms, the combination of haloperidol and behavior therapy (contingent reinforcement) was superior to the combination of haloperidol and non-contingent reinforcement and to placebo and contingent reinforcement, in increasing word acquisition (Campbell et al., 1978).

Clearly, these results should be replicated and research should focus on this type of work. Similar types of studies with pimozide, reportedly an effective drug in this population (Naruse et al., 1982), should be designed.

ACKNOWLEDGEMENTS

Part of this work was supported by NIMH grant MH-32212 and by a grant from the Stallone Fund for Research in Autism (Dr. Campbell). The research was carried out in Bellevue Hospital Center, New York, New York.

REFERENCES

Anderson, G. M., Minderaa, R. B., Volkmar, F., & Cohen, D. J. Monoamines in autism. Abstracts. World Federation of Societies of Biological Psychiatry Regional Congress, Jerusalem, Israel, April 1989.

Anderson, L. T., Campbell, M., Grega, D. M., Perry, R., Small, A. M., & Green, W. H. (1984). Haloperidol in the treatment of infantile autism: Effects on learning and behavioral symptoms. *American Journal of Psychiatry, 141,* 1195-1202.

Anderson, L. T., Campbell, M., Adams, P., Small, A. M., Perry, R., & Shell, J. (1989). The effects of haloperidol on discrimination learning and behavioral symptoms in autistic children. *Journal of Autism and Developmental Disorders, 19,* 227 - 239.

August, G. J., Raz, N., & Baird, T. D. (1985). Brief report: Effects of fenfluramine on behavioral, cognitive and affective disturbances in autistic children. *Journal of Autism and Developmental Disorders, 15,* 97-107.

Birmaher, B., Quintana, H., & Greenhill, L. L. (1988). Case study: Methylphenidate treatment of hyperactive autistic children. *Journal of the American Academy of Child and Adolescent Psychiatry, 27,* 248-251.

Campbell, M. (1975). Pharmacotherapy in early infantile autism. *Biological Psychiatry, 10,* 399-423.

Campbell, M. (1978). The use of drug treatment in infantile autism and childhood schizophrenia: A review. In M. A. Lipton, A. Di Mascio & K. Killam (Eds.), *Psychopharmacology: A generation of progress* (pp 1451-1461). New York: Raven Press.

Campbell, M. (1985). Timed Stereotypies Rating Scale. *Psychopharmacology Bulletin,* Special Feature: Rating scales and assessment instruments for use in pediatric psychopharmacology research, *21,* 1082.

Campbell, M. (1987). Drug treatment of infantile autism: The past decade. In H.Y. Meltzer (Ed.), *Psychopharmacology: The Third Generation of Progress* (pp 1225-1231). New York: Raven Press.

Campbell, M. (1988). Fenfluramine treatment of autism. Annotation. *Journal of Child Psychology and Psychiatry, 29,* 1-10.

Campbell, M., & Palij, M. (1985a). Behavioral and cognitive measures used in psychopharmacological studies of infantile autism. *Psychopharmacology Bulletin, 21,* 1047-1053.

Campbell, M., & Palij, M. (1985b). Measurement of side effects including tardive dyskinesia. *Psychopharmacology Bulletin, 21,* 1063-1066.

Campbell, M., & Schopler, E. (Co-Chairpersons) (1989). Pervasive Developmental Disorders. In *Treatments of Psychiatric Disorders.* A Task Force Report of the American Psychiatric Association. T. B. Karasu, (Chairperson), Washington, DC: American Psychiatric Association, D. C. 1989, 1, 179, 294.

Campbell, M., & Spencer, E. K. (1988). Psychopharmacology in child and adolescent psychiatry: A review of the last five years. *Journal of the American Academy of Child and Adolescent Psychiatry, 27,* 269-279.

Campbell, M., Fish, B., David, R., Shapiro, T., Collins, P., & Koh, C. (1972). Response to Triiodothyronine and Dextroamphetamine: A study of preschool, schizophrenic children. *Journal of Autism and Childhood Schizophrenia, 2,* 343-358.

Campbell, M., Friedman, E., Green,W. H., Collins, P. J., Small, A. M., & Breuer, H. (1975). Blood serotonin in schizophrenic children. A preliminary study. *International Pharmacopsychiatry, 10,* 213-221.

Campbell, M., Small, A. M., Collins, P. J., Friedman, E., David, R., & Genieser, N. (1976). Levodopa and levoamphetamine: A crossover study in young schizophrenic children. *Current Therapeutic Research, 19,* 70-86.

Campbell, M., Andersson, L. T., Meier, M., Cohen, I. L., Small, A. M., Samit, C., & Sachar, E. J. (1978). A comparison of haloperidol, behavior therapy and their interaction in autistic children. *Journal of the American Academy of Child and Adolescent Psychiatry, 17,* 640-655.

Campbell, M., Anderson, L.T., Small, A. M., Perry, R., Green, W. H., & Caplan, R. (1982). The effects of haloperidol on learning and behavior in autistic children. *Journal of Autism and Developmental Disorders, 12,* 167-175.

Campbell, M., Cohen, I. L., & Small, A. M. (1982). Drugs in aggressive behavior. *Journal of the American Academy of Child Psychiatry, 21,* 107-117.

Campbell, M., Grega, D. M., Green, W. H., & Bennett, W. G. (1983a). Neuroleptic-induced dyskinesias in children. *Clinical Neuropharmacology, 6,* 207-222.

Campbell, M., Perry, R., Bennett, W. G., Small, A. M., Green, W. H., Grega, D., Schwartz, V., & Anderson, L. (1983b). Long-term therapeutic efficacy and drug-related abnormal movements: A prospective study of haloperidol in autistic children. *Psychopharmacology Bulletin, 19,* 80-83.

Campbell, M., Adams, P., Perry, R., Spencer, E. K., & Overall, J. E. (1988a). Tardive and withdrawal dyskinesia in autistic children: A prospective study. *Psychopharmacology Bulletin, 24,* 251-255.

Campbell, M., Adams, P., Small, A. M., Curren, E. L., Overall, J. E., Anderson, L. T., Lynch, N., & Perry, R. (1988b). Efficacy and safety of fenfluramine in autistic children. *Journal of the American Academy of Child Psychiatry, 27,* 434-439.

Campbell, M., Overall, J. E., Small., A. M., Sokol, M. S., Spencer, E. K., Adams, P., Foltz, R. L., Monti, K. M., Perry, R., Nobler, M., & Roberts, E. (1989). Naltrexone in autistic children: An acute open dose range tolerance trial. *Journal of the American Academy of Child and Adolescent Psychiatry, 28,* 200-206.

Campbell, M., Anderson, L. T., Small, A. M., Locascio, J. J., Lynch, N. S., & Choroco, M. C. (1990). Naltrexone in autistic children: A double-blind and placebo controlled study. *Psychopharmacology Bulletin, 26,* 1 (in press).

Cohen, D. J., Caparulo, B. K., Shaywitz, B. A., Bowers, M. B., Jr. (1977). Dopamine and serotonin metabolism in neuropsychiatric disturbed children. *Archives of General Psychiatry, 34,* 545-550.

Cohen, I. L., Campbell, M., Posner, D., Small, A. M., Triebel, D., & Anderson, L. T. (1980). Behavioral effects of haloperidol in young autistic children. *Journal of American Academy of Child Psychiatry, 19,* 665-677.

Deykin, E. Y., & MacMahon, B. (1979). The incidence of seizures among children with autistic symptoms. *American Journal of Psychiatry, 136,* 1310-1312.

Ekman, G., Miranda-Linné, F., Gillberg, C., Garle, M., & Wetterberg, L. Fenfluramine treatment of 20 autistic children. *Journal of Autism and Developmental Disorders,* 1989 (in press).

Engelhardt, D. M., & Polizos, P. (1978). Adverse effects of pharmacotherapy in childhood psychosis. In M. A. Lipton, A. di Mascio & K. F. Killam (Eds.), *Psychopharmacology* (pp 1463 - 1469). New York: Raven Press.

Fish, B. Methodology in child psychopharmacology. In D. H. Efron, J. O. Cole, J. Levine & J. R. Wittenborn (Eds.), *Psychopharmacology, A Review of Progress, 1957-1967.* Public Health Service Publication No. 1836. Washington, DC: US Government Printing Office, 1968, pp 989-1001.

Fish, B., Shapiro, T., & Campbell, M. (1966). Long-term prognosis and the response of schizophrenic children to drug therapy: A controlled study of trifluoperazine. *American Journal of Psychiatry, 123,* 32-39.

Geller, E., Ritvo, E. R., Freeman, B. J., & Yuwiler, A. (1982). Preliminary observations on the effects of fenfluramine on blood serotonin and symptoms in three autistic boys. *New England Journal of Medicine, 307,* 165-169.

Gillberg, C., & Svendsen, P. (1983). Childhood Psychosis and Computed Tomographic Brain Scan Findings. *Journal of Autism and Developmental Disorders, 13,* 19-32.

Gillberg, C., Svennerholm, L., & Hamilton-Hellberg, C. (1983). Childhood psychosis and neuroamine metabolites in spinal fluid. *Journal of Autism and Developmental Disorders, 13,* 383-396.

Gillberg, C., Terenius, L., & Lönnerholm, G. (1985). Endorphin activity in childhood psychosis: Spinal fluid level in 24 cases. *Archives of General Psychiatry, 42,* 780-783.

Golden, R. R., Campbell, M., & Perry, R. (1987). A taxometric method for diagnosis of tardive dyskinesia. *Journal of Psychiatric Research, 21,* 233-241.

Greenhill, L. L., Solomon, M., Pleak R., & Ambrosini, P. Thioridazine versus Molindone in Conduct Disorder. Paper presented at the Symposium, Neuroleptics in Children: Efficacy and Side Effects, 140th Annual Meeting of the American Psychiatric Association, Chicago, IL, May 9-14, 1987.

Herman, B. H., Hammock, M. K., Arthur-Smith, A., Egan, J., Chatoor, I., Zelnik, N., Appelgate , K., & Boeckx, R. L. Effects of naltrexone in autism: Correlation with plasma opioid concentrations. American Academy of Child and Adolescent Psychiatry, Scientific Proceedings for the Annual Meeting, (2), 11-12,1986.

Kalat, J. (1978). Speculation on the similarities between autism and opiate addiction. *Journal of Autism and Childhood Schizophrenia, 8,* 477-479.

Leboyer, M., Bouvard, M. P., & Dugas, M. (1988). Effects of naltrexone in infantile autism. *Lancet,* March 26, 715.

Leventhal, B. L. Fenfluramine administration to autistic children: Effects on behavior and biogenic amines. Paper presented at the 25th NCDEU Annual (Anniversary) Meeting, Key Biscayne, Florida, May 1-4, 1985.

Meiselas, K. D., Spencer, E. K., Oberfield, R. A., Peselow, E. D., Angrist, B., & Campbell, M. (1989). Differentiation of stereotypies from neuroleptic-related dyskinesias in autistic children. *Journal of Clinical Psychopharmacology, 7,* 201 - 209.

Minderaa, R. B., Anderson, G. M., Volkmar, F. R., Akkerhuis, G. W., & Cohen, D. J. (1989). Neurochemical study of dopamine functioning in autistic and normal subjects. *Journal of the American Academy of Child and Adolescent Psychiatry, 28,* 190-194.

Naruse, H., Nagahata, M., Nakane, Y., Shirahashi, K., Takesada, M., & Yamazaki, K. (1982). A multicenter double-blind trial of pimozide (Orap), Haloperidol and placebo in children with behavior disorders, using crossover design. *Acta Paedopsychiatrica, 48,* 173-184.

Panksepp, J. (1979). A neurochemical theory of autism. (TINS) *Trends in Neuroscience, 2,* 174-177.

Panksepp, J., & Sahley, T. L. (1987). Possible brain opioid involvement in disrupted social intent and language development in autism. In E. Schopler & G. B. Mesibov (Eds), *Neurobiological Issues in Autism* (pp. 357-372), New York: Plenum Press.

Perry, R., Campbell, M., Green, W. H., Small, A. M., Die Trill, M. L., Meiselas, K., Golden, R. R., & Deutsch, S. I. (1985). Neuroleptic-related dyskinesias in autistic children: A prospective study. *Psychopharmacology Bulletin, 21,* 140-143.

Perry, R., Campbell, M., Adams, P., Lynch, N., Spencer, E. K., Curren, E. L., & Overall, J. E. (1989a). Long-term efficacy of haloperidol in autistic children: Continuous vs. discontinuous drug administration. *Journal of the American Academy of Child and Adolescent Psychiatry, 28,* 87-92.

Perry, R., Nobler, M. S., & Campbell, M. (1989b). Case Report: Tourette-like symptoms associated with chronic neuroleptic therapy in an autistic child. *Journal of the American Academy of Child and Adolescent Psychiatry, 28,* 93-96.

Pickar, D., Vartanian, F., Bunney, W. E. Jr., Maier, H. P., Gastpan, M. T., Prakash, R., Sethi, B. B., Lideman, R., Belyaev, B. S., Tsatsulkovskaja, M. V. A. et al. (1982). Short-term naloxone administration in schizophrenic and manic patients. *Archives of General Psychiatry, 39,* 313-319.

Polizos, P., & Engelhardt, D. M. (1980). Dyskinetic and neurological complications in children treated with psychotropic medication. In W. E. Fann, R. C. Smith, J. M. Davis & E. F. Domino (Eds.), *Tardive Dyskinesia. Research and Treatment* (pp 193-199). Jamaica, NY: Spectrum Publications.

Polizos, P., Engelhardt, D. M., Hoffman, S. P., & Waizer, J. (1973). Neurological consequences of psychotropic drug withdrawal in schizophrenic children. *Journal of Autism and Childhood Schizophrenia, 3,* 247-253.

Realmuto, G. M., August, G. J., & Garfinkel, B. D. (1989). Clinical effect of buspirone in autistic children. *Journal of Clinical Psychopharmacology, 9,* 122-125.

Ritvo, E. R., Yuwiler, A., Geller, E. M., Saeger, K., & Poltkin, S. (1970). Increased blood serotonin and platelets in early infantile autism. *Archives of General Psychiatry, 23,* 566-572.

Ritvo, E. R., Freeman, B. J., Geller, E., & Yuwiler, A. (1983). Effects of fenfluramine on 14 outpatients with the syndrome of autism. *Journal of the American Academy of Child Psychiatry, 22,* 549-558.

Ritvo, E. R., Freeman, B. J., Yuwiler, A., Geller, E., Yokota, A., Schroth, P., & Novak, P. (1984). Study of fenfluramine in outpatients with the syndrome of autism. *Journal of Paediatrics, 105,* 823-828.

Ritvo, E. R., Yuwiler, A., Geller, E., Schroth, P., Yokota, A., Mason-Brothers, A., August, G. J., Klykylo, W., Leventhal, B., Lewis, K., Piggott, L., Realmuto, G., Stubbs, E. G., & Umansky, R. (1986). Fenfluramine treatment of autism: UCLA collaborative study of 81 patients at nine medical centers. *Psychopharmacology Bulletin, 22,* 133-140.

Sananman, M. L. (1974). Dyskinesia after fenfluramine. *New England Journal of Medicine, 291,* 422.

Schuster, C. R., Lewis, M., & Seiden, L. S. (1986). Fenfluramine: Neurotoxicity. *Psychopharmacology Bulletin, 22,* 148-151.

Shell, J., Spencer, E. K., Curren, E. L., Perry, R., Die Trill, M. L., Campbell, M., Lynch, N., & Polonsky, B. Long-term haloperidol administration and intellectual functioning in autistic children. Paper presented at the Annual Meeting of the American Academy of Child and Adolescent Psychiatry, Washington, D.C., October 21-25, 1987.

Strayhorn, J. M. Jr., Rapp, N., Donina, W., & Strain, P. S. (1988). Randomized trial of methylphenidate for an autistic child. *Journal of the American Academy of Child and Adolescent Psychiatry, 27,* 244-247.

Tarjan, C., Lowery, V. E., & Wright, S. W. (1957). Use of chlorpromazine in two hundred seventy-eight mentally deficient patients. A. M. A. *Journal of Disturbed Children, 94,* 294-300.

Walters, A. S., Barrett, R. P., Feinstein, C., Mercurio, A., & Hole, W. The treatment of self-injury and social withdrawal in autism with naltrexone. Paper presented at the Eastern Psychological Association Meeting, Boston, MA, March 1989.

Weizman, R., Weizman, A., Tyano, S., Szekely, G., Weizman, B. A., & Sarne, Y. (1984). Humoral-endorphin blood levels in autistic, schizophrenic and healthy subjects. *Psychopharmacology , 82,* 368-370.

Young, J. G., Kavanagh, M. E., Anderson, G. M., Shaywitz, B. A., & Cohen, D. J. (1982). Clinical neurochemistry of autism and associated disorders. *Journal of Autism and Developmental Disorders, 12,* 147-165.

Autism: Non-Drug Biological Treatments

MARY COLEMAN

INTRODUCTION

In the field of biological treatments of autistic children, therapies tend to fall into two general categories. First are the non-specific therapies which are given to any child who has autistic symptoms regardless of etiology. Dr. Campbell, who has made the major contributions to the field of pharmacotherapy in autism, has reviewed the drugs now available for this patients group. Under this category of non-specific therapies, we will look at the treatments other than drugs which have been proposed for autistic children.

The second general category of biological treatments in autism are those which depend upon specific diagnostic categories - either clinical subgroupings or laboratory classification (Table 1). Discussion of these specific therapies, including case histories, will occupy the bulk of this paper.

Finally, a look at the research literature related to new therapies either currently under unvestigation or recently proposed will be mentioned. For to discuss biological therapies in autism today is to look more to the future than to rest on any laurels of the past - this is how it appears in 1989.

NON-SPECIFIC THERAPIES OTHER THAN DRUG THERAPIES

It is important at the start of this paper to clarify exactly how the terms "specific" and "non-specific" are being used in the context of therapies for autistic children. By the

Table 1. Diagnostic categories with therapies under investigation in 1989.

	Disease entity	Therapy being tried
Laboratory classifications	Fragile X	Folic acid
	Phenylketonuria	Low phenylalanine diet
	Purine autism	Restricted purine diet
		Allopurinol
		Adenosine
	Autism with hypocalcin-uria	High calcium diet
		Calcium supplements
	Autism with lactic/ pyruvic acidosis	Ketogenic diet
		Thiamine
	Seizure disorders diagnosed by EEG-readings	Anti-convulsant drugs

	Symptom(s)	Therapy being tried
Clinical classifications	Ocular self-mutilation (with hypocalcinuria)	High calcium diet
		Calcium supplements
		Anti-convulsants
	Skin discoloration (greenish/yellow palms/ & soles, dark shadows under eyes) (with hyper-uricosuria)	Restricted purine diet
		Allopurinol
	Diarrhoea and increased autistic symptoms with intake of specific foods	Withdrawal of food from diet

term "non-specific", we refer to any therapy which is applied to an autistic child by virtue of the diagnosis itself. Such therapies, theoretically, seek to effect the final common pathway in the central nervous system which leds to autistic symptoms. The hope is that any child with such symptoms would be helped by the therapy regardless of which clinical or laboratory subgroup is used to classify the child. Most drug therapies and the therapies discussed in this section meet this criterion of being "non-specific" therapies.

In contrast, "specific" therapies are targeted therapies aimed at particular clinical or laboratory subclassifications within the autistic group as a whole. These "specific" therapies will be discussed in the next section.

Although the psychoanalytic theory of the etiology of autism still held sway, as long ago as 1961 investigators began studying the biochemistry of autistic patients. In that year Schain and Freedman described the elevation in the blood of a biogenic amine, serotonin, that was known to be present in a number of body tissues including the brain. The group studied were 23 autistic children and six of them were found to have the elevation of this body metabolite. Since then, nine additional studies (summarized in Coleman & Gillberg, 1985a) as well as five more recent studies (Ho et al., 1986; Minderaa et al., 1987; Kuperman et al., 1987; Geller et al., 1988 and Launay et al., 1988) have continued to find elevations of whole blood, platelet or serum serotonins in some autistic children. A much tinier percentage of autistic children were found to have quite low levels of this biogenic amine.

Could an imbalance in serotonin in the central nervous system, as reflected in the blood studies, be related to a final common biochemical pathway in the brain that produced autistic symptoms? One attempt to check this hypothesis by therapeutic intervention was the administration of the precursor of serotonin - 5-hydroxytryptophan (5-HTP) to autistic children with low whole blood serotonin levels (Coleman & Gillberg, 1985b). This was an unsuccessful trial with no useful clinical effect.

Serotonin is thought to be an inhibitory neurotransmitter involved in the pathways that control functioning that can be effected in autistic children - such as sleep disorders. Another pair of transmitters also closely involved in these pathways are the two catecholamines - dopamine and norepinephrine.

Catecholamines are more difficult to study in living patients since we do not have the platelet model system of the type that transports serotonin around the blood stream in a partial model of synaptosome binding. With catecholamines, we more often have to rely on their metabolites in the blood, cerebrospinal fluid or urine for study.

The most consistent catecholamine finding in autism has been an elevated level of homovanillic (HVA), the endproduct of dopamine metabolism, in the urine and cerebrospinal fluid (Cohen et al., 1974; Lelord et al., 1978; Winsberg et al., 1980; Lelord et al., 1982; Gillberg et al., 1983; Garnier et al., 1986; Gillberg & Svennerholm, 1987; Garreau et al., 1988). Studies of the catecholamines themselves, other metabolites such as MHPG and DOPAC and of the catecholamine enzymes - DBH, COMT and MAO - have resulted in more inconsistent and contradictionary results (summarized in Coleman & Gillberg, 1985c; also see Launay et al., 1987).

A depression of the very first enzyme of the catecholamine pathway results in a specific disease entity (phenylketonuria) which is discussed in the next section. Here suffice it to say that the fact of autistic symptoms in some children with phenylketonuria led to consideration of bypassing that step in all autistic children with therapeutic trials of DOPA, the third aminoacid in the pathway which was the immediate precursor of the two catecholamines themselves. (The fact that the endproduct of DOPA - dopamine metabolism (HVA) often was elevated in autistic children was not established at the time these trials were initiated.)

Ritvo and co-workers (1971) first studied the effect of L-DOPA on four hospitalized children. No changes were observed. The second study of the administration of L-DOPA by Campbell and co-workers (1972, 1976) also included the administration of dopamine agonists: D-amphetamine and L-amphetamine. Again, no clinical improvement was found. More recently, Deutsch et al., 1985 tried an L-DOPA provocative test to check the sensitivity of dopamine receptors in the hypothalamus in autistic children. In at least 30 % of the children, they found an alteration in sensitivity which also raised the question of dopamine sensitivity in other sections of the central nervous system as well.

Another approach to therapy of a non-specific type began from studying the tryptophan (precursor of serotonin) pathway in autistic children by Heeley and Roberts in 1965. In the course of a tryptophan loading test in 16 autistic children, they also administered the co-enzyme of this pathway, vitamin B 6, and found improvement in the loading test as a result. This then led to an open trial of the vitamin by Bonisch in 1968 which reported some marked improvements in some patients.

Vitamin B 6 (pyridoxine) also is the co-enzyme of the catecholamine pathway at two sites (effecting the enzymes L-AAAD and DBH) and other amino acid pathways. It is also involved in the biosynthesis of lipids, proteins, carbohydrates, nucleic acids and sphingosine bases in the central nervous system. In the brain, the vitamin is ubiquitous, underlying the non-specific nature of its effects.

Since these early trials, a number of open and double blind studies of the vitamin have been performed (summarized in Coleman & Gillberg, 1985d; Jonas et al., 1984; Martineau and co-workers, 1985, 1986, 1988) and the consensus today is that there is a subgroup of autistic patients who have some improvement of symptoms when they receive pharmacological doses of pyridoxine. It also seems clear that the clinical effects are sustained longer if magnesium is administered with the vitamin. Irritability, sound sensitivity and enuresis are less of a problem if magnesium is given simultaneously (Rimland, 1978).

No one is claiming that pyridoxine therapy totally reverses autism and there are, as yet, a number of unknowns in regard to this therapy. For example, which clinical symptoms are specifically helped by the vitamin and thus, is there anyway to anticipate pyridoxine responders versus non-responders? The role of magnesium needs further work since it may be having a separate clinical effect. Also, since I know from my own work that pharmacological doses of vitamin B 6 raise whole blood serotonin levels, should it be administered randomly in autism or should it be restricted to children with low whole blood levels of serotonin? Should it be restricted to patients with elevations of HVA?

Regarding side effects of pyridoxine, we know that sensory peripheral neuropathy can be a serious side-effect of this therapy (Schaumberg et al., 1983, Coleman et al., 1985). In adults, this may be a serious problem, while in children it is quite rare. In a study in another patients group (Down syndrome children), 0.5 % of the children developed the side effect and it appeared to be directly correlated with niacin deficiency (Coleman et al., 1985). Thus an intermittent administration of niacin during vitamin B 6 therapy is currently recommended.

In summary, none of the non-specific therapies to date have been successful in reversing the autistic syndrome. One of these therapies (vitamin B 6) does appear to help some symptoms in some patients but its precise clinical indications have not yet been worked out.

SPECIFIC THERAPIES WITH CLINICAL OR LABORATORY TARGETING

I. Laboratory indications for biological non-drug therapies

In recent years, specific subgroups of autism have begun to emerge from the general body of patients and, as these subgroups become identified, more targeted therapies become possible. The subgroups have either been identified by specific laboratory testing or, more rarely, by a clinical constellation of symptoms (see Table 1).

Fragile-X cases of autism

Among the patients who are classified by laboratory methods are a group of individuals who have an abnormality in the X chromosome at the site mapping to the vicinity of the band Xq27.3. Prevalence rates for persons with intellectual handicap and the fragile X syndrome in a public school population were 1:2610 for males and 1:4221 for females (Turner et al., 1986). According to Hagerman et al. (1983), almost half (49%) of these patients meet the DSM-III criteria for autism. Looking at the problem the other way around, screening of autistic populations have revealed rates of between 10 to 16 % positive for the fragile X marker (Blomquist et al., 1985; Watson et al., 1984).

Interestingly, a recent report on cerebellar hypoplasia in autism that found diminution of cerebellar vermal lobules VI and VII (when checked by magnetic resonance imaging techniques) did not hold up in many of the patient subgroups. In contrast, the findings in the fragile X males helped confirm the accuracy of the original report, particularly in this patient group (Reiss, 1988).

Thus, if fragile X children have a detectable structural atrophy in one portion of the brain, biochemical approaches to therapy seem less likely to be successful. Nonetheless, because the chromosomal culture yields the fragile X cells in relatively small number only when the cells are grown in a folate - deficient media, trials of oral folic acid have been undertaken in this patient group. A number of studies have been completed and, although the answer is far from clear at this point, it appears that there may be some possible benefit to younger children with virtually no hope of success for therapy started after puberty (Gillberg et al., 1986; Hagerman et al., 1986; Brown et al., 1986; Froster - Iskenius et al., 1986). More double-blind studies pinpointed to particular age-groups are needed before any definitive therapeutic recommendations can be considered.

PKU

Another group of autistic patients who have an error identifiable by laboratory testing are those with the metabolic disease, phenylketonuria (PKU). In these patients, their liver lacks the enzyme necessary to convert phenylalanine to tyrosine. The resulting shunting off of phenylalanine to minor pathways results in a number of compounds quite toxic to the brain.

Most patients with PKU are not autistic but it has been known since 1969 (Friedman) that some children with PKU are mistaken for Kanner autistics. In a recent study of 65 autistic children, who were carefully screened by standard urinary amino acid detection methods, three were found to have phenylketonuria (Lowe et al., 1980).

Since it is now possible in some families to detect PKU in utero by linkage analysis with DNA polymorphisms, this disease may become a preventable form of autism (Antonarakis, 1989). Also, thanks to infant screening, PKU can be detected in the neonatal period and adequate treatment (usually reducing phenylalanine from the diet) can be started (Berry et al., 1979). Unfortunately neonatal screening programmes miss up to 20 % of the liveborn infants in one country (the United States) (Sepe et al., 1979) so that PKU autism is not a disease of the past as it should be under ideal circumstances.

If infants with PKU are not started on treatment in the early weeks of life, they start a deteriorating course which can result, among many other neurological signs, in the development of autistic symptoms. When a child with PKU autism is detected untreated, is it of value to start treatment at such a late date? Starting the diet at later ages may have some behavioral benefit for the older child but major reversal seems out of the question (Lewis, 1959; Gruter, 1963; Lowe et al., 1980).

Purine abnormalities

Purine autism is another medical subgrouping of autistic patients. First described in 1974 in a large study of 69 patients and matched controls, (Coleman et al., 1976) in the United States, the presence ot this subgroup was confirmed in a second study in France in 1986 (Rosenberger-Debiesse & Coleman, 1986). In the American study, 22 % of the patients hade hyperuricosuria (or overexcretion of uric acid in the urine) while 29 % of the French autistic children exhibited this abnormality.

In any individual child, the question arises about whether the overexcretion of uric acid is directly relevant to the child's autistic condition, is a manifestation of a secondary effect from a primary disease process or is an incidental finding. To date, three different enzymes of the purine pathway have been found to be abnormal in one or more autistic children. They are 5-phosphoribosyl-1-pyrophosphate (PRPP) synthetase (Becker et al., 1980) adenylosuccinate lyase (Jaeken et al., 1984) and inosinate dehydrogenase (Gruber et al., 1985). However, the great majority of autistic children, when tested for these three enzymes, are negative suggesting that their disease is not primary or that there are other enzymes in the purine pathway which can be associated with autistic symptoms when the levels are abnormal.

Could it be that errors in the purine pathway will someday become to the autistic syndrome what errors in the amino acid pathway are to mental retardation? We know that purine overproduction in children is often associated with psychiatric symptomatology (reviewed in Coleman & Gillberg, 1985e).

Are there any therapies available to help this patients group? Adenosine, a purine itself, is currently undergoing trials in patients with the adenylosuccinate lyase error. For other patients, the only therapeutic tools under investigation are a diet low or restricted in purine foods or allopurinol, a xanthine oxidase inhibitor which tunes down the entire purine groups of pathways (Coleman et al., 1986).

Although most patients have no irrefutable response to restricting purines from their diet, occasionally a patient does respond. Purine foods constitute about one/fifth of the source of purines used by the body to create the essential constituents of all living cells

- free bases, nucleosides and nucleotides. Hooft and co-workers (1968) reported that a low purine diet resulted in "an undeniable improvement" in a low-functioning child with both autistic features and neurological symptoms such as choreoathetosis/spasticity. There was, however, no crossover phase in this reported case.

I would like to report on one of my cases - an autistic girl of five years of age who had hyperuricosuria of unknown etiology.

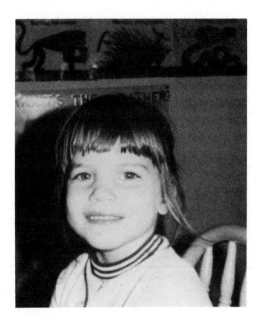

Figure 1. Patient A.

Patient A (Figure 1) had "dada" as an infant but stopped all identifiable words from 12 to 36 months. She began self-stimulations and at one point hit herself on her playpen so hard that she knocked the breath out of herself. She used adult hands as tools and toe-walked. She had refused breast-feeding because she did not like to be held and was bottle fed without being touched. Her eye contact with humans was poor, but she was fascinated by shadows, cracks, shiny objects such as straws or sticks. The child was meticulous and neat and played with toys by lining them up. She began eating glue in school, and developed a pattern of finger motions in front of her eyes.

The patient had a great uncle who is profoundly retarded with no eye contact. Beautiful as a child, he uses his hands as Patient A does so several family members now wonder if this older man might be autistic.

The only abnormality on a medical evaluation of the child was a hyperuricosuria of between 14.5 to 17.5 mg/kg/24 hours with a uric/creatinine ratio of 1.1 - 1.3. She was placed on a restricted purine diet which brought the levels down to between 7.3 - 10.6 mg/kg/24 hours. Clearance studies indicated no kidney dysfunction.

She was placed on a restricted purine diet at five years of age. At that time, her language was described as though she was "speaking from another planet" with echolalia of short phrases with the endings of words incompletely pronounced.

The child's response to the diet was fairly rapid. Only six months later, it was reported she had moved into sentence speech, used the pronoun I, lost her echolalia, began to interact for the first time with her brother, and began playing normally with toys. By one year on the diet, she had begun playing with peers, had moved to paragraph speech, stopped all self-stimulation, and developed excellent eye contact. The child progressed so rapidly that after one and one/half years on the diet, it was decided by the school system to admit her to a normal first grade classroom of 30 children and one teacher.

Because the child lived in the country, her only educational therapy during this period was a once a week speech therapy programme.

The month before admission to first grade, the child was subjected to a crossover where she was placed on high purine foods. The crossover had been planned for ten days but was stopped after three days because "she became hyperactive, like a different personality, and speeded up for days". The family has been unwilling in subsequent summers to repeat the crossover for a second time.

The girl is currently in third grade, a mostly B/C student. She still occasionally has trouble with "s" and "sh" pronunciation. She is intellectually and socially within the normal range. The family maintains her rigidly on the diet, which she likes very much. Urinary levels of uric acid remain within the normal range.

Patient A is the exception; most patients do no respond so dramatically to this diet. Leucocyte and fibroblast samples from this child and 15 other autistic patients with hyperuricosuria are currently under study at the purine laboratory at the University of California, San Diego.

For until we identify the enzyme error underlying the hyperuricosuria it will be impossible to accurately treat most of this patients group.

Hypocalcinuria

In addition to the patients with autism and overexcretion of uric acid, there is another large subgroup of patients who underexcrete calcium in the urine. In a 1976 study of 78 patients and matched controls, there was no statistically significant difference between the serum and urinary calciums in the autistic and control groups. The urinary levels showed a wide variation in both groups, with the pattern more marked in the autistic patients. In 16 of the patients, the urinary value of calcium was below two standard deviations as determined from the results in the non-autistic children (0.7 mg(kg). The lowest value recorded in a control child was 0.9 mg/kg/24 hours. Of the 16 autistic patients who had hypocalcinuria by these criteria, only one (with a urinary value of 0.0 mg/kg/24 hours) had a serum value that was below the normal range (Coleman et al., 1976).

The etiology of the hypocalcinuria in these autistic children remains unknown in spite of multiple studies trying to define its underlying cause. I would like to report on another one of my cases - a boy of five years of age who had marked hypocalcinuria as the main finding of an extensive medical work-up.

Patient B appeared to be a normal infant who developed language at 10 months of age and had phrases such as "bye bye car" and "get bath" by 11 months of age. On the day of his first birthday, he had an operation for strabismus and never spoke again. He became a toe walker, a head banger, and self-stimulated himself watching shadows. He held toys to the sun to watch their shadows rather than playing with them. He used an adult hand to reach items he could not reach. He had great difficulty with changes in routine and tolerating being in crowds of people.

At the time of the evaluation he was able to say a few single words, although he stopped for months at a time and was using a communication board. His eye contact was poor and changes in routine were a major problem. He was almost six years old when he was placed on a high calcium diet and 1800 mg of calcium supplement in liquid form.

With the diet, the child began to improve very rapidly and language accelerated rapidly. He kept being upgraded in the school system and mainstreaming was started. Finally at seven and half years of age, he was put into regular first grade. His first report card showed B/Cs except for math in which he got an A. The only subject he was not really doing well was in language.

This boy is one of eight children (out of more than 100) who were found to have hypocalcinuria and who also responded dramatically to a change in calcium intake. In none of these patients has the etiology of the hypocalcinuria been determined; this is an urgent problem for the future. In all eight cases, crossover off calcium supplementation resulted in loss of clinical improvement on a temporary basis.

Lactic acidosis

In 1985, four patients were described who had autism and the coexistent syndrome of lactic/pyruvic acidosis (Coleman & Blass, 1985). Since lactic acidosis is a non-specific finding which is found in many other disease entities, it was not clear what relevance this finding might have in terms of diagnosis or therapy. In retrospect, one of the four patients (the girl in the group) was diagnosed as having Rett Syndrome.

Just in case the blood finding might be relevant, one of the investigators (John Blass) suggested that either pharmacological doses of thiamine or the ketogenic diet be tried in this subgroup of autistic children. I would now like to describe the effect of the ketogenic diet on one of my patient who was subsequently found to have lactic/pyruvic acidosis.

Patient C was born with only four toes on each foot. His motor milestones were delayed with abdominal crawling followed by a delayed age of walking of 22 months. He first spoke around twenty months of age and developed to short phrases around four years of age. The child developed handwaving, excited jumping up and down, pica, fingers in his ears and poor socialization with peers. He had a savant quality to his auditory memory for stories. When examined, he licked the floor, bit himself and others and had marked haptic defensiveness. Medical evaluation at 5 years of age disclosed lactic acidosis.

The child was placed on the ketogenic diet. After six months, the parent reported that all self stimulation was gone, inappropriate behaviors were gone, language jumped forward, and he was able to attend a summer camp with regular children. The mother said "this child is now tuned into the world".

The child had two crossovers off the diet - one at home and one in the hospital. Marked regression occurred both times. The religious parents described one of the crossovers as "he began acting like he had the devil in him" in contrast to the cooperative normal behavior while on the diet. By seven years of age, the child was partially mainstreamed but not able to attend a regular classroom for a full day.

Again, a great deal of work needs to be done to isolate the specific enzymes which may be relevant to these cases.

Epilepsy presenting as autism

Another laboratory diagnosis that can differentiate a subgroup of autistic children in an epilepsy syndrome associated with an abnormal electroencephalogram. Although the infantile spasm syndrome is often followed by autistic symptoms and, although many autistic patients develop seizures (for review, see Coleman & Gillberg, 1985), Gillberg and Schaumann (1983) published the first cases of epilepsy presenting as infantile autism. In these two initial cases, the accurate diagnosis by EEG resulted in a more successful and appropriate treatment by the use of an anti-convulsant of the type suggested by the EEG readings.

In further studies, this research group did a population-based study of autism and found epilepsy in 20 % of the cases. Although all types of seizure disorders were found, almost 75 % had psychomotor epilepsy (Olsson et al., 1988). These researchers established that epilepsy can occur in autism in the absence of mental retardation.

It is important to clarify that this approach to the treatment of autism differs significantly from the indications for treatment in adult psychiatric disorders where the anti-convulsant, sodium valproate for example, is indicated for a treatment trial by the presence of certain clinical symptoms and the absence of abnormalities on the encephalogram (McElroy et al., 1987)

II. Clinical indications for biological non-drug therapies

Having reviewed the current laboratory indications for specific trials of therapy, we wish to touch briefly on the clinical indications which could lead to specific therapeutic approaches.

Ocular self-mutilation

Ocular self-mutilation is one of the more serious types of self-stimulation seen in autistic individuals. A paper currently in press (Coleman, in press) describes treatment of four autistics who were mutilating their eyes. In two of the patients, one eye was already blinded by the time they came for therapy. All four patients had hypocalcinuria and abnormal EEGs. In all four, a combination of a high calcium intake combined with an anticonvulsant was effective in preventing further self-abuse of the eyes. Patients with this clinical constellation of symptoms should always be studied to determine if they have hypocalcinuria and/or abnormal EEGs. This medical approach can be successful in saving the eyesight of this type of patients in some cases.

Skin discoloration

Another clinical indicator sometimes seen in an autistic indivudual is a subtle yellow/greenish color to the skin most clearly visible on the palms and soles. When this is combined with dark circles under the eyes, purine autism is sometimes found. The treatment, as described above, is a restricted purine diet with or without allopurinol. This therapy is only occasionally successful but is worth a brief trial.

Severe diarrhoea/food sensitivity

Finally, a clinical symptom often seen in autistic children is severe diarrhoea. When other known medical causes have been ruled out, a trial of removing foods such as sugar, milk or wheat has been suggested (Rimland, 1988). Data so far is anecdotal based on parent reporting. In fact, the one scientific study of wheat sensitivity (gluten loading followed by jejunal biopsies - McCarthy & Coleman, 1979) was negative even though the children selected for the study were those whose parents had reported a wheat sensitivity by diet history. However, reports of food sensitivity are a recurring theme throughout the history of autism and not enough studies have been done to put this hypothesis to rest at this time.

CONCLUSIONS

In summary, many biological treatments other than drugs have been suggested for use in autism. Review of the literature suggests that because autism is a syndrome of multiple etiologies, the best medical treatment will be one that is specifically designed for the individual patient based on individual clinical or laboratory criteria. Such approaches, however, are in their infancy. Whole new areas of research, such as neuroimmunology, may enlarge the number of diagnostic categories followed by new research therapies in the future. A chapter on the treatment of autism written ten years from now likely will be vastly different from the minuscule amount of information we have today.

REFERENCES

Antonarakis, S. E. (1989). Diagnosis of genetic disorders at the DNA level. *New England Journal of Medicine, 320,* 153 - 163.

Becker, M. A., Raivio, K. O., Bakay, B., Adams, W. B., & Nyhan, W. L. (1980). Variant human phosphoribosylpyrophosphate synthetase altered in regulatory and catalytic functions. *Journal of Clinical Investigation, 65,* 109 - 120.

Berry, H. K., O'Grady, D. J., Perlmutter, L. J., & Bofinger, M. K. (1979). Intellectual development and academic achievement of children treated early for phenylketonuria. *Developmental Medicine and Child Neurology, 21,* 311 - 320.

Blomquist, H., Bohman, M., Edvinsson, S., Gillberg, C., Gustavson, K. H., Holmgren, G., & Wahlström, J. (1985) Frequency of the fragile X syndrome in infantile autism. *Clinical Genetics, 27,* 113 - 117.

Brown, W. T., Cohen, I., Fisch, G., Wolf-Schein, E. G., Jenkins, V. A., Malik, M. N., & Jenkins, E. C. (1986). High dose folic acid treatment of fragile X males. *American Journal of Medical Genetics, 23,* 263 - 271.

Campbell, M., Small, A. M., Collins, P. J., Friedman, E., David, R., & Genieser, N. (1976). Levodopa and levoamphetamine: a crossover study in young schizophrenic children. *Current Therapies Research, 19,* 70 - 86.

Campbell, M., Fish, B., David, R., Shapiro, T., Collins, P., & Koh, C. (1972). Response to triiodothyronine and dextroamphetamine - a study of preschool schizophrenic children. *Journal of Autism and Childhood Schizophrenia, 2,* 343 - 358.

Cohen, D. J., Shaywitz, B. A., Johnson, W. T., & Bowers, Jr, M. B. (1974). Biogenic amines in autistic and atypical children. Cerebrospinal fluid measures of homovanillic acid and 5-hydroxyindoleacetic acid. *Archives of General Psychiatry, 31,* 845 - 853.

Coleman, M. (1989). A medical approach to self-abuse of the eyes (in press).

Coleman, M., & Blass, J. P. (1985). Autism and lactic acidosis. *Journal of Autism and Developmental Disorders, 15,* 1 - 8.

Coleman, M., & Gillberg, C. (1985). *The biology of the Autistic Syndromes.* New York: Praeger Scientific. Pages cited: a - 77; b - 185; c - 80; d - 182; e - 151; f - 45.

Coleman, M., Landgrebe, M., & Landgrebe, A. (1976a) Purine autism. In *The Autistic Syndromes.* M. Coleman (Ed.), Amsterdam: North-Holland.

Coleman, M., Landgrebe, M., & Landgrebe, A. (1976b). Calcium studies and their relationship to celiac disease in autistic patients. In *The Autistic Syndromes.* M. Coleman (Ed.), Amsterdam: North Holland.

Coleman, M., Sobel, S., Bhagavan, H. N., Coursin, D. B., Marquardt, A., Guay, M., & Hunt, C. (1985). A double blind study of vitamin B6 in Down's syndrome infants. Part I - Clinical and biochemical results. *Journal of Mental Deficiency Research, 29,* 233 - 240.

Coleman, M., Landgrebe, M., & Landgrebe, A. (1986). Purine seizure disorders. *Epilepsia, 23,* 263 - 269.

Deutsch, S. I., Campbell, M., Sachar, E., Green, W., & David, R. (1985). Plasma growth hormone response to oral L-DOPA in infantile autism. *Journal of Autism and Developmental Disorders, 15,* 205 - 212.

Friedman, E. (1969). The autistic syndrome and phenylketonuria. *Schizophrenia, 1,* 249 - 261.

Froster-Iskenius, U., Bodeker, K., Oepen, T., Matthes, R., Piper, U., & Schwinger, E. (1986). Folic acid treatment in males and females with fragile X syndrome. *American Journal of Medical Genetics, 23,* 273 - 289.

Garnier, C., Comoy, E., Barthélémy, C., Leddet, B., Garreau, B., Muh, J. P., & Lelord, G. (1986). Dopamine-beta-hydroxylase (DBH) and homovanillic acid (HVA) in autistic children. *Journal of Autism and Developmental Disorders, 16,* 23 - 30.

Garreau, B., Barthélémy, C., Jouve, J., Bruneau, N., Muh, J. P., & Lelord, G. (1988). Urinary homovanillic acid levels of autistic children. *Developmental Medicine and Child Neurology, 30,* 93 - 98.

Geller, E., Yuwiler, A., Freeman, B. J., & Ritvo, E. (1988). Platelet size, number, and serotonin content in the blood of autistic, childhood schizophrenic and normal children. *Journal of Autism and Developmental Disorders, 18,* 119 - 126.

Gillberg, C., & Schaumann, H. (1983). Epilepsy presenting as infantile autism? Two case studies. *Neuropediatrics, 14,* 206 - 212.

Gillberg, C., & Svennerholm, L. (1987). CSF monoamines in autistic syndromes and other pervasive developmental disorders of early childhood. *British Journal of Psychiatry, 151,* 89 - 94.

Gruber, H. E., Jansen, I., Willis, R. C., & Seegmiller, J. E. (1985). Alteration of the inosinate branchpoint enzymes in cultured human lymphoblasts. *Acta Biochemical Biopsy, 846,* 135 - 144.

Gruter, W. (1963). *"Angeborene Stoffwechselstorungen und Schwachsinn am Beispiel der Phenylketonurie".* Stuttgart: F. Enke Verlag.

Hagerman, R., McBogg, P., & Hagerman, P. (1983). *"The fragile X syndrome: History, diagnosis and treatment",* Colorado: Spectrum, Dillon.

Hagerman, R. J., Jackson, A. W., Levitas, A., Braden, M., McBogg, P., Kemper, M., McGavran, L., Barry, R., Matus, I., & Hagerman, P. J. (1986). Oral folic acid versus placebo in the treatment of males with the fragile X syndrome. *American Journal of Medical Genetics, 23,* 241 - 262.

Ho, H. H., Lockitch, G., Eaves, L., & Jacobson, B. (1986). Blood serotonin concentrations and fenfluramine therapy in autistic children. *Journal of Pediatrics, 108,* 465 - 469.

Jaeken, J., & van den Berghe, G. (1984). An infantile autism syndrome characterised by the presence of succinylpurines in body fluids. *Lancet, 2,* 1058 - 1061.

Jonas, C., Etienne, T., Barthélémy, C., Jouve, J., & Mariotte, N. (1984). Interet clinique et biochimique de l'association vitamine B6 and magnesium dans le traitement de l'autisme residuel a l'age adulte. *Therapie, 39,* 661 - 669.

Kuperman, S., Beeghly, J., Burns, T., & Tsai, L. (1987). Association of serotonin concentration to behavior and IQ in autistic children. *Journal of Autism and Developmental Disorders, 17,* 133 - 140.

Launay, J-M., Bursztejn, C., Ferrari, P., Dreux, C., Braconnier, A., Zarifian, E., Lancrenon, S., & Fermanian, J. (1987). Catecholamine metabolism in infantile autism: a controlled study of 22 autistic children. *Journal of Autism and Developmental Disorders, 17,* 333 - 347.

Launay, J. M., Ferrari, P., Haimart, M., Bursztejn, C., Tabuteau, F., Braconnier, A., Pasques-Bondoux, D., Luong, C., & Dreux, C. (1988). Serotonin metabolism and other biochemical parameters in infantile autism. *Neuropsychobiology, 112,* 1 - 19.

Lelord, G., Callaway, E., Muh, J. P., Arlot, J. C., Sauvage, D., Garreau, B., & Domenech, J. (1978). L'acide homovanilique urinaire et ses modifications par ingestion de vitamine B6: exploration fonctionnelle dans l'autisme de l'enfant? *Revue Neurologique, 134,* 797 - 801.

Lelord, G., Calloway, E., Muh, J. P., & Martineau, J. (1982). Clinical and biological effects of high doses of vitamin B6 and magnesium on autistic children. *Acta Vitaminologica et Enzymologica, 4,* 27 - 44.

Lewis, E. (1959). The developemnt of concepts in a girl after dietary treatment for phenyketonuria. *British Journal of Medical Psychology, 32,* 282 - 287.

Lowe, T. L., Tanaka, K., Seashore, M. R., Young, J. G., & Cohen, D. J. (1980). Detection of phenylketonuria in autistic and psychotic children. *Journal of the American Medical Association, 243,* 126 - 128.

Minderaa, R. B., Anderson, G., Volkmar, F., Akkerhuis, G. W., & Cohen, D. J. (1987). Urinary 5-hydroxyindoleacetic acid and whole blood serotonin and tryptophan in autistic and normal subjects. *Biological Psychiatry, 22,* 933 - 940.

Martineau, J., Barthélémy, C., Garreau, B., & Lelord, G. (1985). Vitamin B 6, magnesium and combined B 6-Mg: therapeutic effects in childhood autism. *Biological Psychiatry, 20,* 467 - 478.

Martineau, J., Barthélémy, C., & Lelord, G. (1966). Long-term effects of combined vitamin B 6-magnesium administration in an autistic child. *Biological Psychiatry, 21,* 511 - 518.

Martineau, J., Barthélémy, C., Cheliakine, C., & Lelord, G. (1988). Brief report: an open middle-term study of combined vitamin B6-magnesium in a subgroup of autistic children selected on their sensitivity to this treatment. *Journal of Autism and Developmental Disorders, 18,* 435 - 447.

McElroy, S. L., Keck, P., & Pope, H. G. (1987). Sodium valproate: its use in primary psychiatric disorders. *Journal of Clinical Pharmacology, 7,* 16 - 24.

Olsson, I., Steffenburg, S., & Gillberg, C. (1988). Epilepsy in autism and autistlike conditions: a population-based study. *Archives of Neurology, 45,* 666 - 668.

Reiss, A. (1988). Cerebellar hypoplasia and autism. *New England Journal of Medicine, 319,* 1152 - 1153.

Rimland, B., Callaway, E., & Dreyfus, P. (1978). The effects of high doses of vitamin B6 on autistic children. A double-blind crossover study. *American Journal of Psychiatry, 135,* 472 - 475.

Ritvo, E. R., Yuwiler, A., Geller, E., Kales, A., Rashkis, S., Schicor, A., Plotkin, S., Axelrod, R., & Howard, C. (1971). Effects of L-DOPA in autism. *Journal of Autism and Childhood Schizophrenia, 1,* 190 - 205.

Rosenberger-Debiesse, J., & Coleman, M. (1986). Brief report: preliminary evidence for multiple etiologies in autism. *Journal of Autism and Developmental Disorders, 16,* 385 - 392.

Schain, R., & Freedman, D. (1961). Studies of 5-hydroxyindole metabolism in autistic and other mentally retarded children. *Journal of Pediatrics, 58,* 315 - 320.

Schaumburg, H., Kaplan, J., Windebank, A., Vick, N., Rasmus, S., Pleasure, D., & Brown, M. J. (1983). Sensory neuropathy from pyridoxine abuse. *New England Journal of Medicine, 309,* 445 - 448.

Sepe, J., Levy, H. L., & Mount, F. W. (1979). An evaluation of routine follow-up blood screening of infants for phenylketonuria. *New England Journal of Medicine, 300,* 606 - 609.

Turner, G., Robinson, H., Laing, S., & Purvis-Smith, S. (1986). Preventive screening for the fragile X syndrome. *New England Journal of Medicine, 315,* 607 - 609.

Watson, M. S., Leckman, J. F., Annex, B., Breg, W. R., Boles, D., Volkmar, F. R., & Cohen, D. J. (1984). Fragile X in a survey of 75 autistic males. *New England Journal of Medicine, 310,* 1462.

Winsberg, B. B., Sverd, J., Castelles, S., Hurwic, M., & Perel, J. M. (1980). Estimation of monoamine and cyclic-AMP turnover and amino acid concentrations in the spinal fluid of autistic children, *Neuropediatrie, 11,* 250 - 255.

Psychodynamically Oriented Psychotherapy in Autism

SHEILA SPENSLEY

INTRODUCTION

Since 1943, a formidable number of research hours have been devoted to the testing of hypotheses concerning autism. Exploratory investigations into its possible causes have been so wide-ranging as to result in propositions as diverse as parental death-wishes towards the autistic child (Bettleheim, 1967) to the presence of abnormalities in his brain (Hutt et al., 1964; Rimland, 1964). In this paper I shall limit my considerations to those theories which concern the psychologial theories of autism. Here, broadly speaking, two lines of thinking can be distinguished; that which restricts itself to formulations concerning conscious and cognitive processes, and that which is pursued by psychologists whose theories include factors deriving from the unconscious mind. It is my view that fewer incompatibilities exist between cognitive and psychodynamic views of autism than are believed to exist and I hope that I may be able to contribute something towards a clarification of the issues and the *apparent* differences which so far have tended to be regarded as irreconcileable.

The development of two disparate lines of thinking about autism, which emanated from Kanner's work, has been unfortunate, yet understandable, and perhaps hardly surprising. In outlining the syndrome in 1943, Kanner drew attention to specific *psychological* phenomena which aroused immediate interest and curiosity, stimulated intense intellectual controversy and have continued to stir not inconsiderable passions ever since. It may not be without its significance that the autistic condition, one of such inaccessability and seeming impregnability, should stir such a degree of curiosity and determination to overcome or remove the enigma.

The drive towards understanding and finding meaning in the world has characterised man since pre-history and his development of knowledge and imagination differentiates him from other animals. Nevertheless, as Immanuel Kant began to expound in the eighteenth century, all of our knowledge of the world and of ourselves rests on the evidence of the senses and is dictated, therefore, by our biological make-up. We get most of our knowledge of the outside world through the eye, whilst hearing gives us a knowledge of other people in the world and how they perceive the environment. The primary significance of the sensory and perceptual apparatus and its integral place in our psychological *and intellectual* evolution is something which deserves re-emphasis in the context of understanding autism. In much of the literature, autism is referred to as a biological handicap (Rutter, 1976) and, I think, care must be exercised to avoid encouraging an implicit assumption that this puts the problem beyond the confines of psychological understanding, as if its biological nature was specific to autism and sufficient to assume a baseline impenetrable to understanding and meaning.

Psychodynamic theories of autism have, as yet, received little serious attention in the world of academic child psychiatry and psychology and are seldom mentioned, except to make passing reference to their fundamental misguidedness. Clinical and experimental evidence abounds to support the view that the autistic child has impairments of a social and cognitive order and it is widely assumed that this is enough to conclude that all theories dealing with intra-psychic dynamics can be eliminated. Such assumptions, particularly prevalent in England, derive from misconceptions about the level of modern psychoanalytic theory and also from generalisations about the clinical practices of child psychotherapists.

In presenting a case for the psychodynamic understanding of autism, a good deal of clarification is required to establish the facts and to dispel the fictions attaching to psychoanalytic theory and practice. Two broad questions will be addressed in this paper - 1. How do psychoanalytic psychotherapists really think about autism? 2. How is their thinking applied in therapeutic practice?

In the first section of this paper, I shall begin by establishing the common ground between cognitive and psychodynamic theories of autism and also take up the more salient criticisms levelled at psychotherapy and psychoanalysis. In the second section, I shall present a brief outline of contemporary and post-Freudian, theoretical developments and their relevance to the understanding of autistic phenomena. Finally, I shall consider the applications of such thinking - to clinical practice in individual treatment, to the problems of management in institutions and also to the further development of the theory of borderline and psychotic conditions.

AREAS OF AGREEMENT

The symptoms of infantile autism appear very early in life and the emotional detachment and social isolation of children with autism, led Kanner to the view that this was a disturbance of affective contact (Kanner, 1943). He described the syndrome as one which distinguished a group of children who "differed markedly and uniquely from anything so far reported". These children did not fit satisfactorily into either of the two possible existing categories - mental retardation and psychosis. Much investigation, research and discussion have subsequently gone into defining autism and it would be inappropriate in this paper to attempt to cover the detail of our decades of work. The main thrust has been towards establishing certain unequivocal criteria concerning developmental delay and this has been positively achieved.

Hermelin and O'Connor (1970) in a variety of experiments demonstrated a degree of retardation based largely on inability to encode stimuli in a meaningful way; and Frith (1970) has shown that children with autism make little use of meaning in their memory and thought processes. Abnormality of language has also been established as an important feature of autism (Ricks, 1975; Martlew, 1987). The accumulating evidence of cognitive and communicative disorder seems to urge the conclusion that the crucial feature in autism is a cognitive deficit and that this underlies all the other impairments of functioning.

Rutter, the most distinguished exponent of this point of view, has argued this diligently and persuasively in many places (Rutter, 1976, 1983, 1985). In a paper entitled Cognitive Deficits in the Pathogenesis of Autism (Rutter, 1983), he has made this position unequivocal.

"All of this research emphasises that much of affect and conation depend on cognitive capacities of one type or another ...... the general idea of interconnections and the notion that cognitive deficits may underlie social or emotional features is not special to autism. Rather, it is a central tenet of developmental psychology and psychiatry". Here, Rutter touches the heart of the matter. Contrary to prevailing belief, there is no dispute between cognitive and psychodynamic psychologists about the existence or extent of cognitive impairment, nor of developmental delay. Psychotherapists, as much as anyone else, can be indebted to empirical research. We cannot but take confidence from the experimental confirmation of intuitive clinical experience. The differences lie, not in conflicting views about diagnosis or definition, but about the predisposing factors, their nature and their order in the developmental disruption. In pursuing the task of identifying "the specifics of connection ...... and the direction in which the causal arrows run" (Rutter, 1983), cognitive psychology would seem to be backing one direction and psychotherapy the other. This creates the danger of a false antithesis, as if cognition and affect were alternative routes leading to different solutions.

With agreement on cognitive deficit and developmental disturbance, I shall turn next to the question of psychosis. Kanner, himself, was interested in the similarities between the withdrawal states of schizophrenia and those found in autism, and he expressed the view that the two conditions would ultimately be linked (Kanner, 1951). Subsequent studies of schizophrenia have not inclined to support the prediction but, instead, have increasingly drawn attention to the many significant differences between the two. Comparisons of the characteristics of onset and distribution, the symptomatology and the course of the illnesses, have established marked differences, sufficient to conclude that they are not the same and that infantile autism is not a form of early onset schizophrenia.

Again, we are in agreement. Psychoanalytic psychotherapists would agree that autistics are not like schizophrenics and that important characteristics differentiate the two. I would add, however, that whilst schizophrenia throws little light on autism, it does not necessarily follow that autism cannot illuminate schizophrenia. I shall return later to consider further this reversal of "causal arrows".

Another major criticism concerns the appropriateness of psychotherapy in the treatment of autism. A commonly held misapprehension is based on the findings that autistic children make little use of imaginative and symbolic play (Wing et al., 1977; Wing, 1980). It is then mistakenly assumed that this rules out a therapy in which fantasy and imagination usually form the core, since it requires mental capacities inappropriate to the developmental level of autistics.

The absence of symbolism and imagination is not in dispute - that much is accepted as an established central feature in autism. However, psychotherapy, as the name implies, is therapy for the psyche; and the psyche's early developmental problems are as relevant to the work of the psychotherapist as are the irregularities of its later functioning.

Psychotherapy is, above all, an observational method of working and it affords the opportunity to study, in minute detail, the characteristics both of relationship *and failure* of relationship. Not all psychotherapists undertake work with autistic children; but the few who do, understand that they are dealing with a level of primitivity which requires its own conceptual framework. The charge that all psychotherapists are naive and attempting to impose on the problems of developmental failure, concepts suited to higher levels of functioning, has to be refuted.

The most distinguished and influential psychotherapist working on the psychoanalytic treatment of autism, is Frances Tustin. She has developed new conceptual formulations to encompass the phenomena of autism and her insights have influenced the work of child psychotherapists internationally. Her writing, rooted in her clinial experience of autistic children, has been widely appreciated also by psychoanalysts working in adult psychosis. Continuing in the tradition of Freud, her own thinking also owes much to the contributions of Klein and Bion.

CONTEMPORARY PSYCHOANALYTIC THEORY

The critics of psychoanalysis seem, almost always, to content themselves with a reading of Freud - and that usually confined to his early work - on which to base their judgements. Outside the circles of practising psychoanalysts and psychotherapists, the steady progress of the thinking which has followed since Freud is virtually unknown. The result has been that contemporary psychotherapists find themselves criticised on the basis of theoretical views which they do not hold; and I would like to say something now in emphasis of the important advances of theory and practice which have been made since 1895.

In a line of development from Freud, the work of Abraham, Klein, Bion and others has clarified and deepened our understanding of intra-psychic processes and, in so doing, the gulf between the concepts of mind and brain has narrowed rather than widened. The "self" is a mind-body concept, consistent with a developmental process which is seen as psycho-biological.

Klein did not address the phenomena of autism although she did describe one child, Dick, (Klein, 1930) in whom the clinical picture certainly suggested a diagnosis of autism. She remained puzzled on the question of diagnosis - which was hardly surprising more than a decade before Kanner's syndrome was discovered. With characteristic percipience, she noted, however, that the condition seemed to be "an inhibition in development and not a regression". Symbolism had not developed, she said, and there was also a lack of any affective relationship to the things around him.

Melanie Klein's major contribution to the theory of psychoanalysis lies in her concept of projective identification (Klein, 1946) and its part in the development of the processes of communication and attachment between mother and infant. This theory has advanced the understanding of psychotic functioning by giving an account of the primitive, infantile object-relationships which characterise the initial dependent feeding situation and have a bearing on the future patterns of behaviour and on the potential for achieving satisfactory personal relationships throughout life. Kleinian theory assumes a degree of relatedness from birth, and Mrs. Klein had difficulty in fitting Dick's pathology to her theory.

Not until the theoretical contributions of Wilfred Bion, building on the work of Klein and Freud, do we have a psychoanalytic theory relevant to the problems of autism. Bion's Theory of Thinking, which encompasses both its normal and disturbed development, does, I believe, have a considerable relevance to the debate concerning the links between cognition and affect. Whether the autistic state is considered in terms of a cognitive deficit (Rutter, 1983), an inability to process stimuli meaningfully (Hermelin & O'Connor, 1970), a failure of object constancy (Anthony, 1958), a lack of empathy

(Hobson, 1986), or the absence of a theory of mind (Baron-Cohen, 1987) - all descriptively accurate - Bion's Theory of Thinking deals with a level of primitive functioning subordinate and, therefore, common to all. Bion regards thinking as dependent on the successful outcome of two main mental developments. The first is the development of thoughts and the second the development of an apparatus for processing them. This may immediately sound odd because it runs counter to the popular conception of thoughts as the *products* of thinking. It is usually assumed that people think thoughts, so it is important to grasp the fundamentally different position from which Bion begins. One does not think a thought, one has a thought that has to be "thunk"! Thinking, he believes, has been brought into existence in the human being as a result of the pressure of thoughts and not the other way around.

Psychopathological developments may be associated with either of the phases, so there might be a breakdown in the development of thoughts or a breakdown of the apparatus for thinking, or both. Thoughts are classified by Bion, according to the nature of their developmental history, into three stages: 1. pre-conceptions, 2. conceptions or thoughts, 3. concepts. Pre-conceptions are really inborn dispositions corresponding to an expectation. You might consider that the baby has an innate expectation that there will be a nipple to go in the mouth or that the male infant might come equipped with a disposition to feel that there is somewhere for his penis to go. Pre-conceptions are a kind of *a priori* knowledge and come close to Kant's concept "empty thought". They do not have to be taught; but when a pre-conception, such as the breast, comes into contact with the breast itself, then the pre-conception is mated with an awareness of the realisation and this is synchronous with the development of a conception. Conceptions will, therefore, be constantly conjoined with an emotional experience of satisfaction. When the pre-conception is mated with a frustration, however, not a realisation, so that the expectation of a breast is matched with no breast available for satisfaction, this mating is experienced as "no-breast" or "absent breast". Depending on the degree of frustration and the capacity to tolerate frustration, this situation leads either to avoidance or evasion when the frustration cannot be tolerated or to the *thought* of "no breast", which can then be thought *about* thus helping to reduce the frustration and bridge the gap between the moment of recognition of need and the moment when appropriate action can result in the satisfaction of the need. The development of thinking thus bridges the gap created by frustration and the capacity to tolerate frustration helps the psyche to develop thinking.

In the relatively mature state of being able to tolerate frustration, the negative realisation of a "no-breast" becomes a thought of the absent breast kept in mind. When frustration is too great, or the capacity to tolerate frustration too weak, what should become a thought becomes, instead, a bad object indistinguishable from a thing-in-itself and fit only to be got rid of - evacuated. This means a major disturbance of the apparatus for thinking and there takes place instead, an accentuation of the use of all the apparatus of projection for the purposes of ridding the psyche of bad objects. Instead of a process of thinking which could be thought of as resembling digestion, the model approximates evacuation and the evacuation of a bad breast becomes synonymous with obtaining satisfaction from a good one. The crux lies in the degree of toleration of frustration and the choice between a digestive model of thinking, accompanied by satisfaction and an evacuative one linked with relief. This is a theory which brings affect into the heart of cognition. When early experiences go well enough for frustration to be tolerable, then normal thinking proceeds on the lines of a digestive process. Commonplace terms, like "taking in", "chewing over", "digesting" and "food for thought" demonstrate the familiarity of this model. If frustration is intolerable, for whatever reason, thoughts are treated as indistinguishable from bad objects and the appropriate machinery, not an apparatus for thinking or digesting thoughts, but one for ridding the psyche of accumulations of bad internal objects.

The potential thought is evacuated, mind is "blown" and identity "spaced out". The dominance of this model confuses the distinction between subject and object and this contributes to the absence of any perception of "twoness". The evacuative model thus impairs the learning capacities and in the absence of satisfaction disposes to repetition. When relief and emptying are equated with taking in and satisfaction, a very different developmental path lies ahead. The prevalence of emptying, pouring, repetitive and ritualistic behaviour in autistics is already well known but the links with obsessional/compulsive disorders deserve more attention.

In schizophrenia, the evacuation of thoughts is apparent in delusions and hallucinations, where the thoughts and percepts are expelled and located elsewhere than in the mind of the patient. However, fragments of an awareness of an "other" remain, in that the projected thoughts are usually enshrined in parts of an"other" like eyes watching , ears listening or voices instructing. For the schizophrenic, then, it is the painfulness of perceptual confusions that he longs to escape from.

At the expense of meaning, the autistic avoids the confusion because he has rid himself of all awareness of the "other". Divorcing himself from auditory and sensual contacts, he no longer differentiates between the animate and the inanimate and is thrown back predominantly on the visual to find a way in a world, not confused or distorted but, instead, random and unpredictable or arbitrary.

The dislocation is not simply an inter-personal one, as between mother and infant, but also an intra-personal bifurcation between mind and body. Frances Tustin has written in detail (Tustin, 1981) about this early failure of sensual communication in which the autistic child's defensive encapsulation against such contact also prevents the development of his own sensual differentiation and integration. The earliest forms of communication, with an infant are established through direct physical contact and this has significance for intra-personal, as well as inter-personal relatedness.

I wish to stress here the primordial level of development which is being addressed in the psychoanalytic theory and treatment of autistic children; also to counter the objections and scepticisms which have sprung from misconceptions that psychotherapists do not appreciate the endogenous nature of the disturbances involved.

PSYCHODYNAMIC PERSPECTIVES ON TREATMENT AND MANAGEMENT

In this section, I should like to look at the applications of psychoanalytic thinking and practice in relation to the needs of autistic children. I shall first of all consider the opportunities for individual treatment and then discuss the ways in which this kind of thinking can also be beneficial to other workers in the field, faced with the day-to-day problems and demands of providing a viable and constructive setting for the long term caretaking of those consigned to institutional care. Finally, I shall refer to the contribution which I think the study of autism is beginning to make to the further understanding of adult pathology.

Treatment

The psychotherapeutic treatment of autistic children has to be lengthy and intense, requiring attendance four or five times per week. The result is that few are treated within the National Health Service in Britain and treatment places are only likely to be found in training institutions like The Tavistock Clinic. It is the view of Frances Tustin, following thirty years experience of treating psychotic and autistic children, that some autistic children respond well to psychotherapy. Particularly when treatment is begun at the earliest opportunity (before four years, if possible), a successful outcome can be achieved in the restoration of the learning function. A number of follow-up accounts have been reported by her of the adult careers of former child patients (Tustin, 1989). Most of the children treated had a diagnosis of autism and some were described as psychotic. Of those she has been able to follow up, she gives individual accounts of their subsequent personal and academic development. The most outstanding among them are two cases of children with diagnosed autism, one treated between six and eleven years. Both have subsequently reached a university level of education. The evidence here of the effectiveness of psychotherapy remains unmeasured but, notwithstanding, it carries enough conviction to merit serious attention.

While early treatment has been found to be the most effective (Tustin, 1981) it is unfortunate that many children are not referred for psychotherapy until parents become desperate. Delay is often unwittingly encouraged by professionals wishing to mitigate the anxieties of parents and supporting beliefs that children may grow out of their peculiarities. Critical opportunities can be lost in this way and, if autistic entrenchments are allowed to continue beyond the age of six or seven years, the child can become increasingly impregnable to the efforts of the psychotherapist. With so much emphasis on educative training in Britain, referral of autistic children for psychotherapy is haphazard. For example, a child brought to me for consultation, very late, at the age of eleven, had earlier been written off as uncooperative and uncommunicative and his parents advised against psychotherapy on the grounds that he would be unsuitable.

In private practice, a few psychoanalysts and psychotherapists treat autistic children along with larger numbers of deeply disturbed children with autistic features. My own experience confirms that of Tustin that many of these children - and the younger the better - do respond to and can be reached by consistent and supportive attention to the disrupted sense of self and to the terrors that they must suffer in experiencing once again their own feelings, without which there is no possibility of self differentation and identity.

Management

It was a lengthy experience of working in an institution for autistic and mentally handicapped children which first drew my attention to the needs of the professional carers in that field, left, it seemed, with an expectation that they should be able to succeed where others had failed. Advice was plentiful but the more instruction and training they received, the more guilty and dispirited they felt when the behavioural methods failed to produce the predicted results. In discussions with staff, it soon became apparent that the psychodynamic way of appraising the problems, which I was introducing, was offering a new perspective which was being found to be both enlightening and practically useful and these discussion groups came to form a model for the current series of Seminars offered at The Willesden Centre for Psychological Treatment, to psychologists working in mental handicap.

One example will serve to illustrate the significance of the change of direction which can take place when understanding of a problem replaces the urgency to remove it or control it.

Attention-seeking behaviour is commonly frowned upon and the following scenario is familiar. Measures are introduced to try to limit a particular child's behaviour because it is deemed attention seeking or it has become a nuisance. The new measures either increase the child's demands or produce more disturbed behaviour, or both. The member of staff begins to feel controlled by the child and increases the pressure. Feelings escalate; the child becomes an increasing problem; the member of staff feels more frustrated and guilty about not being able to maintain control; the child begins to be deemed too disturbed for that setting and recommendations begin to be heard that he needs to be removed to somewhere more suitable. It is an all too familiar sequence which can take a very different direction when time can be spent considering the possibility that an attention-seeker might require attention! It is always feared that this will result in endless demands and never in satisfaction or relief. The universality of this simple misapprehension seems to be astonishing but is rarely appreciated just how powerfully the fears of the autistic get under the skins of those who look after them.

A brief clinical vignette will perhaps emphasise more clearly the change of direction referred to.

An autistic teenager worried nursing staff greatly by his longstanding and recurrent head punching.They tried every kind of distraction and restraint without success. They held on to his hand but he would use the other. They restrained both and he would bang his head on the wall. They eventually resorted to sitting one nurse on either side, sitting on his hands as they tried to distract him with television.

One day when I was present, also feeling highly disturbed by this behaviour, I instinctively put my hands, not on his hand, but on his poor head and the result was dramatic. He stopped immediatley, poised, with his battering hand arrested in mid air.

I do not offer this as an example of a magical solution but solely to exemplify the directional change of approach to a problem which may become possible when sufficient containment of the anxiety aroused, allows for something other than prevention to be considered. To approach this problem from another angle seemed worthy of attention.

APPLICATIONS TO WORK IN ADULT PSYCHOTHERAPY

Although much of the psychotherapeutic work undertaken with individual autistic children is informed by, and dependent on, the developments made more generally in psychoanalytic theory, as I have described them, the benefits have been mutual.

Confusional states, in both children and adults are now relatively well understood and share a basic theory; but in some difficult-to-reach adults, certain problems have remained, defying the theory and creating treatment impasses. The problems concern concreteness in thinking and a level of incomprehension in otherwise intelligent patients; and Frances Tustin's understanding of the encapsulated and unintegrated states in autism is now beginning to have a relevance to these adult states, too.

As the incomprehension begins to be linked with states of mindlessness and non-experience of feeling, pockets of autistic functioning are being identified. The new perspective allows for reformulation of the patient's difficulties; understanding grows and the psychotherapeutic impasses yield to a deeper appreciation of the depth of the problem involved. We have become accustomed to the concept of the borderline psychotic state; but it may soon prove useful to add the borderline autistic state.

There may be some scepticism about the use of the term in this context, particularly among those who would encourage its restriction to a highly defined set of phenomena. On the other hand, one of the most definitive and strikingly demonstrated features of autism, absence of a "theory of mind" (Baron-Cohen et al., 1985), bears a close resemblance to some adult states in which mindlessness is complained of. I have described one such state in an anorectic patient (Spensley, 1988) and it will only be possible here, to give a brief sketch of the conditions referred to, since their illustration would require very detailed analytical descriptions.

I shall quote three patients. The first two share a history of hospitalisation, suicide attempts and marked obsessional behaviour. The third did not require hospitalisation but could not work for over a year during a period of severe depression. She also indulged secretly in self-rocking and head-banging. The diagnoses were, respectively, anorexia, psychotic depression and neurotic depression. All three were highly intelligent and educated women.

The first patient, after some years in psychotherapy, "discovered" that her own feelings had reality and validity and she commented with amazement - " I always thought that reality was what I could see outside, around me. I never thought that what I felt about anything was real or worth taking seriously".

The second patient, at the commencement of psychotherapy, spoke of a conviction that she might have lost her mind. "I feel that it is hollow and empty in my head. I wonder if I have lost my mind or something. I am terrified to let go of any thought because I might never have another - just nothingness, for ever. It is a terrible feeling and I cannot stand it".

In the third case, the patient described the fundamental para noid dilemma. She said that she did not know anything about herself or why she did the things which she, herself, considered to be mad. She then felt herself to be in the impossible position of not knowing whether to accept or reject what I had to say about her and began to feel that she would therefore require an infallible therapist to feel safe! When all the thinking capacities are felt to be in me, she then has the problem of how to know whether I am right.

She was able, herself, to see the nonsense of such a position although the dilemma posed by not knowing what goes on in her own mind remains to be worked on. On one occasion she commented "I hear what you say, but it does not go any further than my ears".

The comparative study of the features of autism and psychosis remains a promising area for research. My own interest in the links between autism and obsessional/compulsive disorder, is focusing on the dominance of the visual mode of perception, which the two conditions have in common and which suggest common origins in a level of primitive functioning which can be resorted to *in extremis*.

CONCLUSION

The psychoanalytic treatment of autistic children, though limited in Britain to the few who find National Health Service or private treatment opportunities, continues to show promise insofar as those concerned are encouraged by the results in individual cases. Whilst a number of parents, teachers and psychotherapists are convinced of the value of psychoanalytic treatment for children with autism, it is clearly not enough to make claims on the basis of belief alone. Not all child psychotherapists undertake such lengthy and demanding work. It requires dedication and courage on the part of the therapist, the parents and the child to sustain the level of highly disturbing work necessary to effect fundamental change. The way is fraught and powerful resistance to experiencing feelings and relationships have to be overcome.

It is true that child psychotherapists have been singularly reluctant to produce the evidence of their work in scientific form and this will have to change. It should not be assumed, however, that the absence of documentation means an absence of scientific rigour in treatment. Psychoanalytic theory has come a long way since 1895 and numbers of psychoanalytic psychotherapists proceed by the method of observation and hypothesis. An inherent problem in communicating results was noted by Bion (1967). Talking of the work of interpretation he said: "Fortunately for psychoanalysis, these events can be demonstrated between psycho-analyst and analysand, but unfortunately for the science they cannot be demonstrated *in the absence of the phenomena*. There is a curious parallel in the plight of the individual who cannot solve a problem of enumeration mathematically but has to resort to manipulation of the objects to be numbered."

Notwithstanding this intrinsic problem, there is reason to believe that psychoanalytic psychotherapy may contribute substantially to the understanding of autistic phenomena and that the primitive mechanisms involved may yet be found to have a universality which will add to the greater understanding of severe psychopathology, in general. In the search for specificity, the necessary diagnostic criteria of autism in children are being gradually reduced. But, to answer the question as to what set of phenomena the term autism may most precisely be applied, the field of enquiry in which the phenomena may be found, may also have to be broadened.

REFERENCES

Anthony, E. J. (1958). An aetiological approach to the diagnosis of psychosis in childhood. *Zeitschrift für Kinderpsychiatrie, 25,* 89-96.

Baron-Cohen, S., Leslie, A., & Frith, U. (1985). Does the autistic child have a "theory of mind"? *Cognition, 21,* 37-64.

Bettelheim, B. (1967). *The Empty Fortress.* New York: Collier-Macmillan London for the Free Press.

Bion, W. R. (1967). *Second Thoughts.* New York: Jason Aronson Inc.

Frith, U. (1969). Emphasis and meaning in recall in normal and autistic children. *Journal of Child Psychology and Psychiatry, 27,* 321-342.

Frith, U. (1970). Studies in pattern detection in normal and autistic children: Immediate recall of and auditory sequences. *Experimental Child Psychology, 4,* 413-420.

Hermelin, B., & O'Connor, N. (1970). *Psychological Experiments with Autistic Children.* London: Pergamon.

Hobson, R. P. (1986). The autistic child's appraisal of expressions of emotion. *Journal of Child Psychology and Psychiatry, 27,* 321-342.

Hutt, S. J., Hutt, C., Lee, D., & Ounstead, C. (1964). Arousal and childhood autism. *Nature, 204,* 908-909.

Kanner, L. (1943). Autistic disturbances of affective contact. *Nervous Child, 2,* 217-250.

Kanner, L. (1951). The conception of wholes and parts in early infantile autism. *American Journal of Psychiatry, 108,* 23-26.

Kant, Immanuel (1781). *The Critique of Pure Reason.* London: Norman Kemp Smith Macmillan Education Ltd.

Klein, M. (1930). The importance of symbol-formation in the development of the ego. In *Love, Guilt and Reparation.* London: The Hogarth Press.

Klein, M. (1946). Notes on some schizoid mechanisms. In *Envy and Gratitude.* London: The Hogarth Press.

Martlew, M. (1987). Prelinguistic Conversation. In W. Yule and M. Rutter (Eds.), *Language Development and Disorders.* London and Oxford: MacKeith Press/Blackwell.

Ricks, D. M. (1975). Verbal communication in pre-verbal normal and autistic children. In *Language, Cognitive Deficits and Retardation.* London: Butterworths.

Rimland, B. (1964). *Infantile Autism.* New York: Appleton Century-Crofts.

Rutter, M. (1983). Cognitive deficits in the pathogenesis of autism. *Journal of Child Psychology and Psychiatry, 24,* 513-529.

Rutter, M. (1985). The treatment of autistic children. *Journal of Child Psychology and Psychiatry, 26,* 193-214.

Rutter, M., & Schopler, E. (Eds.). (1976). *Autism: A Reappraisal of Concepts and Treatment.* New York and London: Plenum Press.

Spensley, S. (1988). *Bridging the Conceptual Gap in Autism Theory.* Paper presented at BPS Annual Conference, Leeds University.

Tustin, F. (1981). *Autistic States in Children.* London: Routledge and Kegan Paul.

Tustin, F. (1989). *The Protective Shell in Children and Adults.* London: Karnac (in press).

Wing, L., Gould, J., Yeates, S., & Brierly, L. (1977). Symbolic play in severely mentally retarded and autistic children. *Journal of Child Psychology and Psychiatry, 18,* 167-178.

Wing, L. (1980). *Autistic Children: A Guide to Parents.* London: Constable.

Comprehensive Treatment Program for Autistic Children and Adults in Denmark

DEMETRIOUS HARACOPOS

INTRODUCTION

The purpose of this paper is to recount our experiences with a group of autistic children and adults who have been receiving a long term comprehensive treatment during the last 25 years. The program is being run at Sofieskolen, a special school for 37 autistic children between the ages of 3 to 18. For some youngsters who have reached the age of 18, residential homes have been established. In order to provide vocational opportunities, sheltered workshops also have been started. In addition, efforts are made to fill leisure time with evening school activities, hobbies, social activities and vacation trips. The principle aim of our program is to provide autistic persons with a life style as near to the normal as possible.

Literature in the field and particularly certain professional practitioners have inspired our work over the years. With regard to the start of Sofieskolen in 1964, we have to remember especially Sofie Madsen in Denmark, a pioneer in the field, and Carl Fenichel from the League School in Brooklyn, New York. We are grateful to Eric Schopler and his colleagues at Chapel Hill, North Carolina for inspiring us with their pragmatic assessment approach and ideas about parental collaboration. Else Hansen, the former Director of Sofieskolen, was the main impetus and driving force behind much of what has happened in recent years in the education and treatment of autistic persons in Denmark. Without the continual support of the Danish National Society for Autistic Persons, as well as a special fund associated to Sofieskolen, it would not have been possible to start our comprehensive treatment program.

THE SOCIAL SYSTEM IN DENMARK

The 1950's marked the beginning of a social system, in which the improvement of services for those in need of it became the cornerstone of its policy. The basic concept was that all provisions should be in accordance with the individual's problems and needs, without creating an economical burden on the family. High level of taxation and new social laws led to the present high quality of services. These new laws and a more humane view of the handicapped led to the emergence of a new way of thinking. The intention was that all type of handicapped children has a right to education and that they should no longer be segregated in large institutions, isolated from the normal society. The five million inhabitants of Denmark live in 14 counties and 279 local districts. Programs are usually organized and administered by the counties. In the following, I will describe our long treatment program which was established in the Copenhagen county.

In Denmark the awareness of the problems and needs of autistic persons emerged parallelly to that abroad. However, a tradition in the treatment of these children began rather early in Denmark. Already in the 1920's, a treatment home for autistic children was established by Sofie Madsen. In the beginning of the 60's, Birthe Hoeg Brask related her concept of childhood psychosis and conducted her well known prevalence study (1972). During the 1960's and the 1970's facilities for autistic children were started including Sofieskolen, other special schools as well as special units and classes in the normal schools. In the late 70's and 80's energy was devoted in initiating programs for autistic adults. Denmark must be considered at the forefront, regarding the provision of facilities for autistic persons. Considering that there are only 5 million inhabitants in the country, we have established, percentage-wise, perhaps more facilities for autistic persons than any other country in the world.

DIAGNOSIS

Today there is a widespread agreement that the causes of early onset autism are primarily the result of some kind of brain abnormality, implicating a range of genetic, biochemical and neurological defects, resulting in cognitive, social and language

252

impairments as well as specific deviant behavioral patterns. Previous opinions suggesting that the causes are faulty parenting, maternal deprivation or psychological trauma are out of date. While attempts are still being made to attain a valid and reliable diagnostic classification system, it is still difficult to differentiate autism and similar pervasive developmental disorders.

The value of early infantile autism as a syndrome is well documented by Kanner (1943) and later by Rutter and Schopler (1987) and Wing (1979). It is useful to distinguish between early and late onset psychosis in terms of symptomatology, course of development, treatment and outcome (Kolvin, 1971). Likewise it is essential to recognize the difference between autism and schizophrenia in childhood. Autistic traits refer to those children who have some of the symptoms which characterize infantile autism. These traits are often seen in conjunction with language impairments, epilepsy, sensory handicap and particularly mental retardation.

In Denmark diagnostic labels such as schizophrenia-like, borderline and late onset psychosis are used with children who have a cluster of symptoms and a personality disorder that are similar or related to adult schizophrenia. In contrast to autism, these children usually have better cognitive, language and social skills. The 130 children who have been or are pupils at Sofieskolen are either autistic or have similar developmental disorders, although we have had a few schizophrenia-like children enrolled in our program. Because of the inadequacies of the present diagnostic system and the individual differences within each diagnostic category, the need for a supplementary pragmatic assessment approach is warranted.

At our program, an assessment is presented in the form of a profile, pinpointing the child's developmental level in areas such as motor skills, receptive and expressive language, imitation, perception, cognition and social skills. The assessment procedure incorporates how much prompting the child needs in the performance of specific skills. In addition, we assess the child's communicative skills, the presence and degree of bizarre and behavioral problems. Finally, we investigate the presence of other handicaps, such as epilepsy, sensory handicap, physical and motor deficiences. These aspects serve as a basis for categorizing autistic persons into 4 groups, namely 1) the profoundly retarded autistic, 2) low functioning, 3) moderately and 4) well functioning autistic persons. This type of assessment facilitates decision-making with regard to placement, grouping, deciding staff resources as well as defining educational and treatment aims.

TREATMENT PROGRAM

Today there is no treatment that can cure autism. Therefore, treatment should be organized on long term perspectives. We base a successful course of development not only on the individual's ability to adjust to the norms of the society. The main goal is to establish a meaningful existence, regardless of the degree and extent of the autistic person's handicap. We prefer to establish sheltered school, work and living environments, where groups of autistic persons can learn, work and live together.

Our treatment approach is eclectic, adapting methods to each individual child's problems and needs. In formulating priorities and goals, we attempt to distinguish between our ambitions and what the child needs in terms of his or her development. This implies that while the autistic person must learn certain rules, norms and behavior, it is important at the same time to respect their peculiarities and individual personalities. Our goal is to promote the child's skills in many developmental areas, enhance their experiences and contact with reality. This improves their chances of functioning in the least restrictive environment and adjust to the normal society.

SPECIAL EDUCATION

Special education is considered the cornerstone of our treatment program. We have found that in working with autistic children and adults, the difference between special education and therapy is largely semantic. When a teacher or parent reduces deviant behavior and at the same time fosters learning and promotes communicative and social behavior, they are doing more than teaching. Such an effort is indeed a therapeutic process. Organized and predictable daily routines, the teacher-child relationship, the use of specific adaptive methods and the activities in which the child becomes involved in, becomes the basic aspects of special education. Recognizing that autistic children reject unexpected changes in their environment, a well organized daily routine is crucial. However, it is important to systematically make gradual changes in the daily activities, so that the child can learn to cope with unpredictable events.

Special education is viewed in a reality oriented and global social context. The idea is to teach the child important functions and behavior, by simulating relevant social situations under clearly defined and controlled conditions. These learning experiences are necessary, before presenting them with the challenge of coping with similar situations in the local community. Such an activity could include setting up a cafeteria in the school, workshop or residential environment and teaching functions and behavior, that one can foresee the autistic person will meet in the local society.

Another important aspect in the special education is providing age-appropriate tasks. Under the assumption that the majority of autistic children function at a low cognitive level, traditional teaching can often result in tedious repetition of the same task. To compensate for these deficits and the child's deviant manner of reacting towards learning, the therapist can choose age appropriate and meaningful task, incorporating the necessary adaptive instructions, methods and materials. Such an approach facilitates the learning of skills and promotes generalization or the transfer of learning to new activities and situations.

TOTAL COMMUNICATION

In conjunction with special education, the development of communicative skills is given high priority. Recognizing that a majority of autistic children have severe communicative problems, such as lack of spoken language and difficulties in comprehending and using social cues, the use of alternative communication systems is practiced. These alternative systems include sign-to-spoken language, pictoral language and written language. For those children with spoken language, group situations are organized among autistic persons, together with the normal and with the family. Here the child is taught how to ask and answer questions, to use critical statements about a particular subject and learning to employ basic rules such as turn taking and not interrupting when someone else is talking.

PARENTAL COLLABORATION

An absolute "must" in our treatment program is the active involvement of parents in defining educational and treatment goals and in supporting them to be more proficient in the upbringing of their own child. In what manner and to what degree the parents are involved, is determined by mutual collaboration. Our work with parents can include grief therapeutic sessions, where a group of parents have the possibility to share and reach a recognition and understanding of the problem of having a severely impaired child. Our collaboration could include teaching parents basic techniques with regard to the enhancement of skills and the reduction of deviant behavioral patterns.

We regard parents as co-therapists and co-partners. This way of working with parents is not only influential in improving the child's development, but it serves as a means for parents to organize themselves into effective basic groups. Parental groups and organizations are important pressure groups for the establishment of treatment programs for autistic persons. In fact, many of the programs in Denmark are the result of a well organized National Society and local parental organizations. In addition, we have recently started sibling groups, where the brothers and sisters of autistic children share the problems of living with an autistic child.

SUPPORTIVE PSYCHOTHERAPY

For those autistic persons who function at a high developmental level, with comparatively good communicative skills, we incorporate in our treatment program family sessions, group talks and individual psychotherapy. Our approach is not psychoanalytically oriented. Rather, we meet the child in their here-and-now situation, dealing with vital problems which preoccupy them. This could include troublesome conflicts or problems with their parents and siblings. Such problems are dealt with by having the autistic child participate in family sessions. In group talks, the initial goal is to teach the autistic person how to communicate in group settings. These sessions are then followed by discussing problems involved in being autistic, about sexual problems or about expectations and fears regarding the future etc. Likewise, individual therapeutic sessions can have the goal to teach the child specific strategies for dealing with actual conflicts.

SPORTS

Our experience with physical training with autistic children and adults have resulted in incorporating this aspect as an integrated part of our comprehensive treatment program. A well planned movement program, promote motor skills and body awareness. Sports such as swimming, jogging and skiing not only give autistic persons a better physical condition and positive changes in body posture and movement, but it also results in marked changes in their deviant behavior. For example, it is apparent that after a 6 to 8 km jog, the autistic person is less hyperactive and shows less deviant behavior and at the same time is more attentive and responsive towards learning. In collaboration with the local sports club, we have also used physical activities as a means for promoting interaction with normal children and youngsters.

PREPARING FOR ADULT LIFE

Recognizing that the majority of autistic persons will continue to need qualified professional assistance in adult life, it is important to plan appropriate activities in the adolescent years, which can serve to prepare the autistic youngster towards a meaningful existence later in life. The improvement of vocational skills and behavior, contribute in helping them to function in a sheltered work shop. In terms of preparing the adolescent to function in a residential home, we emphasize self-help skills, home economics, appropriate social behavior and helping the adolescent to occupy themselves in a goal directed manner when left alone, so that they will be able to enjoy various leisure activities.

ADULT PROGRAM

What is necessary in order to give autistic persons a meaningful existence in adult life? As the children enrolled at Sofieskolen got older, we realized that only a few of them would be able to live, work and thrive among the normal. Therefore the need for continued treatment in adolescence and adulthood became apparent. With the concept "a life as near to the normal as possible", we have established residential homes and sheltered work shops for many autistic adults. In addition, a well organized leisure program has been initiated.

VOCATION

To meet the autistic person's needs for vocational activities and a job in adult life, we have established a variety of work shops, currently for 75 autistic adults in the Copenhagen county. These set-ups are organized so that they appear as near to a normal work situation as possible. The workshops include leather, machine, wood, textile and candlemaking work shops as well as a farm. We strive to involve the workers in the whole work process, from the purchasing of materials, performing different vocational jobs to delivering the finished products. In this way, they can realize that other peoople need the things they produce. The challenge for the staff is to find adaptive materials, instructions and methods, so that each individual can participate actively with the task at hand. Usually the products are the result of a close cooperation between the staff and the autistic youngster. In spite of their handicap and limitations, our experiences show that the majority of autistic persons are able to learn vocational skills, enabling them to produce usable and salable products.

HOMES

We have succeeded in establishing homes for many of Sofieskolens pupils. Some of these homes are for the low functioning, others for those that function at a higher level. In addition, we have recently started homes for youngsters who have reached a level of independence, where they can manage most of the daily chores and skills with only limited professional assistance. Just like in ordinary homes, daily life at the homes for autistics include chores such as housework, washing clothes, shopping, preparing meals, garden work etc. We have avoided employing cleaning and kitchen staff. The daily chores are done jointly by the staff and the autistic residents.

Within this framework, the autistic individual can further develop his skills. They are encouraged to be more responsible for their own person and develop a close relationship to their near environment. Both at home and in the outside world, situations are created, where they can learn new social skills and thereby promote their ability to interact appropriately.

LEISURE

When planning a comprehensive treatment program for autistic youngsters, leisure activities should be an integrated part of it. As many autistic youngsters get older, they are usually more willing to participate in areas of interests chosen for them. However, when left alone, they frequently return to their favorite stereotypical preoccupations. A well planned leisure program, not only serves as a variation and change to daily life's obligations, but it serves to expand their interests and hobbies and encourages them to share these activities with others.

Our leisure program includes organized evening school activities, social activities and vacation trips in Denmark and other countries. Our evening school program includes areas of interests such as dance, sports, music, arts and crafts etc. Our annual ski trips to Norway are today supplemented with summer hikes in the mountains of Norway, Sweden and France as well as enjoyable vacation trips to Greece, Italy, Bulgaria and other European countries.

RESULTS

Results from follow up studies suggest that the majority of children with early infantile autism and similar pervasive developmental disorders have a poor prognosis, (Lotter, 1978; Gillberg & Steffenburg, 1987). Particularly, the use of spoken language and intellectual scores are considered important factors in determining social adjustment in later life. On the basis of these studies, the majority of autistic persons can end up in maximum sheltered environments. This could mean placement in large institutions or hospitals or a life completely dependent on the care of their own families. While these prognostic factors cannot be refuted, the general criteria for these studies emphasize the person's ability to function independently in the normal society. The effect of long term comprehensive treatment has, as yet, not been thoroughly investigated.

Characteristic for many programs throughout the world is intensive help in childhood, with a tendency to terminate treatment and desert these children and their families in the troublesome adolescent years. Since childhood is only a small portion of an individual's life and since most autistic persons will need to live and work in a sheltered environment the rest of their lives, it is important to think in long term perspectives when planning programs for autistic persons. Thus, the question at hand in planning programs is not only to determine if the child has a good, fair, or poor prognosis, but to define conditions and organize treatment, so that each individual, regardless of the extent of his handicap, can have a meaningful existence rather than a miserable one. In effect, a positive personality development can be sustained only if working and living conditions are developed and maintained in adulthood, tailored to each individual's problems and needs.

A preliminary study conducted at Sofieskolen, has shown that it is possible to establish a meaningful life for many of our autistic youngsters and adults. Throughout our 25 years of existence, 93 persons completed their schooling at Sofieskolen. Many of them were pupils throughout their entire childhood. In addition, 37 pupils are presently enrolled at Sofieskolen, meaning that Sofieskolen has given treatment to 130 autistic persons. Of the 93 persons who have finished their schooling at Sofieskolen, we have collected data on 87.

Of these 87, 36 live in homes especially initiated for autistic individuals and 46 work at one of our sheltered workshops. Most of these persons are more or less well placed. A few of them can function in less restrictive environments, while a few need a more sheltered set-up. Of the 51 persons that do not live in one of our homes for autistic persons, 8 live in mini-institutions for the mentally retarded (most of them are well placed), 8 are placed in adult psychiatric clinics, 9 live in their own apartments and 26 live with their parents. The conditions for those who continue to live with their parents vary.

For some, especially those who have a relevant job, their daily existence is satisfactory. Only 4 who are still living with their parents are without some kind of vocational occupation.

For some parents, it is a demanding and strenuous job to have their autistic son or daughter living at home, especially in those families where the parents are old. For those living in their own apartments, many of them would thrive better if they lived together with others of their own age. Obviously, the 8 persons who are placed in adult psychiatric hospitals are in need of an alternative treatment.

Even though we can note a positive development with many autistic adults, it is not unusual that some undergo a serious crisis in their early and middle 20's. For example, it has been necessary to hospitalize 7 residents at an adult psychiatric clinic. Luckily, in all cases, they have returned to their homes. This underlines the importance of creating an adult program for autistic persons. Actually many well functioning autistic youngsters and adults often suffer crises. A well functioning person can, concurrently with a positive development, reach a painful recognition of their limitations. They begin to experience problems in coping with the outside world. They have difficulties to live up to the norms and expectations of society and to realize their inner dreams and wishes - a loving relationship, a job in the normal society and finding and maintaining friendships among the normal. These realities can result in depression, inner turmoil, anxiety and self-isolation.

Nine of Sofieskolens previous pupils are working in the normal society. All of them had good language and cognitive skills as children and were able to develop and use them in adult life. However, a life in the normal society is not synonymous with that this group is doing well. While some of them have jobs, they are living a somewhat lonely and monotonous social life. None of them are married or have established durable friendships or loving relationships. Perhaps these individuals would be functioning better today if we had provided better professional assistance.

CONCLUSION

The results of this preliminary study, suggests that approximately 70% of Sofieskolens previous pupils are living a totally or partially "meaningful" existence. We feel, we have the necessary knowledge and experience to know what needs to be done to create a meaningful program for autistic children, youngsters and adults. However, in order to cover the increasing need of residential and working opportunities for autistic adults, new facilities are demanded. There is also the need to organize a system, including more effective professional assistance, for those autistic persons who can partly or fully manage a life in the normal society. Another problem to consider is how to plan the future for those autistic adults over 40 years of age.

REFERENCES

Brask, B. H. (1972). A prevalence investigation of childhood psychoses. In Nordic Symposium on the Comprehensive Care of the Psychotic child. Oslo: Barnepsykiatrisk Forening.

Gillberg, C., & Steffenburg, S. (1987). Outcome and prognostic factors in infantile autism and similar conditions. A population-based study of 46 cases followed through puberty. *Journal of Autism and Developmental Disorders, 17,* 271-285.

Haracopos, D. (1988). *What about me: Autistic children and adults.* Copenhagen: Andonia Press (printed in Danish).

Kanner, L. (1943). Autistic disturbance of affective contact. *Nervous Child, 2,* 207-250.

Kolvin, L. (1971). Diagnostic criteria and classification of childhood psychosis. *British Journal of Psychiatry, 118,* 381.

Lotter, V. (1978). Follow-up studies. In M. Rutter & E. Schopler (Eds.), *Autism: A Reappraisal of Concepts and Treatment.* New York: Plenum Press.

Rutter, M. , & Schopler, E. (1987). Autism and pervasive developmental disorders: Concepts and diagnostic issues. *Journal of Autism and Developmental Disorders, 17,* 159-186.

Wing, L., & Gould, J. (1979). Severe impairments of social interaction and associated abnormalities in children. Epidemiology and classification. *Journal of Autism and Developmental Disorders, 9,* 11-30.

Exchange and Development Therapies (E.D.T.) for Children with Autism: A Treatment Program from Tours, France

CATHERINE BARTHELEMY, LAURENCE HAMEURY and
GILBERT LELORD

The aim of the proposed method is to promote exchanges between the child with autism and his environment by taking into account the functions of socializing, communication and adaptation (Lelord et al., 1978). It is set within a physiological framework (Lelord, 1989).

Preliminary observations have shown that reeducation of "basic" functions, such as vocal expression, attitude, posture and gait, sensori-motor activity, coordination of movements and of respiration can improve the functioning of young adults with autism who are aloof and inactive (Lelord et al., 1970). These observations have been confirmed in children (Lelord et al., 1975; Barthélémy-Gault & Larmande, 1977).

Results obtained during the past decade have shown that structures exist within the reticular activating system in the brain whose role it is to modulate afferent sensory information and to regulate the processing of this information, as well as of efferent motor output. These dopaminergic innervated structures (Coleman & Gillberg, 1986; Gillberg et al., 1983) participate in the processes of selective attention (Le Moal et al., 1977; Oades, 1982; Bouyer et al., 1986), perception (Sigfried & Bures, 1979; Antelman et al., 1975), association (Miller et al., 1981), intent (Iversen, 1984; Simon & Le Moal, emotions (Thierry et al., 1976; Lavielle et al., 1978; Tassin et al., 1980) and motricity (Kelly et al., 1975; Koob et al., 1984) and even of communication (Rolls, 1981). These structures also assure the constancy of these perceptive, emotional or motor activities over time (Damasio, 1979; Muller, 1985). Such functions are severely disturbed in infantile autism (Lelord and co-workers, 1985, 1986).

The present work describes the functions which are disturbed in autism, as well as the possibilities of reeducating them.

I - Detection and evaluation of dysfunction by clinical and electrophysiological methods

Some methods complement clinical and psychological examinations, others are based on physiological principles.

1. The usual clinical examination includes repeated interviews with the family and careful examination of the child (complementary examinations (vision, hearing, neuromotor function, etc)). The results are entered into a detailed individual observation record of the child and his family. This observation record is updated weekly. The clinical examination comprises an evaluation of autistic behavior (Barthélémy, 1986), cognitive difficulties (Adrien, 1988), language difficulties (Dansart et al., 1988) neurological signs (Garreau et al., 1987a) and psychosocial disturbances (Hameury et al., 1989).

The psychological examination includes the detailed observation of past history and of the behavior of the child (E2 scale of Rimland, Leddet et al., 1986; B.O.S. scale of Freeman, Adrien et al., 1987) plus a series of tests (based on the work of Piaget) which describe sensori-motor and cognitive-social functions (Adrien, 1988).

An evaluation of disturbances affecting the major psychophysiologic functions is carried out based on the behavior summarized evaluation scale (B.S.E.) of Lelord and Barthélémy (Lelord et al., 1981; Barthélémy et al., 1989). The main items of this scale are outlined in Table 1.

2. Electrophysiology contributes to the understanding of dysfunctions shown by children with autism.

"Evoked potentials" are variations in cerebral electrical potential brought about by environmental stimuli. They enable "cerebral electrical behavior" to be observed in response to these stimuli. Using the method of stimuli with different intensities, Bruneau and co-workers (1987) showed two types of perceptive anomalies in autistic children. On the one hand, the amplitude of response was either higher or lower than that of control

Table 1. Psychological functions. The items of the behavior summarized evaluation (BSE) scale (Lelord, Barthélémy, Adrien) are classed, no longer according to the headings adapted from the DSM-III, but according to the main psychophysiological functions including contact and communication.

ATTENTION

23 Unstable attention, easily distracted

IMITATION

26 No imitation of gestures, of voice
28 Lack of sharing emotion

PERCEPTION

4 Abnormal eye contact
24 Bizarre responses to auditory stimuli
29 Odd responses to body contact
15 Auto-aggressiveness

EMOTION

11 Resistance to change and to frustration
17 Soft anxiety signs
18 Mood difficulties
16 Heteroaggressiveness

ASSOCIATION

9 Inappropriate relating to inanimate
   objects or to doll
19 Disturbance of feeding behavior
20 No attempt to control urine and feces

INSTINCT

22 Sleep disturbances
21 Masturbation

INTENTION

8 Lack of initiative, poor activity
13 Agitation, restlessness
10 Uses objects in a compulsive and/or
   ritualistic way

CONTACT

1 Is eager to be alone
2 Ignore people
3 Poor social interaction

TONUS

27 Hypotonia

COMMUNICATION

5 Does not make an effort to communicate
  using voice
6 Lack of appropriate facial expressions
  and gestures
7 Stereotyped vocal and voice utterances,
  echolalia

MOTILITY

12 Stereotyped sensori-motor activity
14 Bizarre posture and gait

TIMING ORGANIZATION

25 Behavioral variability

children. On the other hand, the child with autism did not modulate his response as a function of the intensity of the stimulus.

Martineau and co-workers (1987) showed that the indicator of association constituted by the visual potential evoked by conditioned sound indeed existed in the child with autism, as it did in the normal child, but it appeared later and inconstantly.

Finally, if coupling of stimuli was prolonged, it was seen that the "conditioned potential" was more irregular and more variable in the child with autism than in the normal child.

II - Electrophysiological bases of exchange and development therapies

Electrophysiology can be combined with clinical observations to define mechanisms of "acquisition". We will give three examples of this.

Free "acquisition" (Lelord & Maho, 1969). Pavlov's conditioning couples a stimulus of no specific interest, sound, with a stimulus of particular interest feeding. After coupling these two stimuli, sound acquires the properties of the particular interest and in turn causes salivation: this is the conditioning. Evoked brain potentials can also be conditioned (Lelord et al., 1958), but conditioned cerebral electrical activities are much more flexible than salivation or the conditioned movement of classical experiment. If we supply a stimulus of particular interest and from time to time introduce a stimulus of no interest, no coupling, no repetition, and no particular other conditions, characteristic conditioning responses appear: these are acquired temporary and reflect a very subtle and predominant discrimination in the cerebral cortex (Fig. 1). This is not an unspecific form of conditioning (pseudo-conditioning), but on the contrary a specific process: free acquisition (Lelord & Maho, 1969). This process can be demonstrated not only by electrophysiological methods, but also by detailed observation of behavior (Lelord & Massion, 1963). This is not a particular form of electrophysiological conditioning, but a very general biological process.

Facilitating role of temporal sequences. If two stimuli follow each other at regular time intervals, considerable modifications of the evoked brain potentials are observed. Initially, the amplitude of response to the first stimulus increases. If we then do not present the second stimulus, a "phantom" response appears at the moment this stimulus would have been applied (time conditioning).

The extent of these modifications is substantial when the second stimulus causes motor activity. For example, if we couple sound with percussion on the Achilles tendon (Achilles reflex), the sound causes a slow wave of anticipation (Ragazzoni et al., 1982). There are similarities between the conditioned responses and the free acquisition responses.

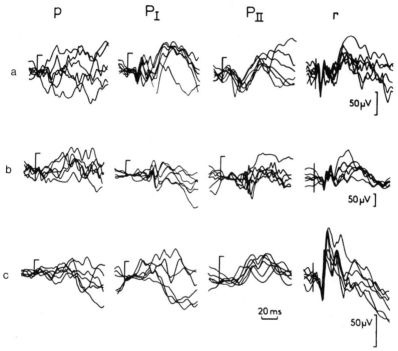

Figure 1. Acquired electrocortical responses. These responses are recorded in the cerebral cortex zone which receive the stimuli constituting a center of interest (region of Pavlov's unconditional stimulus) in 3 different individuals (a, b, c).

p: response to a stimulus without interest applied with no particular protocol (Pavlov's extinction)

r: strong response to an interesting stimulus

p II: response to the uninteresting stimulus after coupling these stimuli with the interesting stimulus (Pavlov's conditional response)

p I: response to the uninteresting stimulus after occasional application of the interesting stimulus (free acquisition).

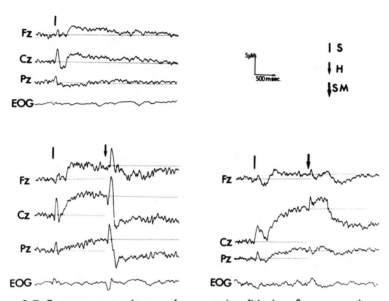

Figure 2. Reflex movement and temporal sequence (conditioning of a movement).

Fz: frontal region

Cz: central region (vertex)

Thin vertical line: sound

Thin vertical arrow: barely painful stimulation of the sciatic nerve

Thick vertical arrow: percussion of Achilles heel

The succession of sound and a stimulation causing a reflex movement (Hoffman's reflex or the Achilles reflex) leads to the appearance of a slow wave on the fronto-central area Fz and Cz, whose preparation is very similar to the premotor wave described in the preparation of voluntary movement. The mechanisms described are similar to those referred to by Schopler (1989) in his description of the structured environment.

There are similarities between the conditioned responses and the free acquisition responses.

One of the interesting clinical correlates in this respect is that gesture can exert an inhibitory effect on sensory influx and thus, for instance on pain. In the dentist's chair, we often clench a fist to diminish the intensity of the pain. This common place experience is "confirmed" by electrophysiology. A gesture, whether it be acquired or voluntary, can diminish or suppress variations in brain potential caused by a sensory and even somesthetic stimulus (Trouche et al., 1963).

Acquisition by mimicry. A free acquisition appears immediately if the child is presented with a filmed or televised sequence showing an actor carrying out a movement (Heuyer et al., 1957; Lelord, 1957; Moron, 1961). It is manifested by electrical activity in the motor region of the brain and appears to accompany the movement of the actor. It is specific to the extent that it depends on both the movement presented by the actor and the individual characteristics of the spectator (Fig. 3).

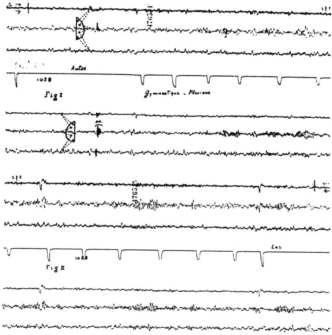

Figure 3. Imitation of movement. Electroencephalogram recorded in a spectator watching a motion picture. The spectator watches the film, in which "neutral" sequences (immobile automobiles, a lake, etc.) alternate with sequences in which an actor carries out a repetitive movement (flexion-extension of the legs or waving both arms). The centroparietal leads include bursts of rhythms at 10 cps beginning at the onset of the movement, accompany it and then stop when it terminates.

Certain principles can be derived partially from the preceding observations. They orient toward a therapy whose exclusive aim is to remedy the difficulties, the confusion and suffering experienced by a child who perceives his environment poorly and who responds poorly to its demands.

Free acquisition. Regardless of the method used, educative, psychoanalytical or neurophysiological, the therapist is present. This presence constitutes a stimulus of particular interest for the child and provides major "reinforcement". The establishment of a good relationship between the child and the therapist in a pleasant atmosphere is a prerequisite which constitutes one of the bases of the medical treatment.

Sequences. Their aim is a better modulation of perceptions and a better regulation of reactions. These sequences may be perceptive or perceptuo-motor. They are most often inserted in games. They require no particular reinforcement, since - as we have seen - the therapist is omnipresent. Certain movements endlessly repeated by the child can be used to trigger these sequences. For example, repeatedly hitting a table starts a game with a drum. Experience has shown that these oriented gestures exert not only an inhibitory effect on the excess of sensory influx, but also a sedative effect on anxiety.

Imitation. The therapist very often has recourse to imitation (gestures, mimic, regard, voice). This imitation is generally expressed during exchanges of objects or movements which familiarize the child with reciprocity.

Therapeutic exercises based on the same physiological principles are defined for each child.

Exercises of attention and modulation of perception. The aim here is to make up for the absence of "filtering" of information, thereby remedying the "cacaphonous" nature of the environment.

Exercises of association. These associations may be perceptive, e. g. association of vision with hearing, or perceptuo-motor (hearing and/or vision are associated with movement).

Exercises of constancy of attention, perception and posture-motricity. Actions are proposed which necessitate a certain continuity in order to reach a goal (construction of a train, a route, bringing the train to a bridge, etc.).

III - Method

This method has been used in the service since 1974 (Barthélémy, 1989).

1 - Examples of exchange and development therapies (E.D.T.) and the educative and therapeutic environment

In most cases, the children referred to the service are afflicted with severe autism corresponding to the criteria of the DSM III (1983), combined with retardation and other disorders, either of known etiology or idiopathic (Sauvage, 1988). In almost half the cases, clinical and neurophysiological examinations reveal neurological signs of variable intensity (Garreau et al., 1984; Lelord et al., 1986).

Various therapeutic measures are introduced either simultaneously or successively: medical and pharmacological, psychological, behavioral, educative, familial and social (Sauvage et al., 1986). Each of these therapies is evaluated (including the use of video taping) and is used intensively in group and individual sessions (Boiron et al., 1988; Dansart et al., 1988; Etourneau et al., 1988).

There are often associated disorders which require antiepileptic and/or psychotropic drugs (Barthélémy et al., 1987), hearing aid, etc. The therapy programme organized for each child also includes participation in educative activities in small groups and individual therapy, especially E. D. T.

2 - Functional analysis and general organization

Various clinical (Barthélémy, 1986; Adrien et al., 1987) psychological (Adrien, 1988; Adrien et al., 1988) and neurophysiological data (Garreau et al., 1987b; Martineau et al., 1987; Bruneau et al., 1987) used to guide therapy are gathered in the step called "functional analysis". At this time, the child is observed intensely in all aspects of life: at home, in the hospital service, taking into account the complex inter-relations which exist around him and with him.

The results of the clinical evaluations and laboratory tests are then compiled, taking into account the different functional sectors previously defined: attention-perception-association, intention-motility, contact-communication, etc. The capacities and deficits of the child in each of these sectors are analyzed. This functional evaluation is then used as the basis for elaboration and surveillance of the therapy program..

At the conclusion of this observation period, a "programming" meeting is held. The following is a list of some of the elements used in the meeting to elaborate the therapeutic program.

The main difficulties of the child are defined not only in terms of behavior disorders, but also functional disorders.

The therapeutic team is composed of two adults who alternate as therapist and observer. Certain operating details planned ahead of time enable stable and coherent markers to be maintained around the child who is horrified of change. For example, the sessions occur if possible every day at the same time and in the same place.

The sequences and games proposed during the sessions are adapted to the child as a function of his capacities, his interests and his particular dysfuntion. Activities adapted to each child correspond to these goals, e. g. exchanging a ball, pantomine songs, musical games.

3 - The sessions

Certain "golden rules" should be observed in order to facilitate selection of information and of actions and to favor the realization of oriented gestures.

First of all, stimuli arising from the environment should be limited in space and in time, in order to favor selection of information and of actions.

The environment is simplified: the room is plain, the main source of attraction is the therapist located opposite the child.

Activities are proposed one by one: when a toy is no longer used, it is discreetly removed by the therapist.

The realization of "oriented" gestures, either spontaneous or imitated, is encouraged. On the contrary agitation, strolling or pacing, disordered movements which are generally not part of the exchange sequences are not encouraged.

These principles can be applied in very different physical settings: seated opposite each other at a small table, but also in a psychomotricity room or in a wading pond.

4 - The evaluations

Each session lasts about 20 minutes. The therapist and observer then get together for a brief discussion. Comments are written in an observation notebook after each session.

The use of video taping enables the session to be observed both directly and at a later time. A video recording is made every month and more often if necessary and is used to score the different behavioral scales.

Behavior disorders are defined and quantitated with the B.S.E. scale (Lelord et al., 1981; Barthélémy, 1986; Barthélémy et al., 1988) (Table 1).

IV - Retrospective study

Fifty-nine children have been treated with E.D.T. in the service. Among these cases, 27 were sufficiently standardized and homogeneous to be used in the analysis of the results.

1 - Children treated (Fig. 4)

27 children (21 boys) between 2 and 8 years of age (21 were between 4 and 6) were included in the study. The population was composed of various clinical sub-groups.

27 CHILDREN (21 boys)

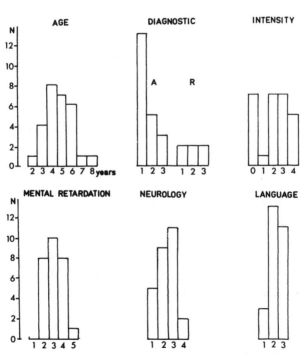

Figure 4. Distribution of the children followed on E.D.T. according to various clinical parameters.   Explanation: see next page.

N: Number of children
Age: Expressed in years
Diagnostic:

A: Autism
1 Autism + mental retardation
2 Mental retardation + autism
3 Atypical pervasive developmental disorder

R: Mental retardation
1 Mental retardation
2 Mental retardation + developmental language disorder
3 Mental retardation + attention deficit disorders

Intensity: severity of the autistic syndrome (maximum score: 4)

Retardation: intellectual quotient 1: > 70
2: 50-70
3: 35-50
4: 20-35
5: < 20

Neurology: neurological disorders 1: No disorder
2: EEG abnormalities
3: Neurological syndrome
4: Neurological syndrome associated with
   EEG abnormalities

Language: 1: normal
2: disturbed
3: absent

DSM III-diagnostic sub-groups: 18 children had autism and mental retardation (autism predominated in 13). Three children had an atypical development problem and 6 had a developmental disorder without autism.

Sub-groups as a function of expert score (intensity of autistic symptomatology). Two psychiatrists in the service attributed a score from 0 to 4 as a function of the overall intensity of the autistic syndrome observed in each child. The six retarded children had no signs of autism (score = 0), while most of the autistic children had high scores of 3 and 4.

Sub-groups as a function of I.Q. The large majority of the children were in the full scale I.Q. range of 20 to 50, i. e. had moderate to severe retardation.

Sub-groups as a function of neurological disorders. In 21 children, there were clear disturbances in the EEG, a neurological syndrome or the combination of both.

Sub-groups as a function of language disorders. Only 3 children spoke normally. Language was absent in 11 children and disturbed in 13.

2 - Distribution of the sessions

There was generally one session per day of presence of the child in the service (or 4 sessions/week). For most children, a total of 50 to 150 sessions were distributed over 1 or 2 school years (Fig. 5).

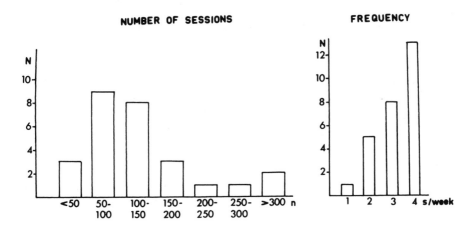

NUMBER OF SESSIONS

FREQUENCY

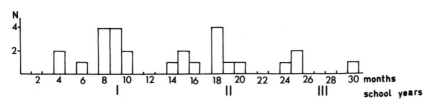

DURATION

N: number of children

nb: total number of sessions.

Frequency expressed as number of sessions per week. Total duration of the E. D. T. expressed in months and school years.

Figure 5. Modalities of application of E. D. T.

3 - Results (Fig. 6)

In each functional sector considered, the mean scores (Sc) for the group were calculated at the beginning and at the end of therapy, in individual and group situations.

In individual E.D.T. sessions (Fig. 6, top) function disorder score all decreased significantly.

When the children were observed in the small groups (Fig. 6, bottom), behaviors in sectors 1 (attention, perception), 4 (contact), 5 (communication), 6 (emotions) all improved moderately. Functions 2 (motility) and 3 (relations with objects), on the other hand, were modified only little or not at all.

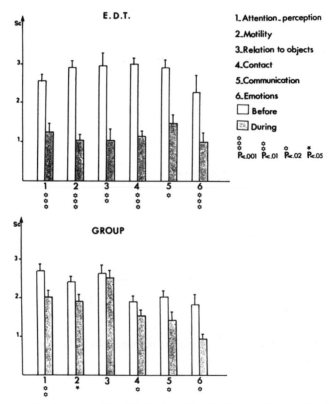

Sc: Mean score for the group (N = 27). Before: Baseline before therapy (beginning of school year). During: Evaluation at the end of the school year (8 months of therapy).

Figure 6. Changes in behavior disorders in the six functional sectors considered in an individual situation (E. D. T.) (top) and in a group situation (bottom).

Figure 7 shows the value and additional efficacy of E.D.T. when it is included in the medical and psychoeducative care program. Clinical improvement (decrease in BSE scores) is more rapid for the children benefiting from an EDT. This is especially true for the signs of autism.

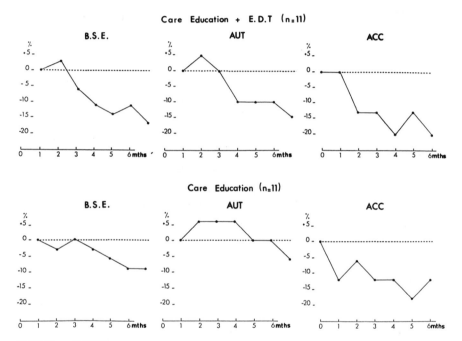

Care Education + E.D.T (n=11)

BSE: Overall BSE score
AUT: BSE sub-score corresponding to specific signs of autism
ACC: BSE sub-score corresponding to "accompanying" signs
Dotted line: Initial score (baseline)
Solid line: Mean of scores for the group of 11 children. Clinical improvement (decrease in scores) is more rapid for the children benefiting from an E. D. T. This is especially true for the signs of autism.

Figure 7. Comparative longitudinal evaluation of BSE scores for two sub-groups of autistic children benefiting from specialized care in the service with E. D. T. (11 children, top) and without E. D. T. (11 children, bottom).

V - DISCUSSION

The combined study of therapy dossiers over the past several years and the analysis of the results obtained confirm certain prior hypotheses and results. Several basic elements of the method are highlighted.

The therapies discussed here concern children between 4 and 7 years of age whose autism is associated with mental retardation. The same method is also applicable to much younger children (Sauvage, 1988). In this case, the therapy program elaborated and coordinated by the medico-educative team and social services can be partly carried out at home.

The E.D.T. sessions must be regular and frequent.

At the onset, the family is informed of the therapeutic project and may also participate in the program.

The functional analysis of behavior patterns enables the relationships between situations and conduct to be described. In order to more efficiently determine the therapeutic goals and applicable strategies to achieve them, it appeared necessary to reconsider behavior disorders as the expression of cognitive and underlying neurophysiological dysfunctions. The evaluation of these functional sectors furnished consistent markers for evaluating the efficacy of the therapy.

The function disorders most specific to autism improved concomitantly, both in individual and group sessions.

CONCLUSIONS

Certain aspects related to the applications of E.D.T. in autistic children need to be emphasized viz.:

- the implementation and organization of E.D.T. can be done only in the context of a specialized service and with the participation of a multi-disciplinary team;

- the difficulties of the child must be precisely evaluated and described in relation to somatic and psychological development;

- the E.D.T. are integrated in a personalized and multi-dimensional program of therapy, in which the family participates at the onset and regularly thereafter.

There are certain similarities between the modes of application of these therapies and the means used by mothers for thousands of years to favor the development of their child.

There are also some resemblances between the protocol of these therapies and the programs proposed by Rutter (1989), Schopler (1989) and Wing (1989).

However, the above therapies are based on physiological grounds. The combination of electrophysiological criteria with clinical characteristics enriches the observation of the child and contributes to the individualization of therapy. Constant reference to physiological data results in the possibility of modifying these therapies as a function of progress made every day in developmental neurophysiology.

ACKNOWLEDGEMENTS

The authors thank Mrs. M. Barre, H. Lehn, D. Lidret and J. Diamond for their technical assistance.

This study was supported by INSERM u316, INSERM - cNAMTS 1989, FRM 1986, Conseil Regional Region Centre and Langlois Foundation.

REFERENCES

Adrien, J. L., Ornitz, E., Barthélémy, C., Sauvage, D., & Lelord, G. (1987). The presence or absence of certain behaviors associated with infantile autism in severely retarded autistic and non autistic retarded children and very young normal children. *Journal of Autism and Developmental Disorders, 17,* 407 - 416.

Adrien, J. L. (1988). L'examen psychologique des enfants autistiques. *Neuropsychiatrie de l'Enfance et de l'Adolescence, 36,* 9 - 18.

Adrien, J. L., Barthélémy, C., Etourneau, F., Dansart, P., & Lelord, G. (1988). Etude des troubles de la communication et de la cognition d'enfants autistiques. Analyse "microscopique" de brèves séquences comportementales a cours de la passation de tests psychologiques. *Neuropsychiatrie de l'Enfance et de l'Adolescence, 36,* 253 - 260.

Antelman, S. M., Szechtman, H., Chin, P., & Fischer, A. E. (1975). Tail pinch-induced gnawing and licking behavior in rats: dependance on the nigrostritial dopa system. *Brain Research, 99,* 319 - 337.

Barthélémy-Gault, C., & Larmande, C. (1977). Les psychothérapies par modification du comportement chez l'enfant autistique. *Acta Psychiatrica Belgica, 77,* 549 - 586.

Barthélémy, C. (1986). Evaluations cliniques quantitatives en pédopsychiatrie. *Neuropsychiatrie de l'Enfance et de l'Adolescence, 34,* 63 - 91.

Barthélémy, C., Martineau, J., Jouve, J., Moraine, C., Muh, J. P., & Lejeune, J. (1987). Méthodologie d'études thérapeutiques contrôlées (vitamine B6, magnesium, haloperidol, folates, fenfluramine) chez l'enfant autistique. In F. Gremy, S. Tomkiewicz, P. Ferrari & G. Lelord (Eds.), *Autisme Infantile/ Infantile Autism.* INSERM, *146,* 265 - 272.

Barthélémy, C., Adrien, J. L., Tanguay, P., Garreau, B., Fermanian, J., Roux, S., Sauvage, D., & Lelord, G. (1988). The behavioral summarized evaluation (B. S. E.). Development and validation of a clinical assessment scale for autistic child (submitted).

Barthélémy, C. (1989). Les thérapeutiques d'échange et de développement (TED). Méthode et application. In G. Lelord, J. P. Muh, M. Petit et D. Sauvage (Eds.), *Autisme et troubles du développement global de l'enfant.* Recherches récentes et perspectives. Expansion Scientifique Française (in press).

Boiron, M., Barthélémy, C., Dansart, P., Etourneau, F., Adrien, J. L. & Langella, B. (1988). Evaluation comparée des troubles de la communication de l'enfant autistique situation individuelle et en groupe. *Actualités Psychiatriques, 4,* 33 - 36.

Bouyer, J. J., Montaron, M. P., Fabré-Thorpe, M., & Rouguel, A. (1986). Compulsive attentive behavior after lesion of the ventral striatum in the cat: a behavioral and electrophysiological study. *Experimental Neurology, 22,* 698 - 712.

Bruneau, N., Garreau, B., Roux, S., & Lelord, G. (1987). Modulation of auditory evoked potentials with increasing stimulus intensity in autistic children. *Electroencephalography and Clinical Neurophysiology, 40,* 584 - 585.

Coleman, M., & Gillberg, C. (1986). *Biologie des syndromes d'autism,* p 277. Québec et Paris: Edisem et Maloine.

Damasio, A. R. (1979). The frontal lobes. In R. M Heilman & Valenstein (Eds.), *Clinical Neuropsychology* (pp 360 - 412). New York: Oxford University Press.

Dansart, P., Barthélémy, C., Adrien, J. L., Sauvage, D., & Lelord, G. (1988). Troubles de la communication pré-verbale chez l'enfant autistique: mise au point d'une échelle d'evaluation. *Actualités Psychiatriques, 4,* 38 - 43.

DSM III - Manuel Diagnostique des Troubles Mentaux. (1983). Paris: Masson

Etourneau, F., Barthélémy, C., Lepape, G., Sauvage, D., & Lelord, G. (1988). Approche éthologique de la communication non verbale chez l'enfant autistique. *Actualités Psychiatriques, 4,* 44 - 47.

Garreau, B., Barthélémy, C., Sauvage, D., Leddet, I., & Lelord, G. (1984). Comparison of autistic syndrome with and without associated neurological problems. *Journal of Autism and Developmental Disorders, 14,* 105 - 111.

Garreau, B., Bruneau, N., & Martineau, J. (1987). Autisme et psychoses de l'enfant. Signe neurologiques et examens complementaires. *Soin Psychiatrie, 82 - 83*, 15 - 17a.

Garreau, B., Bruneau, N., Martineau, J., & Lelord, G. (1987). Etude des potentiels évoqués auditifs du tronc cérébral et de la région frontale chez l'enfant autistique. In F. Gremy, S. Tomkiewicz, P. Ferrari & G. Lelord (Eds.), *Autisme Infantile/Infantile Autism.* IMSERM. *146*, 91 - 100b.

Gillberg, C., Svennerholm, L., & Hamilton-Hellberg, C. (1983). Childhood psychosis and monoamine metabolites in spinal fluid. *Journal of Autism and Developmental Disorders, 13*, 383 - 396.

Hameury, L., Perrot, A., Adrien, J. L., Lenoir, P., Sauvage, D., & Lelord, G. (1989). L'échelle ERPS d'évaluation des facteurs psychosociaux: intérêt de l'analyse descriptive de l'environnement en psychiatrie de l'enfant. *Neuropsychiatrie de l'Enfance et de l'Adolescence* (in press).

Heuyer, G., Cohen-Seat, G., Lelord, G., Rebeillard, M. (1957). Etude EEG d'enfants inadaptés soumis à la stimulations filmique. *Revue de Neuropsychiatrie de l'Enfance et de l'Adolescence, 9 - 10*, 494 - 511.

Iversen, S. D. (1984). Cortical monoamines and behaviour. In L. Descarries, T. R. Reader & H. H. Jasper (Eds.), *Monoamine innervation of the cerebral cortex* (pp. 321 - 350). New York: Alan R. Liss,

Kelly, P. M., Seviour, P. W., & Iversen, S D. (1975). Amphetamine and apomorphine response in the rat following 6 OHDA lesions of the nucleus accumbens septi and corpus striatum. *Brain Research, 94*, 507 - 522.

Koob, G. F., Simon, H., Herman, J. P., & Le Moal, M. (1984). Neuroleptic-like disruption of conditioned avoidance responses requires destruction of both the mesolimbic and nigro-striatal dopamine system. *Brain Research, 303*, 319 - 330.

Lavielle, S., Tassin, J. P., Thierry, A. M., Blanc, G., Herve, D., Barthélémy, C., & Glowinsky, J. (1978). Blockade by benzodiazepines of the selective high increase in dopamine turnover induced by stress in mesocortical dopaminergic neurons of the rat. *Brain Research, 168*, 585 - 594.

Leddet, I., Larmande, C., Barthélémy, C., Chalons, F., Sauvage, D., & Lelord, G. (1986). Comparison of clinical diagnosis and Rimland E2 scores in severely disturbed children. *Journal of Autism and Developmental Disorders, 16*, 215 - 225.

Lelord, G. (1957). Modalités réactionnelles différentes de rythmes moyens et antérieurs à 10 c/s. *Revue Neurologique, 96*, 524 - 526.

Lelord, G., Calvet, J., Fourment, A., & Scherrer, J. (1958). Le conditionnement de la réponse évoquée électrocorticale chez l'homme. *Comptes Rendus de la Société de Biologie, 152,* 1097 - 2000

Lelord, G., & Massion, J. (1963). Etude de la réponse conditionnée de type II et des relations avec les réflexes et les comportements conditonnés. *L'Année Psychologique, 63,* 51 - 83.

Lelord, G., & Maho, C. (1969). Modification des activités évoquées corticales et thalamiques au cours d'un conditionnement sensoriel. II - Evolution des réponses avec les stades du conditionnement. *Electroencephalography and Clinical Neurophysiology, 27,* 269 - 279.

Lelord, G., Martin, A., Etienne, Th., Renaud, P., & Toulemonde, M. M. (1970). La rééducation psychomotrice d'adolescents hospitalisés en psychiatrie. *Pédopsychiatrie,* PUF, 89 - 96.

Lelord, G., Gault, C., Fremaux, T., Adrien, J. L., Larosa, M., & Bitar, F. (1975). La thérapie du comportement dans l'autisme de l'enfant. *Revue de Neuropsychiatrie Infantile, 23,* 267 - 283.

Lelord, G., Barthélémy, C., Gault, C., Sauvage, D., & Arlot, J. C. (1978). Les thérapeutic d'échange et de développement dans l'autisme grave chez l'enfant. *Le Concours Médical, 100,* 4659 - 4662.

Lelord, G., Muh, J. P., Barthélémy, C., Martineau, J., Garreau, B., & Callaway, E. (1981). Effects of pyridoxine and magnesium on autistic symptoms. Initial observations. *Journal of Autism and Developmental Disorders, 11,* 219 - 230.

Lelord, G., Hameury, L., Bruneau, N., Barthélémy, C., & Muh, P. (1985). Aspects somatique de l'autisme infantile. *Bulletin de l'Académie Nationale de Médecine, 169,* 281 - 286.

Lelord, G., Garreau, B., Barthélémy, C., Bruneau, N., & Sauvage, D. (1986). Aspects neurologiques de l'autisme de l'enfant. *L'Encéphale, 12,* 71 - 76.

Lelord, G. (1989). Les thérapeutiques d'échange et de développement dans l'autisme l'enfant. Bases physiologiques et principes. In G. Lelord, J. P. Muh, M. Petit & D. Sauvage (Eds.), *Autisme et Troubles du développement global de l'enfant. Recherches récentes et perspectives.* Expansion Scientifique Française (in press).

Lemoal, M., Stinus, L., Simon, H., Tassin, J. P., Thierry, A. M., Blanc, G., Glowinski, J., & Cardo, B. (1977). Behavioral effects of a lesion in the ventral mesencephalic tegmentum: evidence for involvement of A10 dopaminergic neurons. In E. Costa & G. L. Gessa (Eds.), *Non striatal dopaminergic neurons. Advances in Biochemistry and Psychopharmacology.* New York: Raven Press. *16,* 237 - 245.

Martineau, J., Garreau, B., Roux, S., & Lelord, G. (1987). Auditory evoked responses and their modifications during conditioning paradigm in autistic children. *Journal of Autism and Developmental Disorders, 17,* 525 - 539.

Miller, J. D., Sanghera, M. K., & German, D. C. (1981). Mesencephalic dopaminergic unit activity in the behaviorally conditioned rat. *Life Sciences, 29,* 1255 - 1263.

Moron, P. (1961). Recherche sur la motricité. Corrélations entre données d'électrencéphalographie dynamique et de tests psychomoteurs. Thèse de Médecine, Toulouse.

Muller, H. F. (1985). Prefrontal cortex dysfunction as a common factor in psychosis. *Acta Psychiatrica Scandinavica, 71,* 431 - 440.

Oades, R. D. (1982). Search strategies in a hole beard are impaired in rats with ventral tegmental damage: animal nidel for tests of thought disorder. *Biological psychiatry, 17,* 243 - 258.

Ragazzoni, A., Bruneau, N., Martineau, J., Roux, S., & Lelord, G. (1982). The topography of event related slow potentials during a reflex movement (ankle jerk) conditioning. *Psychophysiology, 19,* 386 - 392.

Rolls, E. T. (1981). Responses of amygdaloid neurons in the primate. In Y. Ben Ari. *The amygdaloid complex* (383 - 393). INSERM. Symposium no 20. Elsevier, North Holland: Biomedical Press.

Rutter, M. (1989). Psychoeducational approaches to the treatment of autistic individuals. In G. Lelord, J. P. Muh, M. Petit & D. Sauvage (Eds.), *Autisme et troubles du développement global de l'enfant. Recherches récentes et perspective.* Paris: L'Expansion Scientifique Française (in press).

Sauvage, D., Barthélémy, C., Garreau, B., Hameury, L., Adrien, J. L., Beaugerie, A., Larmande, C., & Lelord, G. (1986). Autisme de l'enfant. *La Vie Médicale,* numéro special.

Sauvage, D. (1988). Autisme du nourrison et du jeune enfant (0 - 3 ans). Signes précoces et diagnostic. Rapport de Psychiatrie présenté au congrès de Psychiatrie et de Neurologie de langue Française. Luxembourg, 2 - 7 juillet 1984. Deuxième Edition. Paris: Masson.

Schopler, E. (1989). Pedagogical treatment of autism based on an empirical research evidence. In G. Lelord, J. P. Muh, M. Petit & D. Sauvage (Eds.), *Autisme et troubles du développement global de l'enfant. Recherches récentes et perspectives.* L'Expansion Scientifique Française (in press).

Siegfried, B., & Bures, J. (1979). Conditioning composates the reglect due to unilateral 6 OHDA lesions of substantia nigra in rats. *Brain Research, 167,* 139 - 155.

Simon, H., & Lemoal, M. (1985). Influence des neurones dopaminergiques du

mésencéphal sur les processus d'attention et d'intention. *Psychologie Médicale,*
17, 933 - 945.

Tassin, J. P., Hervé, D., Blanc, G., & Glowinski, J. (1980). Differential effects of two
minutes open field dopamine utilisation in the frontal cortices of BALB/C and C
57 BL/6 mice. *Neurosciences Letters, 17,* 67 - 71.

Thierry, A. M., Tassin, J. P., Blanc, G., & Glowinski, J. (1976). Selective activation of
the mesorcortical DA system by stress. *Nature,* 263, 242.

Trouche, E., Santibanez, G., & Lelord, G. (1963). Effets sur l'amplitude des potentiels
évoqués somatiques de la phase active d'un réflexe condtionné défensif classique.
Journal de Physiologie, 55, 283 - 284.

Wing, L. (1989). Psychoeducational approaches to the treatment of autistic individuals.
In G. Lelord, J. P. Muh, M. Petit,& D. Sauvage (Eds.), *Autisme et troubles du
développement global de l'enfant. Recherches récentes et perspectives.* Paris:
L'Expansion Scientifique Française (in press).

The Nature of Behavioral Treatment and Research with Young Autistic Persons

IVAR LOVAAS, KATHERINE CALOURI and JACQUELINE JADA

INTRODUCTION

This chapter discusses some of the main research and theoretical perspectives of the behavioral treatment of autistic persons. Treatment of young autistic children will be emphasized.

Most clinical theory and practice has been derived from social psychology (such as Sullivan), personality theory (such as Freud) or developmental theory (such as Piaget). In contrast, behavioral treatment has been historically associated with experimental psychology and the field of learning and behaviour. The historical antecedents of behavioral psychology can be found in Darwin's work and that of the biologically oriented animal psychologists like Pavlov, Loeb and Watson. Treatment based on behavioral psychology also represents relatively recent developments in clinical practice. The behavioral position has frequently been misunderstood and it is important to define its essential features at the onset.

First, behavioral psychology emphasizes objective and accurate measurement of the clients' observable *behavior* rather than hypothetical constructs thought to underlie these behaviors. Second, the behavioral approach to treatment places a major emphasis on the *experimental manipulation* of the clients' present environment in order to minimize the presence of confounding variables and to establish unambiguous statements of cause and effect between therapy and therapeutic benefits. Third, behavioral work is characterized by an *inductive*, step-by-step research approach. Improvement in treatment technology is considered to occur slowly, but *cumulatively* in the sense that later technology builds on discoveries made at earlier stages of inquiry. Since behavioral treatment is so closely related to its research methodology, an understanding of one will hopefully facilitate one's appreciation of the other. Both will be discussed in this chapter.

Although developed recently, the clinical applications of behavioral techniques have grown rapidly in many areas of medicine, psychology and special education. Medicine has benefited from advances in behavioral therapy by the direct treatment of medical symptoms, like chronic pain and hypertension, and through behavioral medicine, which attempts to modify the detrimental behaviors of the medical patient and his family.

In psychology and psychiatry, behavioral techniques have been used to reduce a number of clinical problems. One of the first psychologists to utilize the theories of learning in a therapeutic setting was Joseph Wolpe (1958). He attempted to alleviate his patients of paralyzing fears, using a technique he called systematic desensitization. Other clinical applications of behavior modification techniques include the treatment of sexual disorders, self-monitoring and behavioral contracts used to control overeating, the aversive conditioning used to combat alcoholism, and the response prevention and cognitive behavior modification used in the treatment of depression and obsessive-compulsive disorders.

Behavioral methods are also widely used in academic settings, to lessen disruptive behaviors of students and to accelerate academic achievements. In addition to being useful with "normal" classroom populations, behavior modification has been a very effective teaching tool for children and adults with developmental disabilities such as mental retardation and autism (for a review of the above, see Kazdin, 1984; Martin & Pear, 1988; & Werry & Wollersheim, 1989).

The behavioral model has provided the framework for numerous studies of the treatment of autistic children. Ferster (1961) was the first investigator to employ learning theory principles derived from experimental psychology to demonstrate that autistic children could be taught that the characteristics of their learning resembled those of the average person. While Ferster's experimental manipulations involved simple and clinically non-significant tasks, the research of Wolf, Risley and Mees (1964) made use of shaping, extinction and time-out to decrease an autistic boy's tantrums and self-injurious behavior and to increase socially meaningful and appropriate behaviors. Lovaas, Berberich, Perloff and Schaeffer (1966) developed techniques based on learning theory to teach mute autistic children to imitate speech. Further approaches were devised to develop functional and meaningful speech in autistic and retarded children (Hewett, 1965; Risley & Wolf, 1967).

Today a wide variety of clients are served by a very large body of research on how to translate learning theory constructs into effective treatment and educational programs. Behavioral treatment has come to be regarded as the most effective for autistic children (DeMyer, Hingtgen, & Jackson, 1981; Werry & Wollersheim, 1989).

BEHAVIORAL ASSESSMENT OF AUTISTIC CHILDREN

In 1943, Dr. Leo Kanner hypothesized that there may be a disorder, infantile autism, which he thought had three main characteristics; one, inability to relate to people, two, an obsessive desire for the maintenance of sameness, and three, problems with language. These are general terms, and considerable effort has been expended in trying to operationally define them to facilitate agreement among observers on the nature and essence of the diagnosis. Most research in autism has followed the simple diagnostic guidelines set by Kanner and other researchers, in accordance with revisions made in the current criteria for diagnosis described in the DSM-III and DSM-III-R (American Psychiatric Association, 1980, 1987). These diagnostic manuals offer a more detailed description of what each of the defining characteristics of autism may be. Despite these additional elements, the DSM-III-R criteria remain general and diffuse.

For research purposes, it is desirable to describe behavior in a way that makes measurement of them easier. One way to achieve this is to describe the child's activities in terms of excessive, deficient and normal behaviors.

Behavioral deficiences include: (1) Gross inattention (apparent sensory deficit). The child may appear to have a hearing or vision impairment. The child may not react to loud noises or painful stimuli, may seem unable to make eye contact, and may behave as if others are not present. (2) Deficient social behaviors may be reflected in an apparent inability to play with other children and a failure to understand commonly accepted rules for conduct in public. (3) Inadequately developed emotional behaviors may be evidenced by an apparent lack of attachment to family members, a resistance to close physical contact, a minimum of common emotions (such as grief, empathy and sadness) and small likelihood of seeking comfort from others. (4) Deficient language may be evident in the areas of production of comprehension of speech, form and content of speech, or conversational skills. Autistic children can range from mute, to echolalic (repeating words) to being able to comprehend others and carry on rudimentary conversations. Language deficiency may also be exhibited in a lack of imaginative activity. (5) Deficient play skills are identified by little or no appropriate to play. (6) There is an absence of play with other children. (7) Self-help skills like dressing and toilet training may be minimal.

(8) Scores on tests of intellectual functioning most commonly fall within the retarded range.

There are two behavioral excesses: (1) Excessive aggression can be exhibited as tantrums, frustration, non-compliance, and anger. The children may physically aggress toward others, or toward themselves. Self-injurious behavior may take the form of head-banging, striking one's own eyes or ears, or biting one's own hands or shoulders. (2) An excessive degree of self-stimulatory behavior may be seen in the form of repetitive, ritualistic, monotonous and stereotyped activities like rocking, flapping hands, gazing at lights, and spinning objects. "Higher level" self-stimulation may include repeatedly singing the same song, lining up objects in a particular order, or recalling birth-dates, numerical quantities, licence-plates, etc.

The children usually exhibit a range of normal behaviors as well. (1) Normal motor development occurs, with the timely occurrence of motor milestones such as walking and an average or above average level of coordination and grace. (2) Memory is normally developed and is often demonstrated in other autistic behaviors like echolalia and insistence of sameness. (3) Special or splinter skills, like an interest in music, math or manipulating objects may also be exhibited. (4) Unusual fears, do sometimes exist, often seen in transitory or less pervasive forms in normally developing children.

BEHAVIORAL POSITION ON DIAGNOSIS AND IQ TESTING

A short note of clarification of the behavioral views on diagnosis and treatment may be helpful at this point. The position of most behaviorists on IQ testing and diagnosis is that both are useful because they sample important aspects of behavior (language, attachment to others, etc) and predict outcome. The diagnosis of autism, given independently and by recognized experts in the field, combined with IQ scores within the retarded range, virtually guarantees that the child will not reach normal functioning without treatment. This stable baseline helps to assure that changes in outcome may be attributed to treatment. A comprehensive pre-treatment evaluation also helps to assure those people from different settings who work with autistic persons that they are addressing similar kinds of clients. Thus, IQ and diagnosis should be obtained as part of a comprehensive pre-treatment assessment. Even so, one can use the diagnosis of autism and the IQ scores in prediction of outcome without addressing the theoretical constructs with which these scores have often been involved. For example, one can use IQ scores to predict educational achievement without hypothesizing that these scores are based on some unitary factor (like "g") which is immutable and resistant to environmental influences. While this hypothesis was a strongly held view in the past (and cherished by those who wished to preserve the status quo), some authorities in the field now consider IQ scores to be based on a multiplicity of separate skills, many to be modifiable by educational efforts (Weinberg, 1989).

Like the "g" factor in intelligence, the construct of "autism" is an inference based on observing the child's behaviors in various situations. The inference that there may exist a "disease of autism" underlying these behaviors is a hypothesis that may or may not be helpful in designing research and treatment efforts. In 1971, we suggested that autism is a construct that may facilitate research or may prematurely freeze or misdirect inquiry (Lovaas, 1971). Rutter (1978), referring to the construct as an "educated guess" (p. 3), holds a similar view. In other words, it is a mistake to claim that "Leo Kanner (was) the discoverer of autism" (Schopler, 1987). An example of how such a misunderstanding can lead to some very erroneous and harmful conclusions is reflected in Schopler and Mesibov's (1988) subsequent statements in which behaviorists are described as having a "disdain for diagnostic grouping .... (to) deny the value of using any diagnostic or assessment procedures" (p. 5) ".... and to foster unrealistic expectations and promises for improvement .... by avoiding IQ testing and comparisons before and after treatment" (p. 6).

The autism hypothesis has motivated a great deal of research to identify the etiology and treatment of the behaviors of autistic clients. Findings to date suggests that we may be faced with a multiplicity of problems rather than one single, all-encompassing one. The data suggests more than one etiology. There is increasing evidence that the behaviors observed in autistic children may also be observed in other diagnostic groups as well as in transitory forms in normal children. Individual differences among children diagnosed as autistic are very large. Research directed at finding the cause and cure of autism as a disease has yielded little information which is useful in treatment (see DeMyer, Hingtgen, & Jackson, 1981). It can therefore be concluded that it is of limited value to be overly concerned about a diagnosis where the functional relationships between etiology and treatment have yet to be identified. At present, the diagnosis of autism could equally well read "the diagnosis of a hypothesis". The "correct way" to diagnose autism in reality reflects different investigators' subjective opinions about what constitutes "true autism". No amount of debate will settle this issue, but future data will. It therefore seems wise to be increasingly flexible, both in our research and treatment approaches to autistic persons and in our predictions about the future for all persons so diagnosed. As was the case with the concept of IQ, perhaps we are confronted with a multiplicity of separate behaviors (language, social, emotional, ritualistic/self-stimulatory, etc.) showing little functional overlap but related to a variety of etiological and treatment interventions in unique and separate ways. Perhaps there are not only a multiplicity of neurological dysfunctions across different clients, but there may be different kinds of neurological damage underlying the different behaviors (language, emotional, social) that we attempt to correct. Some of these hypothetical neurological dysfunctions may not be responsive to pharmacological or surgical interventions, but will require psychological and educational treatments. To illustrate, one may well hope for a medication which teaches an autistic client not to cross the street in heavy traffic, but it is not wise to place too much faith in such a development.

The reservations expressed above about diagnosis and assessment should not be understood to mean that behaviorally oriented therapists and teachers minimize the importance of assessment. Rather, they mean that the diagnosis of autism does not tell a teacher or a behaviorally oriented professional a great deal about how to proceed with a particular client, or how a particular client will respond to a particular treatment. On the other hand, detailed and extensive assessment is possible and most needed after treatment has begun to assess efficacy and to guide further programming. This comes about in part because clients who are labeled autistic show extreme heterogeneity in response to treatment.

STEPS IN BEHAVIORAL TREATMENT

The establishment of a good rapport between child and therapist is critical when starting therapy. To help facilitate this, treatment begins with simple tasks that the child can readily master, and an abundance of rewards, praise and a sense of mastery. Equally important, parents and new therapists are also successful as they begin learning the variables that are involved in teaching. Both the child and the therapist are reinforced from the beginning. Depending on the client's rate of learning (which varies widely across autistic persons), up to twenty different programs may be implemented at one day, selected from the hundreds of programs which are available as treatment progresses. Due to significant differences between clients, treatment must be individualized. A great deal of ingenuity is required on the part of the parent, teachers and therapists who conduct the treatment. It is therefore   important that they maintain continuous communication and receive feedback from each other. The basic steps in treatment may sound simple, but they are based on very abstract laws which are difficult to implement unless one has a basic understanding of the underlying empirical work within learning as well as a good working knowledge of behavioral treatment as applied to these children. While a teacher/therapist can gain some proficiency in behavioral treatment after one or two weeks of close supervision, it may require two years of supervised training to become an expert in this area. It seems a common practice today (in contrast to earlier times) to call one's treatment program "behavioral". We can pose the following questions for deciding whether a program is behavioral or not: (1) Does it contain periodic and objective assessments of clients (before treatment, as well as over the days, months and years of treatment) to determine if the treatment provided has a positive, negative or no discernible effect on the client? (2) Does it employ reinforcement (shaping) procedures and not just stimulus control procedures, and (3) does the staff possess sufficient skill so as to build imitative behaviors and abstract language? A "no" to any of these questions does not justify calling a program behavioral. In any case, it is a mistake to believe that therapeutically meaningful and creative use of learning theory in treatment is either easily or simply attained.

The earliest steps in the treatment program involve the acquisition of elementary receptive language such as "stand up", "sit down", and "go to mommy". Reduction of tantrums and self-stimulation are emphasized. Once a structured learning situation has been established, treatment can proceed.

Autistic clients often do not imitate other persons. This is a critical skill for learning new behaviors and must be taught. This step typically begins with the teaching of nonverbal imitation. The child is taught to copy the therapist's bodily movements. For example, the therapist might say, "Do this," while clapping, raising arms, touching toes or nodding. The child is physically prompted to imitate this behavior and is then reinforced with food or social rewards. Imitation is defined as the establishment of a discrimination where the response resembles its stimulus, and it is built by introducing contrasting stimuli in a discrimination training paradigm. Nonverbal imitation is extended to toy play. The child is taught to imitate throwing a ball, playing with blocks or completing a puzzle. The acquisition of imitation skills allows for larger units of behavior to be mastered, and helps move the teaching away from the more tedious, step-by-step shaping. The acquisition of recreational or play skills serves to replace self-stimulatory behaviors.

Therapy advances to verbal imitation training. Imitation begins with single sounds, then combinations of sounds, then words and eventually phrases and short sentences. Verbal imitation skills are used to prompt early expressive language such as expressive object and action labels. Abstract concepts such as colors, prepositions, pronouns, and sizes are introduced next. Proficiency in verbal communication serves to decrease tantrumous behavior.

Another vital aspect of treatment is the interaction of the autistic children with more typical or average children. The exposure to nursery school is introduced in gradual steps. As with all therapy, the experience in nursery school must be structured for success. The autistic child may join the class for playground play, painting, snack time or even nap time, depending on the strengths of that particular child. The child may initially spend less than a half hour a day in school. The team of therapists decide the preschool activity in which the child may demonstrate the most success. That particular skill is then taught and mastered at home before the child attends the school setting. For example, the child may enjoy some of the simple group games such as Simon Says, Ring Around the Rosie, and Red Light/Green Light. These games are first taught and mastered at home. Thus, when the child actually attends school, she or he will have mastered that particular activity, the main problem which is left deals with the transfer of the behavior from the home to the school environment. As the child achieves success, she or he participates in a greater variety of activities, for a greater length of time.

By the time the children are ready to enter preschool, 6 to 12 months into treatment, the parents know enough about the child's treatment to select and consult with their child's teacher. Depending on how far the child has advanced during treatment, the parents are usually advised not to tell the teacher that their child was once diagnosed autistic. Diagnostic labels often implicate the parents as casual in the development of the child's problems, a destructive element which was common in the past and still exists. Rather, the teacher is informed that the child has a language delay and has had little opportunity to socialize. When the parents are choosing a classroom for their child, it is usually recommended that it be highly structured and organized and that the teacher be willing to collaborate with the parents' educational plans. This is an example of the direct parental involvement which we try to foster in treatment. An ideal therapeutic relationship exists when the parents and the teacher maintain a communicative and supportive relationship in order to exchange information and enhance the child's treatment and functioning (earlier diagnostic labels are likely to be discussed at that time).

Advanced language and formal academic topics (using the past and future tense, reading, etc.) are then introduced into therapy. Treatment soon emphasizes observational learning. Children are taught to learn by observing other children learn. This skill is vital for future school placements where teaching will no longer be on a one-to-one basis. The autistic child is taught to learn from everyday-life situations by observing the behaviors of his or her peers.

Some of the final treatment goals include teaching feeling, caring, and empathy. Therapy can also focus on teaching spontaneity, curiosity and fantasy play.

It must be emphasized that behavioral treatment progresses in very small steps, addresses many behaviors across many situations, and involves many hours of therapy that span years of effort. We consider it a mistake, harmful to both parent and child, to construct a treatment program based on the assumption that there will be sudden and major leaps forward, as is implied when one postulates the existence of a healthy child, waiting to "break out" from inside an "autistic shell". While such a position may seem attractive to many, and was widely held in the past, there is as yet no empirical data to support it.

A detailed presentation of the basic principles and processes of behavioral therapy is beyond the scope of this chapter. The reader is advised to refer to other resources such as Lovaas et al. (1980) for a more thorough presentation of the various treatment programs.

It might be useful to illustrate the structure that optimizes the treatment of autistic children. A fundamental premise is that we must approximate the learning opportunities that are available to a normal child. The normal child learns in all environments and all the time, including evenings, weekends and vacations. A myriad of behaviors is acquired in a large range of situations, taught by many persons, including peers. Autistic children, possessing unusual nervous systems, do not learn in this manner. Therefore, to provide optimal treatment and education, several adults have to be trained to provide instructions to the child for virtually all of his or her waking hours, in the home, school and community. This team initially consists of several novice therapists, one or more experienced therapists, the parents, and eventually peers. The inclusion of the parents, other family members, and peers is vital in order to generalize treatment effects. The parents are taught the techniques used with their children in an apprenticeship model. Parents observe the more experienced therapists, then gradually begin implementing therapy themselves and then teach their skills to others. The therapists provide feedback to the parents and each other on the quality of their therapy. The child learns to use her or his skills with all people in all environments rather than in one setting with one or two teachers or therapists. In addition, the family is well informed about the child's progress, the nature of the treatment and who is providing the treatment. In short, family members are given skills to direct the long-term care of their child as teaching and treatment personnel change or terminate.

YOUNG AUTISM PROJECT

We will use the Young Autism Project as an illustration of a behavioral treatment program (Lovaas, 1987). The elements of behavioral treatment discussed above were utilized to examine the effects of a particularly intense and broad-based approach to the treatment of young autistic children.

Subjects referred to the UCLA Autism Clinic, in the Department of Psychology, were accepted into the study if they met three criteria: (1) diagnosis of autism by an independent diagnostician, (2) chronological age of less than 40 months if mute, and less than 46 months if echolalic and (3) prorated mental age (PMA = 30 x MA/CA) of 11 months or more. Subjects were then divided into an experimental group (n=19) and a control group (n=19). For a period of two years, the experimental group was given forty hours of one-to-one therapy each week, whereas the control group, Control Group I, received about ten hours of one-to-one therapy per week. The assignment into groups was determined solely by the availability of therapists at the time of intake, unless the family lived more than an hour away from UCLA, in which case they were assigned to the control group.

A second control group consisted of 21 subjects who were diagnosed and treated elsewhere, had no contact with the Young Autism Project, but were matched on certain pre-treatment measures. This group primarily served to guard against the possibility that our experimental sample was unrepresentative of those children with the diagnosis of autism.

Twenty pre-treatment measures were obtained for the experimental and control groups to assure that they were comparable at intake. These included tests of intellectual, social, emotional and self-help skills. They were based on standardized psychological tests, behavioral observations and parent interviews. Intelligence tests were administered by graduate students in psychology supervised by clinical psychologists at UCLA or conducted by licensed Ph.D. clinical psychologists at other agencies. The following tests were used (listed in order of frequency of use): The Bayley Scales of Infant Development (Bayley, 1969), the Cattell Infant Scale (Cattell, 1960), the Stanford-Binet (Thorndike, 1972), and the Gesell Infant Development Scale (Gesell, 1949). The relative usage of these scales was similar in each group. The examiner modified typical testing procedures by giving reinforcers for effort and attention. It was hoped that such modifications would result in more accurate assessment of intelligence in children typically uncooperative in testing situations. Although such efforts may have elevated the test scores, three subjects from the experimental group and two from Control Group I were untestable and their mental ages were estimated from the Vineland Social Maturity Scale (Doll, 1953). All scores were converted to PMAs (30 x MA/CA) to adjust for variations in the MA scores as a function of CA at the time of testing.

A behavioral observation was videotaped for each child during free-play. Frequencies of self-stimulatory behavior, appropriate play and recognizable language were recorded and scored by blind observers.

A parental interview included questions about the child's language, toy play, self help, peer play and social interaction skills. Parents were also asked to describe the nature of their child's self-stimulatory and tantrumous behaviors.

These assessments showed that the experimental and control groups were similar before treatment was started. The first follow-up, when the children were seven years of age, assessed the child's intellectual functioning based on an IQ test and school placement. At that time, the experimental group scored higher on measures of level of functioning (IQ score and educational placement) than either control group. Forty-seven percent of the experimental group, or 9 of 19 subjects, achieved a normal level of functioning both intellectually and educationally. Eight subjects (43%) were classified as aphasic, having passed first grade in aphasia classes with a mean IQ score within the mildly retarded to low normal range of intellectual functioning (M=70, range 56-95). Only two children (10%) were placed in classes for autistic/retarded children and scored in the profoundly or severely retarded range (IQ<30). Subjects from the two control groups did not fare as well: only one subject (2%) achieved normal functioning, eighteen subjects (45%) were entered into aphasia classes, and twenty-one subjects (53%) were placed into mentally retarded classrooms. There were no significant differences between the two control groups.

A second follow-up, conducted by McEachin (1987), compared the experimental and Control Group I of the initial study with a group of normal, age-matched subjects. A double blind testing paradigm was used, involving the Wechsler Intelligence Scale for Children-Revised (Wechsler, 1974), the Vineland Adaptive Behavior Scales (Sparrow, Bella & Cicchetti, 1984), the Personality Inventory for Children (Wirt et al., 1981), and a structured clinical interview and rating. Eight of the nine experimental group children classified as normal functioning at age 6 or 7 were not identified as autistic or seriously disturbed in adolescence. They showed normal IQ, did not show emotional disturbances, had adequate levels of adaptive and social skills for their age, and were indistinguishable from a control group, of age-matched normal adolescents, in the subjective clinical impressions of blind examiners.

These findings give strong evidence for the effectiveness of an intensive behavioral treatment of young autistic children. Research by Anderson and Avery (1986) and Strain, Jamieson, and Hoyson (1985) report increases in language and intellectual functioning for young autistic children undergoing behavioral intervention. Their treatment paradigms were similar to ours, but not as comprehensive. Because the outcome from our study is so different from most other results reported in the treatment of autism, and because a more complete replication of our intervention has yet to be carried out, the results of this study are admittedly controversial and in need of questioning. One critisism of this study suggested that positive results were based on skewed subject selection, in appropriate control groups and inappropriate outcome measures (Schopler, Short & Mesibov, 1989). Also, further work is necessary to assess the relative contributions of all the components of the intervention. Nevertheless, certain methodological safeguards were implemented within the design of the study in order to increase the certainty that the improvements demonstrated in the children from the experimental condition were indeed attributable to the treatment.

(1) *Validity of the diagnosis.* To avoid concern that the children were not autistic in the first place, or that they were too young to diagnose, subjects were independently diagnosed by internationally known experts on autism, who have contributed to the formulation of DSM-III. High reliability among diagnosticians was found. Furthermore, outcome data from the control groups, comparable to the experimental group at pre-

treatment, were consistent with those reported by other investigators of young autistic children.

(2) *Assignment to treatment and control groups.* One might suggest that the children would have improved anyway, without treatment. To protect against such a possibility we used control groups: (a) assignment of subjects to control and treatment groups made as randomly as ethically possible. Similar scores between groups on 20 pre-treatment variables suggest that assignments were unbiased; (b) pre-treatment diagnostic and testing procedures were the same for all groups; and (c) subjects stayed in their assigned groups. Similarly, it could be objected that the treatment worked, but only with a select group of intellectually superior children. The subgroup of children who did recover did obviously constitute a select group (by definition), but since the correlation between intake IQ and outcome was only .58, it is unlikely that IQ constituted the most significant or only attribute of that group. Most likely, there is a "good fit" between our intervention and the kind of neurological damage which characterized the best outcome group. There is no reason to believe that present-day behavioral intervention will serve all autistic children (or all organic deviations) equally well.

It may be objected that the children who recovered "held back" during testing, yielding retarded IQ scores, but were in fact intellectually competent and well informed. A very skillful diagnostician would have been able to detect this. While this view of autistic children was widely held in the past, there are to date, no empirical data to suggest that such is the case. Autistic children suffer from major deficiencies across a large range of psychological functioning. But suppose that there existed such an occasional "hidden talent": (a) What would the probability be of assigning 9 such children to the experimental and none to the control group? (b) If the children already possessed so much competence, why did it require a minimum of 2 years of tedious, 40 hours a week, 12 months a year, of 1:1 treatment, for them to achieve normal functioning?

(3) *Spontaneous Recovery.* One could object that the favorable results in the experimental group could have occurred due to factors independent of the treatment, recovered spontaneously so to speak. However, the poor outcomes of the children in the control group who were comparable to the experimental group at intake suggest that spontaneous recovery is unlikely.

(4) *Placebo Effects.* It could be objected that the effectiveness of the treatment condition could be attributed simply to changes in the attitudes, expectations, and relationships of the children to their therapists and parents. This is unlikely for two reasons. First, children from the two control groups did not demonstrate different outcomes, yet one control group had no contact with the project. Thus, it is unlikely that mere contact with the project influenced the treatment effects. Second, most of the

components of the treatment have been shown in earlier research to have specific effects on behaviors, where placebo effects have been ruled out.

(5) *Post-treatment Data.* It could be objected that the outcome data at seven years of age, based on IQ testing and educational placement, do not warrant the label "normal functioning" which we assigned to about half the children in the experimental group. However, the second, more comprehensive, follow-up study discussed above (McEachin, 1987), conducted when the children were an average age of 13 years, was comprised of a large variety of standardized psychological tests and carried out according to a double-blind testing paradigm. This study supports the conclusion of normal functioning. The study has been subjected to critisism by Schopler, Short and Mesibov (1989). Answers to thoses critisism and a more complete discussion of these methodological issues can be found in Lovaas, Smith, and McEachin (1989) and Lovaas and Smith (1988). A film, depicting treatment procedures and outcome, is also available (Lovaas, 1988).

IMPLICATIONS FOR TREATMENT

On the basis of the data which has accumulated to this point, we can draw 4 major implications about how treatment should be constructed.

First, in order for behavioral treatment to work it has to be delivered by all significant persons who interact with the client. This allows treatment to be administered in all of the client's environments and prevents situation specificity in treatment gains. Treatment gain is proportionate to the amount of treatment. Consequently, the involvement of many persons will optimize treatment effectiveness by extending treatment to all of the client's waking hours. This extension allows us to approximate the educational and therapeutic value of the average environment for the average person, an interaction which is functional during all his/her waking hours.

Second, in order to maximize treatment effects therapy must address all significant behaviors. This observation implies that treatment directed at changing selected behaviors, such as speech therapy, pre-academics, music therapy, sensory motor training etc., are likely to show only limited, if any, gains.

Third, it follows that the traditional model of teaching a client in a clinic or classroom setting by a therapist or teacher who is relatively divorced from the parents and other lay personnel may seem obsolete. Either the teacher or therapist would have to work directly with the child's parents and other professionals to introduce educational material within the child's home and immediate community, or the school and clinic would have to be redesigned to resemble a home. Limiting treatment (such as speech therapy) to a few hours a week may well be nonfunctional: Children in Control Group I did no better than

Control Group II children even though the former received up to 10 hours of 1:1 treatment per week while the latter did not. Furthermore, the traditional curriculum for autistic children would have to be drastically revised to include curricula for self-help skills (e.g. dressing, toilet training, proper eating, etc.), community skills, teaching of imitation, observational learning, etc. Teachers have to help children acquire new learning strategies, such as observational learning, to optimize group (classroom) instruction. In short, major innovations in the way teachers are prepared to teach these children need to take place.

Fourth, additional research is needed to identify autistic children as early as possible in order to help find ways to treat them more effectively. Findings to date (Lovaas, 1987) suggest that a large portion of young autistic children may recover and become normal functioning if they receive the intensive treatment described in this chapter. Without such treatment, however, they almost always remain severely disturbed. Unless it is possible to demonstrate that alternate treatments are at least as effective as the behavioral approach, it may be considered ill-advised and unethical not to provide the kind of behavioral treatment described here.

A BEHAVIORAL THEORY OF AUTISTIC PERSONS

A behavioral theory of autistic persons can be best described as comprised of 4 tenets. First, the laws of learning can adequately account for autistic persons behaviors and provide a basis for treatment. Over the last 25 years, several hundred studies have found that excessive aggressive behaviors and self-stimulatory behaviors are lawfully related to the environment in accordance with learning theory paradigms. Similarly, learning theory has formed the basis for remediating the autistic person's behavioral deficiencies such as language, self-help and social skills. An examination of the acquisition curves for these behaviors are shown to match those found in other learning studies.

The second tenet states that the autistic clients demonstrate little or no prior knowledge or experience at pre-treatment. This tenet is supported by 2 observations: First, adequate treatment required that the clients be taught almost everything. Second, there was no evidence during treatment of sudden or qualitative leaps which would indicate a pre-existing set of language or social skills. In particular, we failed to isolate a pivotal response or activate a central construct which would generalize across behaviors or otherwise help the client make sudden and major steps ahead. Related to that, we observed limited stimulus generalization as evidenced by the fact that treatment had to occur in almost all the clients' environments. Finally, data show that many of the behaviors of the autistic persons were functionally related to several different environmental variables. This observation points away from any easily understood, inner organizing construct.

The third tenet implies that autistic children can learn once a special environment is developed for them. At the present time there appears to be no realistic limitation of how much autistic persons can learn, given a systematic exploration of learning environments. Although it it correct that different autistic persons will learn at vastly different rates, this observation must be considered in a context that just 25 years ago, prior to the introduction of behavioral treatment, there was no evidence that the environment could be arranged so as to become therapeutic and educational for autistic persons.

The fourth tenet proposes a mismatch to exist between the autistic persons' nervous system and the average environment. Although the average environment helps teach the person with the average nervous system, it teaches very little to the autistic child. One can think of autistic persons as individuals without learning or experience, like infants in their psychological make-up. The fact that some children do not acquire behaviors in certain environments does not mean that they will also fail in other environments. There is considerable evidence that, with slight changes in the average environment, autistic children can learn like other organisms. Whatever their pathology, they are not prevented from learning once special environments have been explored and activated. A more detailed presentation of this behavioral theory of autistic children is provided by Lovaas and Smith (1989).

RESEARCH METHODOLOGY

Behavioral research has focused on attempting to understand the separate *behaviors* of autistic clients. First, an investigator identifies a behavior (the dependent variable) which can be accurately and sensitively measured. All research on psychological treatment research begins and ends with an assessment of changes in the client's behaviors, be these behaviors emotional, social, intellectual or a combination of these. Sensitive and accurate measures of behaviors are absolutely necessary in research, because changes in these measurements signify whether the client is getting better, worse or staying the same. There is now considerable technology developed for making accurate and objective measures of a large variety of behaviors. Working inductively and without gambling on the discovery of an all-powerful treatment intervention, we were prepared for small changes in the dependent variables. Hence, the added need for sensitive measures. We cannot overestimate how important advances in measurement were in detecting subtle changes in behavior that previously would have gone unnoticed.

Second, the investigator manipulates an independent variable in the child's present and observable environment (i.e. some form of treatment), while observing changes in the dependent variable (i.e. that client's behaviors). By systematically manipulating the treatment variable, such as presenting it and then withdrawing it in an A-B-A- reversal design, or by using an experimental and control group paradigm, we can say with some confidence that the treatment we introduce is in fact producing a specific change. These experimental manipulations reduce the probability of confounded results and make it easier to identify effective treatments and to discontinue those which are not, or those which in fact worsen the clients condition. Over time, several of the environmental variables which controlled the various behaviors of autistic children were isolated. Treatment programs were then developed which helped to reduce deviant behaviors and served to increase language and other appropriate behaviors.

When working inductively and with relatively few theoretical constraints, we are in a position to experimentally manipulate a large range of potential treatment variables. When one works inductively, one does not expect a sudden or dramatic breakthrough. Rather, we work like "pyramid-builders", with the end product, the better functioning individual, seen as comprised of a group of relatively smaller goals. As new relationships in research are discovered, they are implemented into treatment.

One can illustrate both the treatment and the research in the following way. It was relatively easy to discover procedures to help the children look at us, but this did not mean that the children came to see us or became more attentive. However, it was necessary for the client to look at us when we presented them with visual stimuli. Also, children appear a little more normal when they visually attend to others. Teaching a client to imitate gestures does not generalize to vocal imitation, so we researched procedures to help teach both. Once the client could imitate words and gestures, we taught the meanings of these behaviors by relating the behaviors to their appropriate environmental context. A child who was taught to talk and imitate did not necessarily begin to play with other peers. Therefore we had to research and develop explicit programs to help the children interact more effectively with normal peers. If we now add several hundred programs which have been developed over the last 25 years by a large number of investigators working in a variety of clinic/laboratories, it can be seen that the behavioral strategy is *cumulative*. Recent discoveries build directly on earlier discoveries. Sooner or later, enough would be known to help some autistic children reach normal functioning. This attribute of behavioral work is of immense importance in developing effective treatments.

From this inductive paradigm it follows that progress in understanding all persons diagnosed as autistic will occur gradually, in small steps, rather than suddenly as a result of the discovery of one pivotal problem or disease which controls all behaviors of all autistic persons. While behavioral treatment may produce normal educational and intellectual functioning in some children, if started early and given intensively, it does not claim to provide a cure for autistic children. That would require the rectification of a root cause or the problem which is presumably organic. On the other hand, it is possible that future research may show early behavioral intervention to reverse or prevent the further development of certain forms of organic damage. Such a possibility is consistent with the views of Huttenlocher (1984) on the function of increased synaptic density in infancy and early childhood: "Overproduction of synapses may impart plasticity to the brain of young children. This property of developing brain may be exploited for retraining when function is impaired" (Huttenlocher, 1984, p. 488). Numerous and well-controlled studies from William Greenough's laboratory (conf. Sirivaag & Greenough, 1987) do also show that differential experience, such as those requiring problem-solving in the early development (of rats), lead to predictable alterations in underlying and relevant nervous system structures. These developments should be considered in future theories of autism.

Although most behaviorists champion inductive procedures, this does not imply that behaviorists judge those colleagues wrong who pursue the more commonly used hypothetico-deductive approaches to the problems of autistic clients. In science, the two approaches have coexisted and complimented each other in the past. In other words, behaviorists do not rule out the possibility that other investigators who pursue alternate hypothesis (like the disease of autism) may come up with the "big breakthrough". Rather, the complex problem that faces all who work with autistic persons underscores the need to be flexible in our approach so as to better serve these children and their parents. (For a more complete description of the behavioral position on research and treatment of autistic persons, see Lovaas and Smith, 1988).

STRENGTHS AND WEAKNESSES IN THE BEHAVIORAL APPROACH

The major strengths of behavioral treatment with autistic clients can be described as follows: (1) behavioral treatment helps increase socially appropriate behavior, including complex behaviors like language; (2) self-destructive, tantrumous and self-stimulatory rituals can be reduced; (3) the longer the treatment lasts, the larger the gains; (4) intensive early intervention leads to normal functioning in a sizable minority of children; and (5) all clients benefit, but to vastly different degrees.

The major weaknesses of behavioral treatment are: (1) it is very time-consuming, requiring intervention across numerous behaviors by many persons, in many settings; (2) except for a subgroup of autistic children receiving early, intensive intervention, behavioral treatment will not lead to normal functioning and the child will retain the diagnosis of autism; (3) except for the children who achieve normal functioning, treatment gains will relapse should treatment be terminated. These latter observations are consistent with data which we have reported earlier (Lovaas, Koegel, Simmons, & Long, 1973); (4) there is an inherent weakness in the knowledge-base from which the treatment is derived. Empirical learning theory is an open-ended model and represents only one of several potential sources of information about how persons change; and (5) the treatment does not lead to a "cure" for autism. The root cause of autism (which presumably is organic) is not removed. Future research will undoubtedly address ways of making the treatment less cumbersome and more efficient, as well as attempting to answer questions of whether early behavioral intervention may partially arrest or reverse potential underlying organic deviations. The major strength of the behavioral approach was seen to lie in the research design which guides and supports the investigator/therapist.

SUMMARY

This chapter discusses some of the main research and theoretical perspectives of the behavioral treatment of autistic children. The behavioral treatment is characterized by an inductive, step-by-step and cumulative research approach which places a strong emphasis on the measurement of behavior and experimental manipulation of treatment variables so as to isolate functional relationships. A brief history of studies utilizing learning theory principles provide the basis for a discussion of current research.

It was assumed that normal children, possessing an average nervous system, learn from their everyday environment all their waking hours. Autistic children, possessing unusual nervous systems, do not learn from a similar environment. To approximate an ideal learning environment, behavioral treatment should be administered in all environments, by many different therapists, during most of the child's waking hours. Treatment must address all significant behaviors.

Data from a recently completed study was used to illustrate how effective behavioral treatment may be under optimal conditions. A sizable minority of an experimental group of young autistic children who received intensive behavioral intervention achieved normal functioning which was maintained at adolescence. In contrast, a control group of autistic children, similar at pre-treatment, had no recoveries. Strengths and weaknesses of behavioral interventions are discussed.

ACKNOWLEDGEMENTS

The authors wish to acknowledge the support of the National Office of Education (Grant # H133G80103) and the editorial assistance of Greg Buch in the preparation of this chapter.

REFERENCES

American Psychiatric Association. (1980). *Diagnostic and statistical manual of mental disorders (3rd ed.).* Washington, DC: Author.

American Psychiatric Association. (1987). *Diagnostic and statistical manual of mental disorders (3rd revised ed.).* Washington, DC: Author.

Andersson, S. R., & Avery, D. (1986, May). Home-based training for families with pre-school-aged autistic children. In *Parent training: Models and evaluation of outcome.* Symposium conducted at the meeting of the American Association of Mental Deficiency, Denver, CO.

Bayley, N. (1969). *Bayley scales of infant development.* New York: Psychological Corporation.

Cattell, P. (1960). *The measurement of intelligence of infants and young children.* New York: Psychological Corporation.

DeMyer, M. K., Hingtgen, J. N., & Jackson, R. K. (1981). Infantile autism reviewed: A decade of research. *Schizophrenia Bulletin, 7,* 388-451.

Doll, E. A. (1953). *The measurement of social competence.* Minneapolis, MN: Minneapolis Educational Test Bureau.

Ferster, C. B. (1961). Positive reinforcement and behavioral deficits of autistic children. *Child Development, 32,* 437-456.

Gesell, A. (1949). *Gesell developmental schedules.* New York: Psychological Corporation.

Hewett, F. J. (1965). Teaching speech to an autistic child through operant conditioning. *American Journal of Orthopsychiatry, 35,* 927-936.

Huttenlocher, P. R. (1984). Synapse elimination and plasticity in developing human cerebral cortex. *American Journal of Mental Deficiencies, 88,* 488-496.

Kanner, L. (1943). Autistic disturbances of affective contact. *Nervous Child, 2,* 181-197.

Kazdin, A. E. (1984). *Behavior modification in applied settings.* Chicago, IL: The Dorsey Press.

Lovaas, O. I. (1971). Certain comparisons between psychodynamic and behavioristic approaches to treatment. *Psychotherapy: Theory, Research and Practice, 8,* 175-178.

Lovaas, O. I. (1987). Behavioral treatment and normal educational and intellectual functioning in young autistic children. *Journal of Consulting and Clinical Psychology, 55,* 3-9.

Lovaas, O. I. (1988). *Behavioral Treatment of Autistic Children.* Distributed by: Focus International, 14, Oregon Drive, Huntington Station, NY.

Lovaas, O. I., Ackerman, A. B., Alexander, D., Firestone, P., Perkins, J., & Young, D. B. (1980). *Teaching developmentally disabled children: The ME Book.* Austin, TX: Pro-Ed.

Lovaas, O. I., Berberich, J. P., Perloff, B. F., & Schaeffer, B. (1966). Acquisition of imitative speech by schizophrenic children. *Science, 151,* 705-707.

Lovaas, O. I., Koegel, R. L., Simmons, J. Q., & Long, J. S. (1973). Some generalization and follow-up measures on autistic children in behavior therapy. *Journal of Applied Behavior Analysis, 6,* 131-165.

Lovaas, O. I., & Smith, T. (1988). Intensive behavioral treatment in young autistic children. In B. B. Lahey & A. E. Kazdin (Eds.), *Advances in Clinical Child Psychology.* Vol. II (pp 285-324). New York, NY: Plenum Publishing Corporation.

Lovaas, O. I., & Smith, T. (1989). An inductive behavioral theory of autism: A paradigm for research and treatment. *Journal of Behavior Therapy and Experimental Psychiatry, 20,* 17 - 29.

Lovaas, O. I., Smith, T., & McEachin, J. J. (1989). Clarifying comments on the young autism study: Reply to Schopler, Short, and Mesibov. *Journal of Consulting and Clinical Psychology, 57,* 165-167.

Martin, G., & Pear, J. (1988). *Behavior modification: What it is and how to do it.* Englewood Cliffs, New Jersey: Prentice Hall.

McEachin, J. J. (1987). *Outcome of autistic children receiving intensive behavioral treatment: Residual deficits.* Unpublished doctoral dissertation, University of California, Los Angeles.

Risley, T., & Wolf, M. N. (1967). Establishing functional speech in echolalic children. *Behavior Research and Therapy, 5,* 73-88.

Rutter, M. (1978). Diagnosis and definition. In M. Rutter & E. Schopler (Eds.), *Autism: A reappraisal of concepts and treatment* (pp 1-25). New York, NY: Plenum Press.

Schopler, E. (1987). Specific and nonspecific factors in the effectiveness of a treatment system. *American Psychologist, 42,* 376-383.

Schopler, E., & Mesibov, G. B. (1988). Introduction to diagnosis and assessment of autism. In E. Schopler & G. B. Mesibov (Eds.), *Diagnosis and Assessment in Autism* (pp 3-14). New York, NY: Plenum Publishing Corporation.

Schopler, E., Short, A., & Mesibov, G. B. (1989). Relation of behavioral treatment to "normal functioning": Comment on Lovaas. *Journal of Consulting and Clinical Psychology, 57,* 162-164.

Sirevaag, A. M., & Greenough, W. T. (1987). Differential rearing effects on rat visual cortex synapses. III. Neuronal and glial nuclei, boutons, dendrites, and capillaries. *Brain Research, 424,* 320-332.

Sparrow, S. S., Bella, D. A., & Cicchetti, D. V. (1984). *Vineland adaptive behavior scales.* Circle Pines, MN: American Guidance Service.

Strain, P. S., Jamieson, B. J., & Hoyson, M. H. (1985). Learning experiences ... an alternative for preschoolers and parents: A comprehensive service system for the mainstreaming of autistic-like preschoolers. In C. J. Meisel (Ed.), *Mainstreamed handicapped children: Outcomes, controversies, and new directions* (pp 251-269). Hilldale, New Jersey: Erlbaum.

Thorndike, R. L. (1972). *Manual for Stanford-Binet intelligence scale.* Boston, MA: Houghton Mifflin.

Wechsler, D. (1974). *Manual for the Wechsler intelligence scale for children -revised.* New York: Psychological Corporation.

Weinberg, R. A. (1989). Intelligence and IQ: Landmark issues and great debates. *American Psychologist, 44,* 98-104.

Werry, J. S., & Wollersheim, J. P. (1989). Behavior therapy with children and adolescents: A twenty-year overview. *Journal of the American Academy of Child and Adolescent Psychiatry, 28,* 1-18.

Wirt, R. D., Seat, P. D., Broen, W. E., & Lachar, D. (1981). *Personality inventory for children.* Los Angeles, CA: Western Psychological Services.

Wolf, M. M., Risley, T., & Mees, H. (1964). Application of operant conditioning procedures to the behavior problems of an autistic child. *Behavior Research and Therapy, 1,* 305-312.

Wolpe, J. (1958). *Psychotherapy by reciprocal inhibition.* Stanford, CA: Stanford University Press.

Treating Autistic Children at Home: A London Based Programme

PATRICIA HOWLIN and PAMELA YATES

INTRODUCTION

The range of management problems faced by the parents of autistic children is considerable. Not only do families have to cope with the specific difficulties associated with the disorder, notably social and communication deficits and ritualistic and obsessional behaviours, but also with many non-specific problems of the sort that are common to children with a variety of handicaps. Moreover, although the types of problem may seem similar across children (language abnormalities, social problems, routines and obsessions, toiletting and feeding difficulties, disruptive behaviours, overactivity etc.) the ways in which these need to be tackled will vary according to the skills and deficits of the individual child and his or her family circumstances.

Before embarking on any programme to alter behaviours or to improve the child's level of functioning it is essential to carry out a functional analysis of these difficulties. Such an analysis needs to take account not only of the circumstances in which problem behaviours occur and of antecedent and subsequent events but must examine carefully the functional role of these behaviours for an individual child. It is easy, for example, to dismiss self injurious behaviours as "deviant" or "inappropriate" but if they are the child's only effective means of communicating distress or dissatisfaction then attempts merely to eliminate such problems are unlikely to be successful.

In the discussion that follows I shall attempt to give a "flavour" of the types of techniques that we have found effective in dealing with, particularly, the more "syndrome specific" problems faced by families with an autistic child at home.

COPING WITH LANGUAGE PROBLEMS

Almost by definition, language deficits of some sort are found in every autistic person. These can vary from very severe impairments in understanding and almost total lack of verbal ability, to excessive and repetitive speech, to much more subtle defects in interpreting and using abstract or non-verbal forms of communication.

For children with the most severe forms of linguistic impairment, that is, they can neither use nor understand speech, our experience (Howlin & Rutter, 1987) in common with other research findings, has indicated that even the most intensive efforts to increase their repertoire of speech sounds are unlikely to meet with great success. Although a few sounds may be acquired by behavioural methods, functional use of such verbalizations is almost always severely limited. Instead, treatment can focus more usefully on the establishment of simple comprehension skills that may help the child to make at least a little sense of the world around him. Physical prompting and shaping techniques can be used to teach the child to respond first to commands involving gross motor acitivities and later to more complex instructions. At all times it is essential that the activities involved are ones that are relevant to the child's daily environment. For instance, building comprehension training into mealtime or playtime activities, or making it an integral part of "life skills" programmes, is likely to be far more valuable, and effective, than teaching in isolation (McGee et al., 1983, 1985).

Expressive language programmes with this more globally impaired group of children will also need to take careful account of individual profiles of skills and weaknesses. As noted above, spoken language is unlikely to be acquired with ease but various alternatives exist. Signing is probably the most commonly taught although systems involving symbols (Bliss, Rebus etc.), pictures or written language may also be of value. Very often such systems are chosen as a sort of "second best" to speech, following the failure of verbal training, rather than as a result of deliberate teaching strategies. However, there is sufficient experimental evidence available to provide guidance before therapy begins as to what systems may be most appropriate for an individual child. This requires assessment of the child's level of skills in a variety of different domains and Table 1 indicates the sorts of alternative communication systems that might be chosen according to the child's patterns of skills and deficits (Howlin, 1989).

Table 1. Choice of alternative system according to individual child characteristics

Child characteristics	Level of ability			
Speech	-	-	-	-
Comprehension	-	-	-	+-
Non-verbal I. Q.	-	+-	-/+-	+
Motor imitation	-	-	+-	+-
Social motivation	-	-	+-	+-
Systems to try	Pictural	Symbols (Bliss etc)	Signs	Written (Type, Computer)

Key: -   = low ability lewel
     +   = high ability level
     +-   = moderate ability

Perhaps "alternative" is the wrong term here, as, clearly, all non-speech systems will be less flexible and more restrictive (in terms of audience) than verbal communication. However, as augmentative systems, that is as adjuncts to spoken language, they have a number of advantages. Most non-verbal systems make fewer demands on memory and processing skills; they are simpler to prompt and, in that they are presented more slowly and involve less redundancy, it may be easier for the child to make the connection between their use and the achievment of his needs. Any non-verbal system will have its own merits and drawbacks and these too need to be kept in mind when selecting the most appropriate method for an individual child.

Table 2 summarises the main advantages and disadvantages of the most commonly used alternatives to speech: signing and symbols.

Controversy still exists regarding the teaching of augmentative systems to autistic children; for example, are iconic signs easier to acquire than more abstract ones; is multi-modal teaching more successful than teaching in a single modality, and under what circumstances is the acquisition of non-verbal communication likely to generalize to the use of spoken language (see Howlin, 1989; Kiernan, 1983). Nevertheless, although better controlled experimental studies are required in order adequately to answer such questions, clinical experience suggests that the successful use of even very basic communication aids, such as simple signs or sets of pictures, can have beneficial effects in many areas. Not only may receptive or expressive abilities be enhanced but many improvements in behavioural problems may also occur once the child is able to gain greater control over his environment by these means.

Table 2. Relative advantages and disadvantages of signs versus symbols

	ADVANTAGES	DISADVANTAGES
SIGNS	Good for spontaneous requests etc Syntactically flexible Unlimited lexicon No special equipment required	More demands on: Motor/ imitation skills Cognitive and sequencing ability Long term memory Limited use/understanding by others
SYMBOLS/ PICTURES	Fewer demands on: Long term memory Sequencing ability Easier for audience Simple to prompt Individually tailored vocabulary	Limited vocabulary Restricted grammar Slow to process Slow in use Restrict spontaneity

Non-verbal systems are generally used with more severely impaired children. For those who already have some useful understanding of speech, show some imitative abilities and possess a repertoire of sounds that might be shaped into words or word approximations, intervention tends to focus instead on the development of communicative speech. At this level of teaching both developmental and motivational factors play a crucial role. It is essential to tailor programmes appropriately to the child's developmental level, whilst at the same time taking account of the functional value of what is taught (Howlin, 1989).

In general, attempts to teach basic verbal skills tend to be most successful with younger children (those under the age of severn or so). Although some useful speech may be achieved through behavioural intervention with older children, this is rarely as flexible or as spontaneous as when language is aquired earlier in life (Howlin & Rutter, 1987).

For children of higher levels of linguistic competence, who show relatively good use of syntax and semantics, therapy may focus instead on the teaching of social aspects of language, such as conversational skill, or on the development of abstract linguistic concepts. Here, programmes may extend from the teaching of simile and metaphor, to the use of drama techniques and these more sophisticated programmes can be used to enhance the communication skills of relatively competent individuals at any age. Details of the various types of procedures that may be effective in increasing spoken language at different levels are described by Howlin (1987).

Whatever the ability level of the child, problems of generalization and maintenance may interfere with the success of any training programme. Such difficulties may be most successfully reduced if therapists (be they parents or professional) steer clear of the notion of "language training sessions". After all, normal children do not acquire language by having daily half hour sessions of exposure to their native tongue. Instead, communication training needs to be intrinsically linked to the teaching of other daily living skills so that it becomes part of a general "habit chain" (McGee et al., 1983, 1985). Naturalistic or incidental approaches to training, combined with structured teaching programmes when necessary, tend to be more successful than teaching in artificial settings (Carr et al., 1987; McLean & Snyder-McLean, 1978).

It is crucial, too, that the skills taught are ones that will give the child more effective and rapid control over his environment so that motivation to use them is enhanced and is independent of any extrinsic reinforcers (Goetz et al., 1983). Analysis of existing communication skills allows new functions to be built onto existing forms, so that the child's current abilities can be most effectively developed. Detailed assessment of the child's gestures or word approximations can be used to develop "communicative profiles" which may then serve as a basis for developing higher level language skills (Wetherby, 1986).

With some autistic children the problem is not so much that they do not speak, but that they do so too much (as in obsesssional questioning or constant repetitions) or that they do so in inappropriate ways. For example, they may use echoed rather than generative speech or they may use words, notably swear words, or repetivitve phrases ("How far is it from New York to Madrid?"; "Do you like primrose yellow cars?"; "You're not going to be a naughty girl are you") that are calculated to irritate, annoy or in some other way gain attention.

Many parents, who have worked, perhaps for years, to encourage their children to speak are anxious that if they attempt to correct such utterances the child may again cease to communicate. In fact, by ensuring that the linguistic input is not at too high a level for the child, by correcting him each time he uses inappropriate means (eg. echoed or stereotyped utterances) and by supplying him instead with more appropriate ways of communication, such abnormalities of speech can be much reduced. It is important, nevertheless, to recognise that certain "deviant" aspects of speech, such as echolalia, may serve an important communicative role for many autistic children. Rather than dismissing such utterances as inappropriate and automatically attempting to eliminate them, successful therapy should aim to analyze the communicative functions of these forms of speech and to replace them with equivalent but appropriate verbal responses (Durand & Crimmens, 1987).

If echolalia on repetitive questioning reflects the child's lack of comprehension on the poverty of his social language then intervention can best focus on increasing skills in these areas. Many children also tend to use stereotyped or unacceptable speech because of the reactions this achieves from others. Making loud, personal and derogatory comments about people on the bus or shouting loudly in shops is almost sure to result in a fair amount of attention. Dealing with these behaviours in public can be very difficult for parents, and the contingent cessation of outings or removal of treats, whilst effective in principle, may not always be feasible in practice. However, if such behaviours become very disruptive, parents may need to restrict their outings with the child to ones that can be readily terminated should difficulties arise. Meanwhile, ignoring such utterances at home, and ensuring that the rest of the family do so too, whilst at the same time giving the child the maximum encouragement for talking appropriately, can help greatly to reduce the frequency of inappropriate speech.

DEALING WITH SOCIAL PROBLEMS

Autistic children show a wide range of social difficulties and merely to describe them as "withdrawn" is to give much too simplistic a view of their problems. Intervention programmes need to focus on many aspects of social development and, more importantly, the interrelationships between these. Reinforcing and increasing "eye contact" by autistic individuals, for example, is not a particularly difficult task. However, unless attention is given to the multiplicity of factors influencing the normal, social use of eye gaze, all such programmes are likely to procude in the disconcerting use of fixed or prolonged stares. It is the meshing together of social responses and signals and the continuous modification of these according to the changing demands of social circumstances that are the crux of social relationships. Unfortunately, the teaching of highly complex patterns of skill may prove much more problematical than the teaching of discrete behaviours.

When very young, autistic children may try to avoid contact with others and will often prefer to engage in solitary, ritualistic behaviours. At this stage deliberate intrusion into solitary activities and insistence that the child takes part in some social interactions with others is important. Otherwise solitary activities of this kind may become very persistent and entrenched. Physical activities, games or even the child's ritualistic behaviours can be used as the basis for some degree of social cooperation. At certain times the child's access to such activities can be made dependent on his sharing of cooperating with others, and deliberate instrusion of this kind has proved to be of considerable benefit in breaking down solitary patterns of behaviour (Rutter & Sussenwein, 1971).

As autistic children grow older most do demonstrate an interest in other people, escpecially the adults in their environment, and may try hard to communicate with them. Unfortunately, their lack of social skills and their failure to empathise with others' feelings mean that such interactions are often fraught with problems. They may well try to engage the interest of ANY adult whom they meet, regardless of whether they know them or not. They may bombard complete strangers with obsessional questions, or details of the intimate lives of their families, or go into the tedious minutiae of some particular interest of theirs. Non-verbal communication, such as smiles or eye contact, is likely to be used quite inappropriately, sometimes giving totally misleading "messages" to those with whom they are interacting. They may also be totally unaware of the effects that certain behaviours will have on other people. Thus, they may quite innocently take off their clothes in public (for example, in the middle of an apartment store because they are feeling hot); they may indiscriminately approach or even hug or kiss strangers because when younger they had been encouraged to do this with family members; or they may indulge in manneristic or stereotyped activities with no regard for people's reactions to these.

Some help can be given to reduce the more disruptive of these problems. For younger children basic rules about who or what NOT to talk to or about can be helpful, as are strict instructions about not undressing in public, not approaching strangers, and restricting physical contact to family members only. Simple social skills training, using role play and feed-back from video or audio tapes, can help improve very obvious deficits in eye contact or facial expression or tone of voice. Basic conversational skills can be taught using similar techniques, and may also be effective in reducing the ritualistic questioning which many children use to greet both strangers and familiar adults.

We have encouraged some older children to join special drama groups and this has sometime proved very effective in improving social skills. Overt practice and role play in HOW to behave correctly can also help to avoid future difficulties after particular problems have been experienced.

It is clear that with appropriate help and practice older children can generalize the skills they have learned during training sessions to other settings. The main problem lies in their failure to appreciate when behaviours should be modified according to the changing demands of social interactions. One young man, for example, having made good progress during sessions designed to teach him how to approach girls at his special club, then decided to put his new skills into practice outside the local ladies' lavatories. Another intelligent 12 year old, having been warned by his parents not to talk to strangers, then refused to carry out his regular trips to the paper shops because he insisted that this would involve talking to people he did not know.

Intervention techniques also have their limitations when it comes to dealing with more fundamental deficits, such as lack of empathy, difficulties in reciprocal interactions and inadequacies in dealing with abstract concepts or nonverbal communication. Although help may result in superficial improvements, the basic handicap remains and much greater research is needed in this area if therapy is to be of real benefit.

RITUALISTIC AND OBSESSIONAL BEHAVIOURS

Although once thought to be secondary to the social and communication deficits that characterize the disorder, it is now recognised that the obsessionality and resistance to change shown by autistic children is very much a core part of the conditon. Moreover, they continue to result in many problems for even the most able autistic individuals throughout their lives.

In the early years, rituals and routines may seem relatively mild and innocuous, so that parents give in to them for the sake of pacifying children who are so often distressed. However, with time, these behaviours may grow to such an extent that they can severly affect normal family functioning. Complex rituals and routines may involve not only the child but also other family members. Ritualistic questioning can come to dominate all the child's verbal interactions. The resistance to change may result in extreme restrictions on family life or in severe and prolonged distress if changes have to be made. Abnormal attachments to objects may interfere with the child's abilities to learn or to play more appropriately. Obsessional tendencies can also result in problem behaviours related to toiletting, feeding and sleeping.

The longer such behaviours are left to "take hold" the more resistant they will be to subsequent intervention. The only truly satisfactory way of dealing with these problems is to ensure that parents are given adequate help and support in the early years, in order to avoid obsessional traits gaining control. It may not be possible or even advisable entirely to overcome obsessional tendencies (after all, autistic individuals are so lacking in normal ways of occupying themselves that in can be quite wrong to deprive them of all their interests). However, with guidance, parents can be helped to reduce such behaviours to a level where they are no longer disruptive. Once this is done there is no reason why the child cannot indulge in some of his obsessions at times when he is not otherwise occupied. There is also some evidence that obsessional interests, if under appropriate control, can be employed as very effective reinforcers for more appropriate activities. They may also form the basis of skills or interests that can eventually be developed into useful social or occupational activities. For example, Kanner (1973), in his long term follow up of autistic individuals, found that those who had made most progress socially were those who had obsessional interests that allowed them access to normal social groups. Table 3 shows some ways in which we have utilized obsessional interests as the basis of a number of more practical skills.

Table 3. Use of obsessional interests in developing other skills

INTEREST/SKILL	OUTCOME
Dates	Exams in history/geography
Directions	Careers in cartography, horology etc.
Clocks	Skills in orienteering, route planning etc.
Weather	
Timetables	Membership of special interest groups etc.
Transport	Train spotting clubs
Music	Membership of musical/art groups etc.
Art	Possibility of self-employment
Design	
Spelling	May help improve social status at school
Numbers	Development of skills in chess/computing etc.
Patterns	

Once obsessional behaviours have been allowed to take hold they can be very resistant to intervention. However, with GRADUAL intrusion into such problems, steady improvements can be brought about with minimal distress to the child or his family. Table 4 illustrates the type of approaches that we have found helpful in the modification of

Table 4. Modifying obsessional behaviours

OBJECT ATTACHMENTS
GRADUALLY REDUCE: Amount of time spent with object. No. of places in which object allowed. Size of object itself.

RITUALS
GRADUALLY REDUCE: Amount of time spent in activity. No. of places where/people with whom ritual allowed.

RESISTANCE TO CHANGE
Help individual to PREDICT change. Deliberately but gradually introduce changes into daily routine.

GENERALLY:

TREATMENT SHOULD AIM TO
    MODIFY - NOT ELIMINATE OBSESSION
    UTILIZE OBSESSION AS EFFECTIVE REWARD
    SHAPE OBSESSION INTO MORE SOCIAL/FUNCTIONAL ACTIVITIES

obsessional behaviours. In general, our aim has not been to eliminate such behaviours entirely, as this is likely to prove an impossible task. However, with care, time and patience such behaviours may be reduced to a level at which they no longer interfere with family functioning. They may then be used as a basis for encouraging more useful and socialised activities. Table 5, for example, illustrates the use of this graded change approach in the reduction of obsessional collecting of objects.

Table 5. Graded change in the reduction of obsessional collecting.

PROBLEM: Collecting and storing teddy-bears in armchair

SOLUTION:	WEEK 1	Removal of single bear short distance from chair. Child reinforced for alternative activities.
	WEEK 2	Second bear removed from chair. First bear left in child's bedroom.
	WEEK 3-4	More bears distributed around house. Used in pretend play.
	WEEK 5	All bears removed. Parents able to sit in chair.
	WEEK 6	Imaginative play with bears developed. No further collecting allowed.

As noted above, obsessional traits may also be responsible for sleeping, toiletting or feeding difficulties. Table 6 illustrates how graded change was used to improve sleeping problems in a 7 year old boy who refused to sleep alone.

Table 6. Graded change in the reduction of sleeping problems.

PROBLEM: Refusal of child to sleep alone - mother in bed with him each night

SOLUTION:

	WEEK 6	Mother sleeps on inflatable mattress next to child's bed.
	WEEK 2	Mattress moved few inches from bed.
	WEEK 3	Distance increased, but mother still able to reach out and touch child.
	WEEK 4	Mother no longer in reach of child.
	WEEK 5	Mattress at door of child's room.
	WEEK 6	Mattress in hallway.
	WEEK 7	Mattress at door of parents' bedroom.
	WEEK 8	Mother returns to own bed.

N. OF PARENTS EXPRESSING SATISFACTION WITH TREATMENT

STAGE

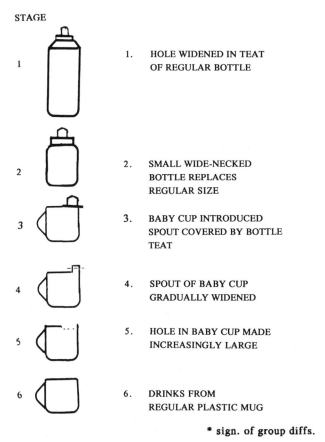

1.   HOLE WIDENED IN TEAT
OF REGULAR BOTTLE

2.   SMALL WIDE-NECKED
BOTTLE REPLACES
REGULAR SIZE

3.   BABY CUP INTRODUCED
SPOUT COVERED BY BOTTLE
TEAT

4.   SPOUT OF BABY CUP
GRADUALLY WIDENED

5.   HOLE IN BABY CUP MADE
INCREASINGLY LARGE

6.   DRINKS FROM
REGULAR PLASTIC MUG

* sign. of group diffs.

Figure 1

Stages in Reduction of Attachment to
Drinking Bottle

317

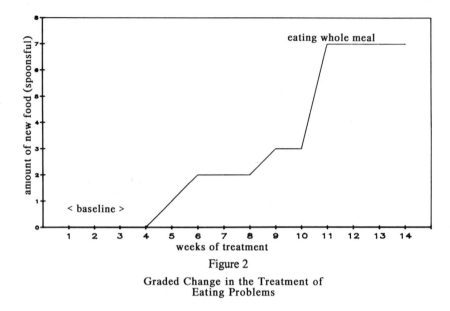

Figure 2

Graded Change in the Treatment of
Eating Problems

Figure 1 shows how a 4 year old boy's attachment to a drinking bottle was gradually reduced, thereby allowing him to move on to the consumption of solid food. Finally, Figure 2 shows how refusal to eat anything other than a very restricted range of food was improved by gradually, but firmly insisting on the child's consumption of minute quantities of more varied foods.

DEALING WITH OTHER PROBLEM BEHAVIOURS

The purpose of this chapter has been to focus on ways of dealing with the SPECIFIC difficulties shown by autistic children, that is with their characteristic social, communicative and obsessional problems. However, parents will also have to cope with a whole range of other problems, which, although not specific to autism (in that they are common to many other groups of children), nevertheless present many problems of management. Moreover, they may be additionally difficult to deal with because of the autistic child's lack of social motivation and awareness. The rigidity of behaviour patterns may also mean that once behavioural problems have become established they tend to be much more difficult to eliminate. For these reasons it is crucial that families are provided with early help to develop effective management techniques and to prevent such behaviours becoming too entrenched. The sort of management techniques employed will not necessarily differ in kind from those needed with other groups of children.

Desensitization and relaxation procedures, developed for use with normal young children, are often equally effective in dealing with the fears and phobias that are typical of so many autistic children. Differential reinforcement and "Time Out" or extinction procedures may frequently be successful in reducing disruptive behaviours. However, before embarking on any programmes involving reduction of attention, or removal of privileges etc., our work with families has focused on an assessment of why the child may be engaging in such behaviours and in particular what it is they are trying to communicate by such means. As the work by Prizant and Wetherby (1985) or Durand and Carr (1987) has indicated, the most successful way of reducing "inappropriate" speech or behaviours, even those of a self injurious nature, may not be to try to modify these directly. Instead, it may be much more effective to assess the functional role of such behaviours and then to supply the child with more acceptable means of achieving the same goals. Alternatively, if disruptive behaviours occur as a result of the child's obsessional behaviours or because of fears or phobias, the aim of treatment will be to reduce the obsessional demands or phobic behaviours that may be producing the temper tantrums.

When there is a need to teach self help or occupational skills, the same techniques of prompting and shaping that are effective with learning disabled children will prove beneficial. Improvements in these areas may then, in turn, have positive effects on other behaviours, such as overactivity or non compliance.

As noted above, whatever the problems and whatever the most effective ways of dealing with these, the crucial need for all families with an autistic child is for early help and support. Dealing with the behavioural problems of a 3 year old can present problems enough - managing the same sorts of difficulties in a 13 year old may present an almost insurmountable task.

PRESENT RESOURCES

Our work with the families of autistic children was developed initially in the context of a research programme, with 16 families in treatment and similar sized groups as the short and long term controls (Howlin & Rutter, 1987). At that time our work was entirely home based and we employed two full time research workers, with additional help from consulting professionals, to carry this out. Because of the need to work with fairly homogeneous groups for research purposes, the age range was limited to children between 3 and 10 years of age, with I.Q.'s of 60 or above. We were lucky enough to receive some continuation of funding once the research project came to an end, but with greatly decreased resources (approximately 2 half time workers) and, over the years, greatly increased demands.

Table 7. Current patterns of referral

TOTAL NUMBER OF CASES 108		SOURCE OF REFERRAL	
% Autistic	67 %	Greater London area	43 %
(excluding severe retardation)		South East England	35 %
% Severe handicap	15 %	South West England	3 %
% Language disorder	7 %	North & East England	3 %
% Other	11 %	Wales	10 %
		Abroad	6 %
AGE GROUP		TYPE OF INVOLVEMENT	
2 - 5	23 %	Single assessment or	
6 - 11	31 %	consultation only	40 %
12 - 15	15 %	Follow up assessment	16 %
16 +	31 %	Ongoing work	44 %

Table 7 documents the types and source of cases seen over the preceding year. One hundred and eight cases were seen in total, with referrals coming mostly from the south east of England, but with several from Wales and some from the north or east of the country. The youngest age at which children tend to be referred is still around 3 but the upper limit is now 39. Indeed, work with older, more able individuals is steadily growing and this group now comprises 30 % of all cases seen. Only around 50 % of our work is now home based, with much less frequent contact than we had been able to offer in the past. Much now has to be done on a consultancy basis, with schools and other agencies, to establish appropriate support systems and then to ensure that these continue to try to meet families needs.

Although, unfortunately, time spent in face-to-face contact with individual families has been reduced, one aspect of our work that has expanded is direct involvement with older autistic individuals. This has required a move away from straightforward behavioural interventions to greater use of cognitive methods and self control strategies as well as greater emphasis on social skills training and contingency contracting between autistic individuals and their families.

We are now also much more involved in work with employers who have taken on autistic individuals. This may take several different forms: explaining about the autistic condition; helping staff to understand the reasons behind some, at least, of the abnormal social behaviours and avoiding misinterpretation of these, and advising about the best ways of dealing with difficulties. For example, the young autistic man who questions every secretary about the colour of their underwear, fails to observe the usual rules about "body space" and smiles sweetly at every new male who enters the office is not likely to be either a potential rapist or homosexual, just poor at picking up normal social cues. Direct feedback will need to be given about the behaviours that cause disruption or offence. It may also be necessary to draw up simple contracts so that the autistic individual is provided with clear guidelines to follow and so that staff have appropriate expectations of his behaviour.

It can be difficult sometimes for colleagues to deal in an unembarrassed way with such situations, not wishing to "talk down to" someone who may be considerably more skilled than they are in particular fields such as computing or accounting. However, the autistic person himself is rarely perturbed by such advice and is most likely to appreciate it, especially if it results in his experiencing greater acceptance and more opportunities to take part in social activities.

SUMMARY

A variety of ways of dealing with the specific problems shown by autistic children are discussed. Appropriate management techniques will vary according to the individual circumstances of each child and his family and hence careful assessment of the child's skills and deficits is necessary before embarking on treatment programmes. However, one of the most essential elements of treatment, if behavioural disturbances are not to escalate, and possibly become beyond parents' control, is early diagnosis and emotional and practical support from practitioners who are aware of, and skilled in dealing with, the very special needs of autistic children.

REFERENCES

Carr, G., Kologinsky, E., & Leff-Simon, S. (1987). Acquisition of sign language by autistic children. 111. Generalized descriptive phrases. *Journal of Autism and Developmental Disorders, 17,* 227 - 234.

Durand, V. M., Carr, E. (1987). Social influences on "self stimulatory" behaviour: Analysis and treatment applications. *Journal of Applied Behavior Analysis, 20,* 297 - 308

Durand, V. M., Crimmens, D. (1987): Assessment and treatment of psychotic speech in an autistic child. *Journal of Autism and Developmental Disorders, 17,* 17 - 28.

Goetz, L., Schuler, A., & Sailor, W. (1983). Motivational considerations in teaching language to severely handicapped students. In M. Hersen, V. van Hasselt & J. Matson (Eds.), *Behavior Therapy for the Developmentally and Physically Disabled.* New York: Academic Press.

Howlin, P. (1987). Language and Communication Training. In W. Yule & J. Carr. (Eds.), *Behaviour Modification for People with Mental Handicaps.* (2nd Edition) London: Croom Helm.

Howlin, P. (1989): Changing approaches to language training with autistic children. *British Journal of Communication Disorders, 24,* 151 - 168.

Howlin, P., & Rutter, M. (1987). (With Berger, M., Hemsley, R., Hersov, L., Yule, W.) *Treatment of Autistic Children.* Chichester: Wiley.

Kanner, L. (1973). *Childhood Psychosis: Initial Studies and New Insights.* New York: Wiley.

Kiernan, C. (1983). The use of non-vocal communication systems with autistic individuals. *Journal of Child Psychology and Psychiatry, 24,* 339 - 376.

McGee, G., Krantz, P., Mason, D., & McClannahan, L. (1983). A modified incidential teaching procedure for autistic youth. Aquisition and generalization of receptive object labels. *Journal of Applied Behavior Analysis, 16,* 329 - 338.

McGee, G., Krantz, P., & McClannahan, L. (1985). The facilitative effect on incidental teaching on preposition use by autistic children. *Journal of Applied Behavior Analysis, 18,* 17 - 31.

McLean, L., & McLean, J. (1974). A language training program for non-verbal autistic children. *Journal of Speech and Hearing Disorders, 39,* 186 - 193.

McLean, J., & Snyder-McLean, L. (1978). *A Transactional Approach to Early Language Training.* New York: Charles E. Merrill.

Prizant, B., & Wetherby, A. (1985). Intentional communicative behaviour of children with autism: Theoretical and practical issues. *Australian Journal of Human Communication Disorders, 13,* 25 - 65.

Rutter, M., & Sussenwein, F. (1971). A developmental and behavioral approach to the treatment of pre-school autistic children. *Journal of Autism and Childhood Schizophrenia, 1,* 376 - 397.

Wetherby, A. (1986). Ontogeny of communicative functions in autism. *Journal of Autism and Developmental Disorders, 16,* 295 - 316.

The REBECKA-Project:
A Short Summary

LENA ANDERSSON

RFPB (Riksföreningen för Psykotiska Barn), the Swedish National Society for Psychotic Children, was founded in 1973 by a group of parents. Today the RFPB has about 2000 members in 20 counties. Half of the members are relatives, the others are professionals. There has always been a close collaboration between parents and professionals in our society. On the board there are members of both categories.

In 1976 the Swedish government wanted to revise the existing act for the intellectually handicapped. The same year the RFPB succeded in passing a motion in parliament calling for an official report on the situation of persons with autism in Sweden. As a result the government appointed a committee whose brief was to consider a new act for the mentally retarded (Ministry of Health and Social Affairs, 1987), persons with "childhood psychosis" and persons who have, as a result of brain injury caused by external violence of physical disease, incurred a significant and permanent intellectual impairment.

In 1981 the committee report was presented to the government and as is customary, it was sent out to a number of involved authorities and organizations, including the RFPB, for comments.

The committee's primary suggestion was a new habilitation organization at the county level with several local branch offices for all types of handicaps. It was proposed that schools for the mentally retarded, hitherto organized at a county level become the responsibility of the local authorities, who also organize schools for normal children. The underlying philosophy was one of decentralization with the provision of services/facilities near the home: a nonspecialist and a nondiagnostic approach. One talked about children and adults with special needs rather than people with, for instance, autism.

The RFPB in their critique concluded that the suggested habilitation team, with nonspecialized medical, psychological, educational and social competencies, would never be able to recognize the special features of autism or identify the special needs of people with autism.

Instead the RFPB among others proposed five regional centres throughout Sweden, which would encompass enough children with autism to maintain "know-how" in the field and to which parents, teachers, doctors, schools and even the suggested habilitation team could turn for help.

The RFPB also concluded that, during the ages up to 20, the class-room is a very important part of any individual's life. The committee had no significant suggestions regarding special education for children with autism. The RFPB held that this could only be developed through practical expericence in schools for children with autism. This does not mean that the RFPB claims that all children must go to special schools. However, in such schools one can develop methods, knowledge and expericence, which can be applied even to mainstreamed pupils with autism.

However, in the early 1980's, the views held by the RFPB were regarded as "backward thinking", and did not become part of the new law.

Nevertheless, the critique was considered to be so valuable that the government contacted the RFPB to see if the ideas on developing and coordinating services for persons with autism could be put into practice with funding from the government. This resulted in the introduction of the so called REBECKA-project in 1984. (REBECKA because that was the name of the day when the project started.)

The RFPB chose to locate the project in Göteborg and four surrounding counties because this area has a population large enough to motivate a diagnostic center and a school for children with autism. The area was appropriate because of the intense research activity at the Department of Child and Adolescent Psychiatry and the leading authorities' positive attitude to the RFPB. In addition, the Göteborg university was at that time the only place in Sweden that offered courses in special education for autism/childhood psychoses, which would be useful when developing a school. Lastly Göteborg had and still has an active parent group (Riksföreningen för Psykotiska Barn, 1988).

The project was divided into five "working" areas:

* Early diagnosis
* Family support
* Education
* Adults
* Coordination

It was based on three main principles:
- the parents were to provide suggestions for what was to be done,
- the evaluation was to be done from the children's and the parents' point of view,
- the RFPB should, if possible, run things in cooperation with the authorities ordinarily responsible (that is to add money, knowledge and initiative to an already existing system).

The Early Diagnosis Project

The first step in this project was to initiate investigations into the early signs of autism - looking for screening devices. We started to video-tape autistic toddlers and we did one retrospective study comparing the behaviour of normal, mentally retarded and autistic children during the first two years of life (Dahlgren & Gillberg, 1989).

The second step consisted in educating The Well Baby Clinics in the region. Today we have held ten educational seminars for about 1 000 professionals in this field.

The most important goal was to establish a diagnostic centre for autism/childhood psychosis. This was, in a way, the easiest part of the project, because the RFPB and Christopher Gillberg had the same vision of the aims of such a centre: the responsibility for providing an accurate diagnosis and a medical work-up, for providing information to the parents and for setting up a preliminary treatment plan.

The diagnostic centre is now, a few years later, a national special clinic, to which children from all over Sweden can be referred.

The Family Project

This project began with interviews of families with autistic members living in the Göteborg area. A report called "61 families" describes the living conditions of these families. It concludes with a list of the practical and psychological services that these families asked for:
* Short-term care homes
* Meaningful occupation for adults
* Suitable living facilities for adults
* Some sort of information centre for the family to turn to, where their child's needs will be well understood
* Better education for teachers and caregivers
* Psychological and practical advice for the parents

The need for short-term homes for persons with autism was obvious. The RFPB bought a house and staffed it with personnel who either had, or were willing to acquire, special knowledge of autism. Today the home can take care of four children at a time and is used by approximately 40 families. The routines are one weekend a month for certain families and one or two days a week for others. The maximum stay allowed is two weeks at time. From the evaluation which has been performed it appears that the parents are very satisfied - but also that we need many more of these facilities so that the families can get the "free time" that they need.

The Education Project

In this case too we began the project with an interview survey. This time teachers and assistents, working with children, adolescents and adults with autism in and around Göteborg, were interviewed about their teaching experiences, their own education and their present needs.

As a result of these interviews, the need for an educational centre was outlined and so the Bua School (where three classes for autistic children had already been started by Christopher Gillberg, Helen Schaumann and Margareta Kärnevik) was expanded. The school is situated next door to the primary school. Today it has seven classes ranging from pre-school up to vocational training. The total number of pupils is 25. After school-time the leisure personnel take over. The school is open 12 months a year, but during vacation periods it is run by "substitute" and leisure time personnel.

All personnel at the Bua-school are given educational supervision and guidance in their work. The parents of children at Bua have available to them the services of a parent consultant. A child psychiatrist is also linked to the school.

In accordance with the needs outlined by the teachers, a network of educational supervisors from the whole area has been developed, to supervise teachers with isolated special classes or with individual autistic pupils integrated in ordinary classes. These supervisors meet at least four times a year to discuss questions about supervision and to support each other in starting up educational centres in their counties.

The Adult Project

Finding suitable living and working conditions for adult persons with autism currently constitutes one of the greatest problems in the field of autism in Sweden. For several years we have looked abroad for good examples of how to care for them. Although the official attitude in Sweden is that living and working should be separated from each other, many of the parents in our interviews had a vision of small residential communities with farming or gardening, as well as weaving, woodwork etc.

The RFPB found a suitable house in the country where a little community could start to grow. The county council in this area, and the National Board of Health and Welfare approved the activity for three years and today four young adults have their home and daily activities in this place. Similar facilities are being established in other parts of Sweden.

Coordination

One result of the Rebecka-project is that the RFPB will propose that the Ministry of Health and Social Affairs organize the services for people with autism at different levels:

* National level
  At least two special centres for diagnosis and investigation

* County council level
  A specialist team for persons with autism of all ages (with doctor, psychologist, social worker, special teacher, speech therapist and physiotherapist) whose purpose it is to:
  - plan for the future of the person with autism, together with the family and responsible authority
  - provide "know-how" and information for parents and staff
  - coordinate the different activities.

* Local level
  Facilities adapted to the needs of persons with autism (pre-schools, schools, short-term care homes, boarding homes, group homes etc).

The RFPB hopes that adoption of its proposals will lead to significant improvements in the coordination and quality of the services, offered to persons with autism and their families, in the near future.

REFERENCES

Dahlgren, S-O., & Gillberg, C. (1989). Symptoms in the first two years of life: A preliminary population study of infantile autism. *European Archives of Psychiatry and Neurological Sciences, 386,* 1 - 6.

Ministry of Health and Social Affairs, International Secretariat. (1987). *Special Services For Intellectually Handicapped Persons Act and Act Concerning the Implementation of Special Services for Intellectually Handicapped Persons Act.*

Riksföreningen för Psykotiska Barn. (1988). A Government Grant to develop and describe services for autistic children and adults in Sweden. *REBECKA-report* no 7. (In English. Obtainable from the RFPB, Bondegatan 1D, 116 23 Stockholm.)

Habilitation for Children with Autism: A Swedish Example

CHRISTOPHER GILLBERG

INTRODUCTION

Any treatment or habilitation programme for childhood autism relies upon an accurate diagnosis, which in itself often constitutes part of the treatment. The notion that diagnostic and treatment strategies are generally based on specific theories or at least in some essential way related to theoretical constructs is a common one. Few of us realize the extent to which treatment is often pragmatic and initially unrelated to theoretical frameworks. Autism provides a good example of how theory-generated diagnosis and treatments have failed the test of time, whereas non-theoretical pragmatic models have prevailed and have influenced the theories instead.

Early causation theories had it that autism (often ill-defined on the basis of obscure constructs and "feelings" on the part of the "therapists" that the child had various kinds of "egodysfunction") resulted from specific deficits in parental care and interaction with the child. Consequently children were diagnosed as being influenced by parents' personalities and problems. Psychotherapy with the child, the parents or both became the most widely accepted mode of therapy. With time, it has become apparent that the psychogenic causal theories were unsupported by empirical evidence (McAdoo & De Myer, 1978). Diagnosis and treatment based on such premises were inadequate and - by and large - unsuccessful.

Meanwhile, more "atheoretical" therapists specializing in autism maintained that educational measures and behavioural treatment programmes for autism were useful. They have left their mark on the nomenclature in that autism is no longer regarded as a form of psychosis, but rather as a developmental disorder (Rutter, 1985). Empirical progress in other fields, such as in research on the neurobiological correlates, (Coleman & Gillberg, 1985), on rating scales (Brand Teal & Wiebe, 1986) and the gradual delineation of more specific psychological deficits (Baron-Cohen et al., 1985, 1986; Baron-Cohen, 1989) has also contributed to this changed perspective on autism.

TREATMENT OR HABILITATION

The current state-of-the-art in the field of autism does not provide us with the tools for rational treatment in all cases of autism. To the contrary, the concept of autism is now emerging as a diagnostic label similar to cerebral palsy; it is increasingly becoming recognized as a not quite specific (Reichler & Lee, 1987), behaviourally defined syndrome (Rutter & Schopler, 1987) with varying etiology (Gillberg, 1988). This in itself suggests that a unitary treatment of autism is unlikely - even in the long run. Specific treatments depending on underlying etiology may well be available in some cases of autism ten years from now, but so far developments in this area are only just beginning (if, that is, we don't count PKU and lactic acidos - and perhaps we should). Developmental aspects need to be taken into account and educational and behavioural modes of help for the child seem to be those with the best potential at the present stage. Therefore, on a balance, I would suggest that until such time as we have progressed further in respect of specific treatments, we should be speaking about habilitation rather than treatment in the field of autism.

"AUTISM" VERSUS "AUTISTIC"

Before we proceed I would like to say just a few words about the use of the term "autistic". Of late, I have come to realize just how problematic this term is. By saying "autistic", consciously or not, you suggest that the child is the disorder. It removes you from current thinking in the field, which conceptualizes autism as a handicapping condition in the child and not a mystical all-absorbing "state". Without further elaboration of this negative implication of the use of the word "autistic" - which actually merits an "in-depth" analysis - I would like to make a plea for talking about "people with autism" rather than "autistic people". A "child with autism" sounds like an individual; an "autistic child" on the other hand sounds like one of a group of identical children.

TABLE 1. Special autism services in the Gothenburg area in May, 1989

Service	Age group (years)	Catchment area	Authority
Diagnostic centre	0-20	Sweden (8.5 million)	Health (East hospital)
Furuhöjd in-patient treatment centre (10 "beds")	0-18	Western Swedish region (2.0 million)	Health (East hospital)
Habilitation team	0-25	Gothenburg (0.5 million)	Health (East hospital)
Boarding homes for children (2x4 beds)	0-21	Gothenburg	1) BPSMR
Pre-school groups 1x3 children + 1x6 children	0-6	Gothenburg Western Swedish region	Social welfare Regional habilitation (Bräcke Östergård)
Respite care home (30-40 families)	0-20	Gothenburg	1) BPSMR
Class-rooms (6x4 pupils) (including 1 for children with normal IQ)	7-21	Gothenburg	School
Boarding homes for adults (2x4 adults)	22+	Gothenburg	1) BPSMR
Day centres (2x4 adults)	22+	Gothenburg	1) BPSMR
"Autism community" (4 adults)	22+	Western Swedish region	1) BPSMR

1) Board for Provisions and Services to the Mentally Retarded

THE GOTHENBURG EXAMPLE

In Gothenburg in the early 1970s, we had a behavioural treatment centre (Furuhöjd) for autism within the Department of Child Psychiatry (Table 1). This was the only specialized service for children - or adults - with autism in the whole region. The city itself is inhabited by c 0.5 million people and the region (including Gothenburg itself) is about 2.0 millions.

From 1977, we have been a small group of specialists who have tried to develop a "habilitation chain" for autism; that is a set of services for people with autism ranging from a diagnostic centre for young children to group homes and day-centers for adults. The "team" has consisted of a social worker, two nurses, a teacher, two psychologists and myself. Our work has never been planned once and for all, but rather has grown out of continuously felt needs for change and development. We have tried to influence administrators and politicians around us, often without success, but, in the long run, with considerable progress as a result. Even before the era of the "Rebecka-project" (Lena Andersson's chapter) the services were developing at a reasonable rate. During the "Rebecka-era" more and more services have come into existence (Table 1). Some of these services are provided by the health authorities, others by the local educational system and others still by the local Board for Provisions and Services to the Mentally Retarded (BPSMR). At the moment there exists about a dozen different facilities tailored to meet the special needs of people who suffer from autism.

TABLE 2. The habilitation chain in autism. Essential features.

Essential feature	
1	The first evaluation: assessment and diagnosis
2	Neuropsychiatric work-up
3	"Crisis" intervention
4	Work with the family
5	Practical and financial support for the family (including respite care)
6	Education for the patient (including special autism class-rooms)
7	Physical education
8	Pharmacotherapy
9	Psychotherapy
10	Behaviour modification
11	Long-term perspective
12	Integration of approaches: the autism habilitation team

4-11 can sometimes be provided in special autism "treatment centres"

The Habilitation Chain

In my opinion, a good habilitation programme for individuals with autism has to contain a number of elements, the most important of which are outlined in Table 2. In order to provide a habilitation programme of this kind, facilities of the magnitude presented in Table I represent less than what is really needed. A major analysis of the special needs for children, adolescents and adults with autism in Gothenburg in the early 1980s showed that about double the amount of services shown in the table would be required for a minimum acceptable standard to be reached.

The details as regards diagnosis and the first evaluation have already been presented in preceeding chapters. In the following, I shall briefly comment on the various parts in the suggested habilitation chain.

The First Evaluation: Assessment and Diagnosis

An early diagnosis of autism has many advantages. It creates a possibility for the parents to face a crisis in which they can begin to come to terms with the experience of having lost a healthy child. It gives everybody involved the benefit of realistic prognostic speculation (for instance: "It is not likely that he will grow up to be free of handicap"). It enables the treating physician to proceed with a reasonable medical work-up and provide counselling as regards causes, genetic risks and, sometimes, specific treatment. It serves as an impetus to design the best possible educational programme for the child and to provide the general outlines for a longitudinal habilitation programme (including practical help) for the child and his family.

Neuropsychiatric Work-Up

Once a diagnosis of autism is seriously considered it is essential to refer the child to somebody knowledgeable in the field. Psychiatrists and psychologists not very familiar with autism should not, in my opinion, start what will mostly turn into an amateurish search in the dark for diagnostic labels, reasonable assessment tools and adequate interpretation of symptoms, signs and neurobiological data. Autism is a difficult field, growing and diversifying every day, and should - in the initial stages - be left to those who have abundant clinical experience. This may mean having to refer the child and family to an expert team hundreds of miles away. In these days of community-based services and decentralization someone might take offence and suggest we leave matters like these to the

G P or the non-specialized child psychiatrist. However, we don't leave cerebral palsy or childhood epilepsy to the non-specialist at the time of diagnosis. Autism is more complicated than such conditions and it should go without saying that it is a specialist concern.

There are various "autism diagnostic tools" in use (e g the CARS (Shopler et al., 1980), the E-2 form (Rimland, 1964) and the ABC (Krug et al., 1980)). Now, for the psychiatrist or psychologist (or for that matter social worker or teacher) familiar with autism, such devices are not necessary for arriving at a correct diagnosis. However, they can be very useful in the longitudinal follow-up of the child as a "base-line", in treatment trials and in clinical research. I have found the CARS and the ABC to be helpful, simple and not too time-consuming instruments within that group of checklists/rating scales.

It is essential that the child's cognitive level and style be assessed in some detail. IQ is the single most powerful predictor of outcome in autism, and education needs to be geared to a level appropriate to the child's developmental age. There is no such thing as an "untestable case of autism". It is always possible to arrive at some sort of estimation of the child's functional cognitive capacity. It has been repeatedly shown (e g Clark & Rutter, 1979; Rutter, 1983) that the cognitive deficit in autism is real and not due to "lack of motivation", "withdrawal into the autistic shell" or some such similar reason. It is not the child who is untestable, but sometimes (indeed rather often) the psychologist doesn't have the skills and experience to manage testing! The Leiter test, the Vineland Social Maturity Scale, a language test (such as the Reynell's) and, in school age children of relatively high IQ, the Wechsler scales are the ones most commonly used in my department. The Griffiths scale is also much used but really adds very little to the experienced clinician's global assessment. Some sort of evaluation of the child's capacity to impute that other people have minds, feelings and perspectives of their own, is often helpful. Simple tests in this field have been suggested by Frith and co-workers (Baron-Cohen et al., 1985, 1986; Leslie & Frith, 1988; Baron-Cohen, 1989).

Additional medical (including dental), neurological and psychiatric handicaps must be discovered and attended to in the early stages of the disorder. Hearing deficits, refraction errors and other visual problems, epilepsy and depression are all common in autism and need careful consideration and differential treatment. Dental care is as important in autism as in normality, but is a sadly neglected area which needs much more attention in the future.

The absolute minimum in respect of neurobiological work-up required in every autism case in which the etiology is not readily apparent would be: thorough medical/physical examination (e g to diagnose hearing and visual deficits, skin signs of tuberous sclerosis or neurofibromatosis, auricule or genital signs of the fragile-X-syndrome), a CAT or MRI-scan of the brain (early signs of tuberous sclerosis, toxoplasmosis etc), an EEG ("subclinical" epilepsy, see Gillberg & Schaumann, 1983), a spinal tap with CSF-electrophoresis (early signs of a neurodegenerative disorder) and a chromosomal culture in a folic acid depleted medium (fragile-X-syndrome, applies both in boys and girls, Gillberg et al., 1988). Depending on the situation and the specific symptoms and signs in the individual case, a host of other neurobiological assessments may need to be used (Coleman & Gillberg, 1985).

Crisis Intervention, Work with the Family and Practical and Psychological Support

Families with children who have autism, just as much as families with children who suffer from cerebral palsy or epilepsy, are in need of long-term contact with a small group of medical, paramedical and education people who are knowledgeable and skilled in the particular field represented by the child's handicap. This group of specialists needs to constitute a collaborative professional team, not necessarily working within the same four walls, but cooperating on a regular basis. They need to work much, if not all, of their professional time, in the field of autism. Based in child psychiatry, pediatrics or developmental medicine depending on regional characteristics, such teams cannot be expected in all towns or rural areas, but should be available within a hundred miles or so from the family. There may also be the need for regional expert diagnostic centers to help promote the development of early screening measures and basic and clinical research. The psychological support that is inherent in the very fact that the specialists really know something of what the child and family are going through can hardly be over-estimated. The feeling that: "At last I don't need to explain everything to puzzled "experts": finally there is someone who can tell me something" is usually a great relief for the parents.

Many people surmise that a family faced with a diagnosis of autism will necessarily find themselves in an acute crisis which requires psychotherapeutic intervention. Although this may be, and sometimes is, the case, very often no such crisis occurs. In such cases, the family members have usually been living in a state of "chronic crisis" for several months or years. The child's behavioural abnormalities, sleep problems and the lack of an adequate diagnosis have put a severe strain on the family's coping abilities. What is usually called for in such situations is practical help. Providing opportunity for respite care outside of the family, adjusting the family's house or apartment to some of the most extreme needs of the child, prescribing appropriate "sleep-inducing" medication, or helping the parents to apply for societal economic support are only a few examples of what might be done. Such things, rather than classical psychotherapeutic measures, all have psychotherapeutic effects.

Psychotherapy should never be offered on a tone of: "We know that this is what you need", but rather be seen as a, sometimes important, adjunct to a range of facilities offered to the family. It is essential to note that professionals tend to judge families as more stressed by the child's symptoms than do families themselves (Bebko et al., 1987). In my experience, less than one in five of all parents with young children with autism need formal psychotherapy. In the majority of cases practical help and psychological support will go a long way in relieving some of the tensions and confusion which may be prevailing and feelings of guilt which afflict all parents of children with autism (as well as parents of children with other handicaps and normal children).

Sibling problems are often overlooked in the field of autism, usually because of the enormous physical and emotional strains put on the parents, and the mother in particular, which makes for a situation with little time or emotional strength left over for the brothers and sisters. The "habilitation team" will need to be aware of such matters and take appropriate steps to prevent psychiatric breakdown in siblings. Information about autism in general and in the particular case, as well as psychotherapy with the brother or sister, parents or conjointly and pharmacological treatment (usually antidepressant) may all have their place.

Education and Behaviour Modification for the Patient

To put it briefly, the kind of special education and behaviour modification required for a child with autism encompasses a number of crucial elements. First, there is a need for a high teacher: child ratio (1:3 to 1:1 being necessary depending on the child's degree of handicap). Second, a substantial degree of structure is important, but, as Rutter (1985) points out "the needs may well vary according to the autistic child's age and developmental level". Third, the essence of any autism education programme, in my opinion is continuity as regards person, room and time, or, if you wish, something like "the same teacher should try to train or teach the same thing in the same child in the same place on the same weekday (at the same time of the day)". This minimizes the child's need to impose routine and rituals and provides a feeling of a "safe frame-work" for the educational process. Nevertheless, the child's problems as regards generalizing educational and behavioural gains, makes it necessary to teach the child how to use acquired skills in various settings, and, in the case of the relatively gifted children, teach them verbally and in other ways that the new skill is for use in more than the specific educational setting. Here it is essential to involve the parents at an early stage. Trivial settings, indeed almost all settings are appropriate for training and generalizing skills taught in the classroom.

Education and behaviourally oriented programmes have to be applied for several hours a day. A class-room (or sometimes a residential setting within an autism treatment centre) is often the most appropriate place, both for the very young and somewhat older children. Whether or not this has to be an "autism" classroom depends on the needs of the individual child and the environmental opportunities. It is sometimes claimed that all children with autism need the interaction of normal children. I am not sure that I agree in this respect. One of the central symptoms in autism is the lack of a good capacity to interact reciprocally with age-peers. I know a few bright young men with autism who have told me that the best thing that ever happened to them was when they could leave school and have an isolated job of their own in which human interaction (with age-peers) was kept to an absolute minimum. If a child who is said to have autism needs the social interaction of age-peers more than anything else (as is repeatedly claimed by some administrators and theorists: rarely, if ever, by those with practical experience of both "mainstreaming" and "specializing units for autism") the diagnosis may be mistaken. What the child with autism (especially when very young) needs most of all is the dependable, well-organized, consistent adult who can provide everyday skills and tools for "social survival". These may range from dressing to controlling bladder and bowel functions in the very young age group and from learning to ski and skate to being in a crowd of people in the school age group.

In summary it has been my contention that education and treatment for children with autism, at least in an urban area, in many cases is best provided within the setting of a special autism education unit which must maintain a very close contact with the child's parents. Regular, at least monthly, home-school meetings at which the behavioural/educational programme is reevaluated and reformulated, are required. However, one must not, in the individual case assume that a special autism unit is always preferable. There is, however, a need for such units for most autistic children, not least in the pre-school period. I have seen tragic examples of how children with autism, "integrated" in normal pre-schools (much to the delight of some politicians and administrators) have been deprived of adequate stimulation and developmentally appropriate skills - even when they have had the benefit of a full-time special assistant who has received skilled counselling at regular intervals. Special units have the advantage of a concentration of special skills on the part of the teachers and they provide a good base for involving the family in all sorts of education/treatment planning and strategies. Nevertheless, especially in the more intellectually able children and those with milder variants of autism, placement in ordinary daycare nurseries or ordinary schools, may sometimes be the most suitable solution for everybody involved.

Clearly then, there is a great need to regard all people with autism as individuals who share a common problem, viz autism, but who can never be reduced to copies of each other. It goes without saying that children and adults with autism come in as many shapes as there are persons with that diagnosis. No one treatment can be expected to fit all, and that goes for everything from pharmacotherapy to education and need for special units.

Education and behavioural treatment of children with autism make most difference in the behavioural domains, some difference in the fields of language competence and usage and probably no difference whatsoever with respect to general intelligence (Howlin & Rutter, 1987). Claims for more revolutionary results (which are constantly offered by therapeutic enthusiasts) by far exceed what can in fact be realistically attained (Rutter, 1985).

Children with autism will not be cured by education and behavioural treatment programmes. This goes for all other currently used treatment methods, too. However, this factual state of affairs should not inspire pessimism. Indeed a lot of worthwhile things can be achieved through appropriate treatment, but children, parents, teachers, other personnel and administrators/politicians will benefit from realistic insight and rational suggestions as to what might best be accomplished rather than by repeatedly being disillusioned by the many self-elected magicians in this field.

Pharmacotherapy

Psychopharmacology has no major role in the treatment of young children with autism. In adolescence and sometimes in adult life, however, severe behaviour problems often necessitate a trial of neuroleptics, lithium or antidepressants. They may occasionally be of great avail in cases with disorganized behaviour, aggressiveness, motor overactivity and sleep problems. Lithium, in particular, may have a role in those cases of autism who show severe mood and/or behaviour "swings" (Steingard & Biederman, 1987; Kerbeshian et al., 1987). Self-destructiveness, in my experience, is not particularly responsive to any of these drugs. Opiateantagonists (Small & Campbell, 1989), B-vitamins (in particular B6) (see Rimland 1987 for a review) and folic acid (Gillberg et al., 1986) and beta-blockers (Ratey et al., 1987) may all prove to be worthwhile in future studies, but so far the evidence for any of them is equivocal or lacking altogether. Current psychopharmacological treatment methods do not seem to affect the basic course of the disorder (Howlin & Rutter, 1987). However, as in all other fields, this should not be taken to mean that pharmacotherapy should never be used. Medical treatments rarely cure, but can be very useful in ameliorating short term crises (see also Magda Campbell's chapters in this book).

Most of us want to refrain from using drugs in the treatment of young children as far as possible. Nevertheless, no autism treatment team can do without psychopharmacological expertice.

Antiepileptic pharmacological treatment may be essential in some cases (carbamazepine and valproate being drugs of choice because of the usually limited negative effects on behaviour (Gillberg, 1989)), but deleterious in others (barbiturates and benzodiazepines often contributing to deterioration in behaviour according to clinical expericence). In the future, antiepileptic surgery may achieve an important role in the field of autism and epilepsy.

Fenfluramine, an anorexogenic drug launched as somewhat of a miracle drug in autism, probably has no place in the treatment of the disorder. This was shown for instance in one of the few systematic "treatment studies" from our centre (Ekman et al., 1989).

Physical Education

Clinical and empirical experience both suggest that physical activity - leading to physical "fatigue" - very often has positive effects as regards negative/destructive behavioural symptoms in autism (McGimsey & Favell, 1988).

Psychotherapy

Individual psychotherapy (analytically oriented) does not seem to have a clear place in most cases of young children with autism (Howlin & Rutter, 1987). However, relatively brighter, and in particular verbal autistic adolescents may benefit from individual psychotherapeutic approaches. These should not (indeed usually cannot) be of the classical psychoanalytical kind, but rather geared to conveying long-term "empathy" and constructive guidance in a setting acknowledging the young person's specific handicaps. Unwarranted hopes for cure should not be conveyed.

Some parents need psychotherapy. In my experience this applies in less than 20 per cent of autism cases. This may take the form of short-term crisis intervention at the time of diagnosis, long - term individual support for one or both parents or conjoint family therapy (without the child with autism present). Non-experts often claim that all parents with a handicapped child experience severe guilt feelings. Clearly, not all of them do. Support for the parents (and brothers and sisters) cannot be fitted into any one overriding particular model but rather needs to be attuned to the varying practical and emotional needs of each individual family. There is nothing whatsoever to support the popular view that family psychotherapy (or indeed parental psychotherapy) by itself can do anything to positively affect the handicaps associated with autism, either in the child or the secondary strains imposed on the family. In fact, I have seen dozens of families with "autistic children" who received nothing but family therapy (10 - 80 sessions) for several years, until the child was given a correct diagnosis of Rett syndrome, tuberous sclerosis or fragile-X-syndrome by an independant doctor. Not one of these families got anything but increased guilt feelings (and became increasingly confused) by this procedure.

Long-term Perspective, Integration of Approaches and Provision of Services

The following is my suggestion for optimal provision of services in the field of autism.

Any catchment area of 2 - 4 million people will need to have a regional central diagnostic/assessment team for autism consisting of child neuropsychiatrist, clinical psychologist, child psychiatric social worker, speech-therapist and teacher. All children raising suspicion of suffering from severe problems in any of the three "main" fields suggestive of autism should be referred for evaluation to this team, preferably before age 3 years, but later if no clear diagnostic consensus has been reached before that age. This team needs to work in close collaboration with neuropediatricians and other "neuro-specialists" in order that "modern" neurobiological work-up in each individual case be achieved at an acceptable level.

Another team, consisting of a consultant child psychiatrist, psychologists, social workers, speech therapists and teachers should constitute a long-term follow-up central habilitation-team, working in close collaboration with the diagnostic team. Treatment programmes and follow-up should be designed by this team, which might itself provide the treatment in certain cases and "inspire" treatment by other specialists in other cases.

Smaller local habilitation teams should be provided in the community depending on size of population and frequency of handicap. One of the main tasks for this team would be to provide family-based intervention programmes, such as recently succintly summarized in Howlin and Rutter (1987).

Personal assistants receiving regular counselling from experts, preferably in groups, may be one of the most important pillars of treatment in certain cases, particularly if and when the child is integrated in non-specialized units. Almost all children with autism outside of special schools or treatment centers, in my opinion, should be assigned such a full-time personal assistant.

It has been my clinical experience (based on several hundred cases who have received either "segregated" or "integrated" education/treatment or both) that a majority of children with autism benefit most from treatment and education in special units. Special pre-school-groups and special classes (within special or comprehensive schools) as well as residential treatment centres, in my opinion, need to be provided at a rate covering 50 - 75 per cent of the population of children with autism.

Adolescents and adults with autism (Asperger syndrome not included), will need some kind of specialized service in at least 75 per cent of the cases. Special group homes (3 - 10 individuals), which may well be localized in sets of 2 or more and special work day-centers are both essential elements in any comprehensive service for autistic people.

If one is to make optimal use of these special services, one should not blindly accept the diagnosis of autism as the only criterion for suggesting this or that kind of special service. Age, personality characteristics, language level, degree of behaviour problems, IQ and family background are but some of the characteristics one will need to consider in each individual case before an optimal decision is reached.

"NEW HOPE FOR A CURE"?

In autism, as in most severe handicapping conditions of childhood, enthusiastic claims for miraculuos cures are often voiced. In 1988 I surveyed a majority of all the cases of autism (n = 152) and autistic-like conditions (n = 72) under age 15 years that I had personally examined in some detail up until then. Altogether at least 18 of these 224 families had been promised or led to believe that their child would be cured if they would enter a particular treatment. Ten of these had had their children (high and low IQ cases included) in regular psychoanalytically oriented therapy for at least 2 years at least once a week (except holidays). The remaining 8 had "gone through" holding therapy for at least one year. A further 14 had received rigorous operant-conditioning treatment in in-patient settings for att least two years (often more). The outcome status 1 - 15 years later is shown in Table 3. The outcome categories are those used in Gillberg and Steffenburg (1987) and are similar to those used by Lotter (1974). Although no conclusions as regards treatment effects can be drawn from these figures, it is clear that the various approaches had not led to cures. Interestingly, some of the very few extremely good outcomes I've seen myself in the field of autism have been in cases who haven't received any particular kind of treatment.

TABLE 3. "Outcome" at ages 5 - 25 years in the 1 - 15-year perspective in 224 cases of autism and autistic-like conditions seen by author when they were under age 15 years. Outcome versus various treatment models. All outcomes at least one year after "completion" of therapies.

Treatment strategy	Good or fair outcome	Intermediate	Poor or very poor outcome
° Various approaches (education, family support, medication behaviour modification psychotherapy)	30	36	128
° Rigorous operant	3	1	10 1)
° Psychoanalytical			10 2)
° Holding therapy		1	7

1) including 3 cases considered "cured" by therapist, yet scoring >70 on ABC (all 3 had no speech (school-age) and 2 had tested IQ-levels <30)

2) including 2 cases considered "cured" by therapist (both living in institutions, with no speech (now school-age) and tested IQ-levels <30)

CONCLUDING REMARKS

Treatment, or rather, habilitation in autism, although progressing, is far from satisfactory in most cases at the present stage. Usually, there is no cure within reach. Autism should be accepted as a - possibly life-long - handicap with great individual variation as regards severity and course, much along the lines of prevailing views in the fields of cerebral palsy and mental retardation. Therapeutic (over-) enthusiasts usually do much more harm than good. There is a basis for cautious, realistic optimism. Good treatment can lead to clearly enduring positive effects as regards behaviour and every-day skills and to slight and moderate improvement in the field of communication. IQ and life-time course do not seem to be affected by treatment (Howlin & Rutter, 1987). However, life-quality for the family and the child can probably be changed into a positive direction by using appropriate treatment strategies.

REFERENCES

American Psychiatric Association (1987). *Diagnostic and Statistical Manual of Mental Disorders. DSM-III-R (3rd rev ed.).* Washington, DC: Author.

Baron-Cohen, S., Leslie, A. M., & Frith, U. (1985). Does the autistic child have a "theory of mind"? *Cognition, 21,* 37 - 46.

Baron-Cohen, S., Leslie, A. M., & Frith, U. (1986). Mechanical, behavioural and intentional understanding of picture stories in autistic children. *British Journal of Developmental Psychology, 4,* 113 - 125.

Baron-Cohen, S. (1989). The Autistic Child's Theory of Mind: a Case of Specific Development Delay. *Journal of Child Psychology and Psychiatry, 2,* 285 - 297.

Bebko, J. M., Konstantareas, M. M., & Springer, J. (1987). Parent and professional evaluation of family stress associated with characteristics of autism. *Journal of Autism and Developmental Disorders, 17,* 565 - 576.

Bettelheim, B. (1966). *The Empty Fortress:* Infantile Autism and the Birth of Self. New York: Free Press.

Brand Teal, M., & Wiebe, M. (1986). A Validity Analysis of Selected Instruments Used to Assess Autism. *Journal of Autism and Developmental Disorders, 4,* 485 - 494.

Campbell, M. (1987). Drug treatment of infantile autism - the past decade. In H. Y. Meltzer (Ed.), *Psychopharmacology: The Third Generation of Progress* (pp 1225 - 1232). New York: Raven Press.

Clark, P., & Rutter, M. (1979). Task difficulty and task performance in autistic children. *Journal of Child Psychology and Psychiatry, 20,* 271 - 285.

Coleman, M., & Gillberg, C. (1985). *The Biology of the Autistic Syndromes.* New York: Praeger.

DeMyer, M. K., Hingtgen, J. N., & Jackson, R. K. (1981). Infantile autism reviewed: a decade of research. *Schizophrenia Bulletin, 7,* 388 - 451.

Ekman, G., Miranda-Linné, F., Gillberg, C., Garle, M., & Wetterberg, L. (1989). Fenfluramine treatment of 20 autistic children. *Journal of Autism and Developmental Disorders* (in press).

Garreau, B., Barthelemy, C., Sauvage, D., Leddet, I., & Lelord, G. (1984). A comparison of autistic syndromes with and without associated neurological problems. *Journal of Autism and Developmental Disorders, 14,* 105-111.

Gillberg, C. (1989). The Treatment of Epilepsy in Autism. *Journal of Autism and Developmental Disorders* (submitted).

Gillberg, C. (1988). The neurobiology of infantile autism. *Journal of Child Psychology and Psychiatry, 29,* 257 - 266.

Gillberg C., Olsson V. A., Wahlström, J., Steffenburg, S., & Blix, K. (1988). Monozygotic female twins with autism and the fragile-X-syndrome (AFRAX). *Journal of Child Psychology and Psychiatry, 29,* 447 - 451.

Gillberg, C., & Schaumann, H. (1983). Epilepsy presenting as infantile autism? Two case studies. *Neuropediatrics, 14,* 206 - 212.

Gillberg, C., Steffenburg, S., & Jakobsson, G. (1987). Neurobiological findings in 20 relatively gifted children with Kanner-type autism or Asperger syndrome. *Developmental Medicine and Child Neurology, 29,* 641-649.

Gillberg, C., Wahlström, J., Johansson, R., Törnblom, M., & Albertsson-Wikland, K. (1986). Folic acid as an adjunct in the treatment of children with the autism-fragile-(X) syndrome (AFRAX). *Developmental Medicine and Child Neurology, 28,* 624 - 627.

Howlin, P., & Rutter, M. (1987). *Treatment of Autistic Children.* Chichester: Wiley.

Kerbeshian, J., Burd, L., & Fisher, W. (1987). Lithium carbonate in the treatment of two patients with infantile autism and atypical bipolar symptomatology. *Journal of Clinical Psychopharmacology, 7,* 401 - 405.

Krug, D. A., Arick, J., & Almond, P. (1980). Behaviour checklist for identifying severely handicapped individuals with high levels of autistic behaviour. *Journal of Child Psychology and Psychiatry, 21,* 221 - 229.

Lane, H. (1976). *The Wild Boy of Aveyron.* Cambridge, Massachussetts: Harvard University Press.

Leboyer, M., Bouvard, M. P., & Dugas, M. (1988). Effects of naltrexone on infantile autism (letter). *Lancet March* 26, 1 (8587), 715.

Leslie, A., & Frith, U. (1988). Autistic children's understanding of seeing, knowing and believing. *British Journal of Developmental Psychology 6,* 315 - 324.

McAdoo, W. G., & DeMyer, M. K. (1978). Research related to family factors in autism. *Journal of Pediatric Psychology, 2,* 162 - 166.

McGimsey, J. F., & Favell, J. E. (1988). The effects of increased physical exercise on disruptive behavior in retarded persons. *Journal of Autism and Developmental Disorders, 18,* 167 - 179.

Ratey, J. J., Bemporad, J., Sorgi, P., Bick, P., Polakoff, S., O'Driscoll, G., & Mikkelsen, E. (1987). Open trial effects of beta-blockers on speech and social behaviors in 8 autistic adults. *Journal of Autism and Developmental Disorders 17,* 439 - 446.

Reichler, R. J., & Lee, E. M. C. (1987). Overview of biomedical issues in autism. In E. Schopler & G. Mesibov (Eds.), *Neurobiological issues in autism.* New York: Plenum Publishing Corporation.

Rimland, B. (1964). FORM E-2: Diagnostic Check-List for Behaviour-Disturbed Children (AUTISTIC-TYPE CHILDREN). San Diego, California: Institute for Child Behaviour Research.

Rimland, B. (1987). Megavitamin B6 and Magnesium in the Treatment of Autistic

Children and Adults. In E. Schopler & G. Mesibov (Eds.), *Neurobiological issues in autism.* New York: Plenum Press.

Rutter, M. (1983). Cognitive deficits in the pathogenesis of autism. *Journal of Child Psychology and Psychiatry, 24,* 513-531.

Rutter, M. (1985). The treatment of autistic children. *Journal of Child Psychology and Psychiatry, 26,* 193-214.

Rutter, M., & Schopler, E. (1987). Autism and pervasive developmental disorders: concepts and diagnostic issues. *Journal of Autism and Developmental Disorders, 17,* 159-186.

Schopler, E., & Mesibov, G. B. (1985). *Communication Problems in Autism.* New York: Plenum Press.

Schopler, E., Reichler, R. J., DeVellis, R. F., & Daly, K. (1980). Toward objective classification of childhood autism: Childhood Autism Rating Scale (CARS). *Journal of Autism and Developmental Disorders, 10,* 91-103.

Small, A. M., & Campbell, M. (1989). *Pharmacotherapy in Autism: Research Perspective and Update.* Paper read at World Congress of Biological Psychiatry, Jerusalem.

Steingard, R., & Biederman, J. (1987). Lithium responsive manic-like symptoms in two individuals with autism and mental retardation. *Journal of the American Academy of Child and Adolescent Psychiatry 26,* 937 - 938.

Steps Towards the Organization of Services for Autistic Children and Their Families: The Responsibility of Child Psychiatry

MICHAEL BOHMAN, INGA LILL BOHMAN and EVA SJÖHOLM - LIF

IMPEDIMENTS TO THE TREATMENT AND EDUCATION OF AUTISTIC CHILDREN

Since Kanner's first description of infantile autism almost fifty years ago (Kanner, 1943) there has been a prolific and increasing number of both scientific and popular publications about this syndrome. Persons with autism have also been personified in many plays, films or on television. Truffaut's *L'enfant sauvage* (based on Itard's (Itard, 1932) description of Victor, the wild Boy of Aveyron), Hertzog's *Kaspar Hauser* or more recently, Barry Levinson's *Rain Man* (with Dustin Hoffman) are but a few examples of the strong fascination which the phenomenon of autism arouses in the general public. There seems to be no limits to the growing interest in this mysterious condition (which is certainly out of proportion to its relatively rare occurrence) among both specialists and laymen.

Delay of diagnosis and treatment

It is a paradox that in spite of this widespread interest in autistic phenomena it is still very common that parents of autistic children meet with great difficulties when they are seeking help for their children. Their reports and anxieties about their children's symptoms are seldom taken seriously by doctors or other personnel in the health system. The diagnosis and assessment of the autistic handicap is very often postponed for several years, sometimes indefinitely. Parents are being referred to different specialists but it can take years before somebody takes responsibility for a proper action leading to treatment and habilitation. This situation is still prevailing in many places in our country according to recent investigations. We suspect that Sweden is by no means an exception concerning this paradoxical delay of identification and treatment of children with autism. There are at least three important reasons for this seemingly contradictory situation.

The frequency of autism

First, autistic syndromes are rather rare phenomena and not so easy to recognize during the child's early years. The general practitioner or pediatrician may not encounter enough cases in his lifetime to be well accustomed to the special signs and symptoms which are characteristic of early infantile autism and other pervasive developmental disorders. But we don't believe that the rarity of these syndromes in the most important cause of the delay of diagnosis and treatment of autism. There are admittedly other equally rare conditions, beginning in infancy or childhood which are promptly identified in the present health system.

The confusion about etiology

A second reason for the still prevailing delay of diagnosis and treatment of autism is probably related to the controversies about the etiology of autism which started already with Kanner's own vacillation between organic and psychological theories. For many years etiological theories were dominating which regarded autism as a disorder caused by deficiencies in the parents' abilities to give the child a good enough emotional contact during the first years of life. These etiological theories or beliefs were embraced by famous international experts in child psychiatry and psychoanalysis. They were widely accepted as dogmas by many child psychiatrists and other professionals in the field and had a profound and negative influence on the treatment policies and the attitudes towards the parents of autistic children. According to recent investigations such misconceptions are unfortunately still prevailing among some professionals. The confusion about etiology and scapegoating of parents of autistic children were probably strong reasons behind the delay of implementations of services for autistic children at a time when such services were being widely organized for most other disabled children. Comprehensive screening procedures for early diagnosis of autistic disorders were seldom if ever organized by the public health system nor were educational and training programmes developed as was usual for other children with various mental or physical handicaps.

The fragmentation of services

A third, important factor behind the lack of success in the treatment and education of autistic children is due to the present prevailing fragmentation of services for all children with handicaps. In our modern welfare society parents with sick and handicapped children have to meet with at lot of different specialists and helping services with different responsibilities or mandates. Such public services are working fairly well for children with specific handicaps (i e deafness, cerebral palsy, diabetes etc) because responsibilities for the handling of every case are almost always clear and approved in the public system services. In contrast, autistic handicaps were for a long time nobodys responsibility. The controversies about the nature and etiology of autism created an unclear, ambiguous situation for these children in the public health and welfare systems. The consequence was that no speciality or organization was given a clear mandate to take the responsibility for the identification, treatment or education of these children. They were often classified as mentally retarded and referred to various hospitals, institutions or treatment homes for severely mentally retarded people. Many ambitious projects have been born with the optimistic aim of helping or even curing autistic children but most have failed and gone astray in a chaotic jungle of bureaucracy. Overlapping organizations have been eager to offer different kinds of treatment or education, in a competition which has left parents in a state of confusion and despair.

WHAT SHOULD CHILD PSYCHIATRY DO?

We do not believe that the delay of diagnosis and treatment of autistic children which is still a common phenomenon in our country is due to lack of resources, money, personnel or expertise in our present public health system. On the contrary we have reason to believe that at least some of the failures has been due to deficiencies in the organization of services and unclear, ambiguous regulations about responsibilities for persons with autistic handicaps.

There is perhaps a change in a positive direction by the implementation of a new Swedish law from 1986 which regulates public services for mental retardation. This law guarantees services for children and adults with childhood psychosis which by and large corresponds to the English term pervasive developmental disorders, including autistic disorders. According to this law the county's organization for the mentally retarded has the overriding responsibility to offer care, education and other kinds of support also to persons with childhood psychosis. With this law there is reasonable hope that in the future services for autistic persons and their parents will be better organized in Sweden.

However, early identification and diagnosis of handicaps, including autism are necessary conditions for treatment and planning of the children's future. This must still be the responsibility of the public health system, i e the primary health care, pediatrics and child psychiatry. It is obvious that a programme which has the ambition to organize services for *all* autistic children and their families in a catchment area will still meet with many difficulties and impediments for those reasons we have put forward here.

Child psychiatry, which is a part of the public health services, has been but one of many public or private organizations supposed to be in charge of autism. In the preparation for the afore-mentioned law from 1986 child psychiatry has recently been given an important role in the early identification, diagnosis and treatment of autistic handicaps. But this role has never been obvious or selfevident, even among child psychiatrists themselves. The aim of the present paper has been to try to define some of the tasks which should be the responsibility of child psychiatry in the present public health system in our country.

Having encountered difficulties for many years in our clinical work with autistic children we decided in the beginning of the seventies to develop a programme for early diagnosis and treatment of autistic children at the department of child psychiatry in Umeå, Västerbotten County. Here we will briefly describe our experiences from this work during about a decade.

STARTING SERVICES IN A NORTHERN SWEDISH COUNTY

The county of Västerbotten has about 240 000 inhabitants and is situated in the north of Sweden south of the Arctic Circle. About 69 000 are under the age of twenty.

During the seventies there were no special services for autism and other pervasive developmental disorders in this county, the catchment area for the department of child and youth psychiatry at the University Hospital in Umeå. Delay of diagnosis was a rule with few exceptions and in many cases autism was never identified. Most older children with autistic handicaps known to us were living with their parents and were registered by the organization for the mentally retarded. But there were no special services which provided education, training or other occupational activities for autistic children.

The county has public pediatric services and well baby clinics. There is also an organization for the education and care of the mentally retarded which is independent of the Public Health Services. Children with various developmental disorders were as a rule referred to the department of child psychiatry from other departments for assessment and diagnostic evaluation.

The deplorable condition of many autistic children who were referred to our department promted us to take a look at the total situation of autism in the county and try work out some basic principles, goals and guidelines for a comprehensive organization of services for children with autistic handicaps.

Mainstreaming in normal schools

As mentioned, most autistic children lived with their parents, very few were staying in institutions. The county is very thinly populated and there are practical difficulties to arrange special services for autistic children because of the very long distances between cities and villages. For practical reasons children had to be integrated in their local school or nursery. In our own work we were encouraged to find that some autistic children could successfully be integrated among normal children both in nursery schools and ordinary normal classes in the comprehensive school if special arrangements were made.

AN EPIDEMIOLOGICAL SURVEY

A necessary condition for the planning of services for children with handicaps is knowledge of the number of cases in a catchment area. As we had no clear idea about the size of the autistic population in the county and the actual need for services we started with an epidemiological survey. Methods and results have been described elsewhere (Bohman et al., 1983) and here we will only report some of the most salient findings.

We identified 39 children among 69 000 in the age-group 0-20. The prevalance of "childhood psychosis" which in our investigation fairly well corresponds to autism or autistic syndromes (according to the DSM III R) was 5.6:10 000 (Table 1). The highest prevalence was found in the age-group 7-9 years which is considerably higher than was found in earlier investigations (Gillberg, 1984).

Table 1. Prevalence of childhood psychosis (=DSM III R autism): by sex and three-year age-groups (pop. 69 000 0-20 yrs).

Age-group (years)	Boys	Girls	Boys + Girls	Prevalence per 10 000
0-3	2	0	2	1.7
4-6	2	3	5	5.0
7-9	9	3	12	12.6
10-12	5	3	8	7.8
13-15	2	3	5	4.6
16-17	3	0	3	4.6
18-20	1	3	4	4.1
Total	24	15	39	5.6
Boy-girl ratio 1.6:1				

Delay and neglect of diagnosis

Among the 39 cases identified as childhood psychosis, 20 cases had never been previously diagnosed. Among the 19 children who had been properly identified and diagnosed prior to the study, only two had been so before 30 months of age. Nine cases were recognized between 4 and 6 years. Table 2 confirms the assumption that delay or neglect of diagnosis of autism was still a very common phenomenon in the Swedish public health system as late as in the beginning of the eighties. There are indications that the circumstances are still far from satisfactory.

Table 2. Age (in years) when diagnosis was made.

Age (years)	< 1	1-2	2-3	3-4	4-5	5-6	6-7	>7
Number	0	0	3	0	6	3	2	5

Diagnoses made : 19
Not made previously: 20

The value of "broad information" about autism

One important condition for the realization of our epidemiological survey was a close cooperation with the personnel in the public health services, the organization for the mentally retarded, the local comprehensive schools, and the nursery schools. There was very little knowledge about autistic syndromes among this personnel or among people in general at the time of the survey but the intensive information drive, which was a part of the investigation, increased the general interest in autism and other developmental disorders in children all over the county. The result was an increasing number of referrals for assessment of small children with various disturbances much younger than previously. A consequence of this increasing number of referrals was improved diagnostic skills among the staff at the department. It is also probable that the intensive and repeated information to the "grass-root level" was an important reason for the relatively high prevalence of autism in our study compared to other earlier investigations.

The natural history of autism

The survey of an almost total population of autistic children from early childhood to adolescence made it possible to study the natural history of autistic syndromes. As others before us we found that autism is a chronic and heterogenous disorder which in most cases has a poor social prognosis. However, there were large differences with regard to the degree of impairment. Intellectual abilities varied between severe mental retardation and normal levels. Table 3 gives an account of different types of schooling among 37 children (two cases were beyond school age).

Table 3. Childhood psychosis 0 - 20 years. Type of schooling by sex.

School	Boys	Girls	Boy + Girls
Nursery school	9 (6) *	4 (1)	13 (7)
Comprehensive school	8 (6)	1 (1)	9 (7)
School for mentally retarded	2	3	5
Training school	2 (1)	5	7 (1)
Special school for autistic children	2	1	3
Total	23 (13)	14 (2)	37 (15)

*Numbers in brackets: the child has a personal assistant. Two children beyond school age.

More than 50 % of the children were integrated in a normal school or a nursery school. The majority of these children had a personal assistant (numbers in brackets), who helped and trained the children during lessons or leisure-time. As a matter of fact a personal assistant (a kind of tutor) was a necessary condition for a successful integration among normal children. As a part of our treatment programme these assistants hade some training and supervision from the department of child psychiatry.

It is also obvious from the table that a much higher proportion of girls, compared to boys, were attending schools for the severely mentally retarded. This reflects the well-known fact that autistic girls, although much rarer than boys, are often much more severely handicapped or brain damaged (Tsai et al., 1981).

Treatment and prognosis

There seems to be a general agreement that autistic handicaps are lifelong and that they seriously restrict the social functioning also in adult age. Ten or at most twenty per cent of autistic children might be able to support themselves as adults and to live an independent life (Lotter, 1978). The crucial question is if there are any possible interventions or treatment methods which may cure or prevent autism. There are many who have reported promising methods and results (Bettelheim, 1967; Tinbergen &

Tinbergen, 1983) but so far scientific proof is lacking. However, there is growing evidence that autistic children do develop less severe symptoms and improve in social skills if diagnosis is made early and followed by training and education in a structured milieu (Howlin & Rutter, 1987).

Our own experiences also indicate that some autistic children who had got early training and support of an assistant very much improved their social skills after some years. In one case, diagnosed as "classic" autism at three years of age we found a remission of all typical symptoms some years later. But it may be wise not to expect too much an improvement or "cure" from a treatment programme. Prevention of self-destructive and other severe stereotypic behaviours may be important first-hand goal. Progress in learning or social skills is generally very slow. Most important may be practical, stress-relieving arrangements and support to the parents which may permit them to have room for some life of their own.

BASIC PRINCIPLES FOR TREATMENT

Both the epidemiological survey and our clinical work gave us experiences from which we could develop some basic principles for child psychiatric services to autistic children and their parents. Our ambition was to give both practical and psychological support to parents, organize training of children during their first years in connection with diagnosis and assessment and last but not least give assistance and consultations to other services for children. Our work was largely founded on common sense principles. The budget of an ordinary child psychiatric department seldom permits long-term individual psychotherapies. Instead the principle must be to organize services starting from those resources already existing around the child: parents, relatives, neighbours, school etc.

Our treatment programme did not contain anything extraordinary which couldn't be carried out by any child psychiatric department. However, what is needed is some kind of stubborn determination among the staff to be ready to take over the responsibility for the identification and assessment of pervasive developmental disorders in all children in the catchment area. It often means hard work with only very little spectacular success and require much patience.

In the following section we will comment upon our experience and summarize some leading principles in our programme.

1. The First Contact

In general parents were referred to the clinic by paediatricians, child well-fare clinics or district medical officers. In most cases they had already had many different contacts with doctors or psychologists with discussions about their child's problem. It is important that the staff shows respect and understanding for the deep anxieties which is connected with their childrens deviant development. A trustful relation between parents and the staff should be established already from the beginning. This may be a difficult task because parents are often not only anxious but also suspicious and disappointed after several earlier consultations and investigations. During this initial stage we try to make a preliminary diagnosis on an out-patient basis. Some cases may already at this stage be dismissed if it is quite obvious that autism or other pervasive developmental disorders are out of the question.

2. Clinical Investigation

If we have reasons to believe that the child is suffering from an autistic syndrome we try to motivate the parents to collaborate in a four-week clinical investigation at our family ward. The family ward is arranged as an ordinary flat. The staff is working only during daytime and weekdays, the family leaving the hospital during weekends. It is important that the parents are given enough time to think over the proposal, which may increase their anxiety and confirm their fears that their child has a serious disturbance. But most parents have been able to accept this offer.

A clinical observation during several weeks gives unique possibilities to get hold of the entire complicated situation which arises in a family with an autistic child. It is possible to observe the child in an almost "natural" setting, at meals or bed-time, with parents or other children in different play situations. It is also important to involve parents in the observations, to take advantage of their own experience and knowledge of their children and to invite them to be active participants in the investigation. One goal should be to develop a working alliance with the parents which is one important condition for a stable, longstanding future cooperation.

Most parents who are seeking help at the clinic have been living in protracted state of crisis, anxiety and uncertainty. One aim of the observation is to try to convey some realistic information to the parents about the child's handicap and the consequences this may have for the future. This is a difficult task. It takes a long time for the parents to get through their deep disappointment and bitter feelings. Some parents react with denial, others with aggressiveness when confronted with realities about their child. As in the case of other childhood handicaps it may take a very long time for the parents to accept information and realities. The staff which is confronted with these problems must have learnt to show understanding, patience and empathy. It is wise not to force information upon parents who are tired, depressed and worn out after years of distress, and last but not least lack of sleep. Their first need is usually concrete help to solve practical questions concerning daily life: some stress relieving arrangements, financial support etc. Psychotherapeutic interventions to relieve depression and feelings of guilt may be indicated at a later stage of the contact with the parents.

a)   Neuropediatric investigation

In cooperation with the pediatric department every child gets the usual neuropediatric assessment, including metabolic screening, chromosome analyses, EEG, investigations of hearing and sight, and in some cases brain tomography or PET-scan. Though causal explanations of the child's handicap are found only on a minority it is important not least for the parents to get a clear opinion of the child's biological conditions (Coleman & Gillberg, 1985).

b)   Assessment of developement

Various observations methods and tests are used to assess the child's abilities i e the Griffiths' Developmental Scale, the Vineland, the BRIAC-scale and Wing's "Schedule of Children's Handicaps, Behaviour and Skills" (Wing, 1971). Special attention is payed to the child's communication abilities. The results of observations and tests are summarized in a developmental profile.

3. Planning of Treatment and Support

One of the goals of the four-week observation is to work out a preliminary plan for measures and treatment in collaboration with the parents. For psychological reasons it is important that the parents who have until then lived in uncertainty about the prospect of their children, should get at least some grounds for how to manage the future. What are the possibilities to get practical help to relieve the immediate stress in daily life? What can parents do themselves to improve their own and their childrens situation?

Our planning covered four main points or measures to be taken by the staff responsible for the management of autistic children: 1: regular support of parents, 2: regular follow-up of the child, 3: information about the child's handicap to teachers and other people in charge of the child, 4: training and supervision of the child's personal assistant.

(a) Support to parents

Parents generally have a difficult time during their stay at the hospital and they are seldom ready to face the real consequences of the diagnosis. It takes a long time to reconcile oneself to a fact which has for a long time been suspected and feared but denied. In spite of information about the handicap denial may still be there, which implies an impediment to the future treatment process. These parents are afraid of further contact with the staff and may perhaps try other treatment alternatives. But we think that it is important to insist on fixed regular contacts with the staff soon after discharge from the hospital. This will help the parents face a difficult situation, accept realities and to work constructively to help their child. As a kind of "ombudsman" for the child and his family the staff may also be in a good position to help them in their struggle for the rights they are entitled to according to the mental retardation law. In general we succeed in our efforts to develop a working alliance with the parents during several years even after the responsibility for education and care has been taken over by the organization for the mentally retarded.

(b) Follow-up of children

The child is seen by the staff at regular intervals, often in connection with visits to the child's class or nursery school. With the permission of the parents members of the staff receive regular information from teachers or other personnel in charge of the child. As the child is growing and developing its behaviours and problems are also changing. In discussions with the teachers the goal of training and treatment has to be adjusted to new situations.

(c) Information to other services

The staff also has regular cooperation with other public services in charge of training and education of handicapped children as for instance the organization for the mentally retarded. In addition, it is necessary to give a more general information about autistic handicaps at regular intervals to personnel in charge of children (teachers, nurses etc) because the turnover of personnel in the public services tend to decrease the knowledge about autistic disorders.

(d) Training and supervision of the assistant

The assistant was a necessary condition for the successful training and education of autistic children in normal classes or nurseries. In most cases they had no previous experience with autistic children. Supervision and continuing instruction about autism was accordingly an important part of our programme. Supervision was given by one of the psychologists from the staff twice during a month. Seminars and lectures about autism and similar handicaps were also arranged for assistants and teachers.

THE ROLE OF CHILD PSYCHIATRY

Recently the conditions for preventive services for children have been somewhat affected by changing public health policies in Sweden implying later referrals of children with autistic disorders. On the other hand the public services for the mentally retarded have graudally started to develop more services for children with autistic handicaps in accordance with the Mental Retardation Act from 1986. These changes may have some consequences for the services of child psychiatry.

In the future the task of child psychiatry will probably be limited to: 1: the early identification and diagnosis of autistic handicaps (in close collaboration with the pediatric services), 2: initiate training and education in cooperation with the parents, and 3: be responsible for training and supervision of different categories of personnel working with autistic children.

FOLLOW-UP AND EVALUATION

The programme described here was gradually developed during several years, in close cooperation with the parents. Our approach to the various problems we encountered were largely atheoretical and pragmatic. We were often forced to make adjustments to local condtions and to work out solutions suitable for every single case. As a rule parents wanted to keep their children at home and there was seldom or never the option of institutional care or other arrangements far from home. To be able to help parents of autistic children we had to work out a programme that met the needs and wishes of both children and parents and which did not go beyond budgetary requirement. Thus, integration of autistic children among normal children was a consequence of the lack of other options, not of a preconceived plan or idea.

In order to get more systematic information about the experiences and results of our programme we made an evaluative study of 15 cases (13 boys and 2 girls), who had taken part in our programme at the time of the survey (1980) with the support of a personal assistant. By interviews with parents, teachers and personal assistants a couple of years after the survey we got information on various aspects of the treatment programme, with special regard to the integration of autistic children. In order to minimize subjective biases interviewers were chosen who had not previously been involved in the project.

The majority of these cases were younger children who had been identified in our diagnostic programme during several years. In general these 15 children were also less mentally retareded than the other children in the survey. Older children with autism and severe mental retardation had as a rule been taken care of by the organization for the mentally retarded previous to our survey.

Parents, teachers and assistants were surprisingly positive in their opinion about the programme. However, parents and teachers were unanimous that the personal assistant was the essential condition for the realization of the programme. The assistants emphasized the importance of regular, continuous supervision as a necessary condition for their work. It was also reported by teachers that the class mates displayed a predominantly tolerant and caring attitude towards autistic children.

Needless to say our follow-up study cannot answer the question if "normalization and integration" is superior to other treatment principles. One may argue that autistic children hardly benefit from the company with other children as they seldom interact or play with them. Under such conditions "integration" may seem to be an empty word. But it was obvious that the children in our study did learn a lot of valuable social skills from being with normal children.

It should be emphasized that the study clearly indicates that the parents were living under hard strain. Our treatment programme may have lessened their burden to some extent but they were still left with many severe problems. Sometimes we thought that they payed too high a price for keeping their children at home.

In summary we found that individual integration among normal non-autistic children in many cases had been an adequate solution for education and training. But it could only succeed with the continuous support of a skilled personal assistant. Social developement of autistic children was positively influenced and stimulated by their contact with normal children. These experiences of mainstreaming are in agreement with recent reports from the USA and Great Britain (Lovaas, 1982; Strain et al., 1985).

REFERENCES

Bohman, M., Björk, P. O., Bohman, I. L., & Sjöholm, E. (1983). Childhood psychosis in a northern Swedish county: some preliminary findings from an epidemiological survey. In H. Schmidth & M. H. Remschmidt (Eds.), *Epidemiological Approaches in Child Psychiatry.* Stuttgart-New York: George Thieme Verlag.

Bettelheim, B. (1967). *The Empty Fortress - infantile autism and the birth of the self.* New York: The Free Press, Collier-MacMillan.

Coleman, M., & Gillberg, C. (1985). *The Biology of the Autistic Syndromes.* New York: Praeger.

Gillberg, C. (1984). Infantile autism and other child psychoses in a Swedish urban region. Epidemiological aspects. *Journal of Child Psychology and Psychiatry, 25,* 35 - 43.

Howlin, P., & Rutter, M. (1987). *Treatment of Autistic Children.* Chichester: John Wiley & Sons.

Itard, J. M. G. (1932). *The wild boy of Aveyron.* New York: Century.

Kanner, L. (1943). Autistic disturbances of affective contact. *Nervous Child, 2,* 217 - 250.

Lovaas, O. I. (1982). *An overview of the young autism project.* Paper presented at the meeting of the American Psychological Association, Washington, D. C.

Lotter, V. (1978). Follow-up studies. In M. Rutter & E. Schopler (Eds.), *Autism: A Reappraisal of Concepts and Treatment.* New York: Plenum.

Strain, P. S., Jamieson, B., & Hoyson, M. H. (1985). Learning Experiences. An alternative programme for preschoolers and parents: A comprehensive service system for mainstreaming of autistic-like preschoolers. In C. J. Meisel (Ed.), *Mainstreamed handicapped children: Outcomes, controversies and new directions.* Hillsdale: N. J. Erlbaum.

Tinbergen, N., & Tinbergen, E. A. (1983). *Autistic Children. New hope for cure.* London: George Allen & Unwin Ltd.

Tsai, L., Stewart, M., & August, G. (1981). Implication of sex differences in the familial transmission of infantile autism. *Journal of Autism and Developmental Disorders, 11,* 165 - 713.

Wing, L. (1971). *Schedule of Children's Handicaps, Behaviour and Skills.* London: Medical Research Council.

State-of-the-Art Programming in Massachusetts:
A Brief Description of the May Institute

STEPHEN C. LUCE and WALTER P. CHRISTIAN

STATE-OF-THE-ART PROGRAMMING IN MASSACHUSETTS

The May Institute is a private, non-profit human service agency serving persons with autism and other severe developmental disabilities. The Institute began as the parents' School for Atypical Children in 1955 and was founded by Dr. and Mrs. Jacques M. May as a center dedicated to the understanding and rehabilitation of autism. Dr. May, who was famous as a physician, author, and researcher with the World Health Organization, established the program in the town of Chatham about 145 km. from Boston on scenic Cape Cod in Massachusetts. Having fathered twin autistic sons, Dr. May was interested in establishing a treatment center focusing on study of the autistic child which contrasted to the treatment of the day which was parent-centered. The Mays found such an approach which linked autism to parental personality traits, counter productive.

During the first 23 years of its existence the May Institute grew to a size of about 38 children under the leadership of the Mays and a series of Directors who ran the agency after both Dr. and Mrs. May died. In 1978 a new Executive Director, Walter P. Christian, Ph.D., was hired in an attempt to re-establish the agency as the kind of innovative treatment center that the Mays had envisioned. Dr. Christian, who is a behavioral psychologist, immediately set out to institute the kind of state-of-the-art programming advocated by leaders of the field at that time: specifically, "special educational programs using behavioral methods and designed for specific individuals" (Ritvo & Freeman, 1977).

The process by which Christian and his colleagues re-programmed the May Institute has been thoroughly documented (Christian, 1983), and it is therefore unnecessary to describe in detail here. During that process several questions relating to service delivery were answered (see Anderson et al., 1987; Dyer & Peck, 1987; Luce, 1987; Luce & Christian, 1981). Perhaps the greatest contribution of the May Institute staff was the work done to establish 1) *a technology of transitional programming across a continuum of services* and 2) *a technology of staff training and supervision that assures that clients are provided the best possible services.*

Transitional Programming: Moving Autistic Clients through a Continuum of Services

The last two decades have witnessed an enormous growth in knowledge about and interest in autistic persons in the United States. This increase is functionally related to the promising practices that have been developed in the same period (e.g., Koegel, Rincover, and Egel, 1982). While autism remains a life-long severely debilitating condition, the advances of late have made it possible for the vast majority of autistic youth to live in communities with their families. While the technology of care for autistic persons is beginning to focus on the care of older persons exhibiting autistic behaviors, for most of these older clients, and a significant number of the youth described as severely autistic (Coleman, 1976) or low functioning (DeMyer, 1979), programming in the community is found to be insufficient.

In her study of autistic children and their families, DeMyer (1979) found that many parents sought residential care as their child became stronger and more difficult to manage. Fifty-eight percent of the autistic children she studied with a mean age of 15 years were living away from their families. It has been suggested that as much as 75% of those clients with a diagnosis of autism are placed in full residential care and of the remaining

25%, extensive community support is necessary and often includes short-term residential placement. Of relevance here is the concept of *continuum of services* widely discussed in North America. It recognizes that autistic persons exhibit a wide variety of individual needs and to serve them all, many different program types are needed. Those program types that are substantially removed from the natural community are referred to as more *restrictive.*

As the advances in treatment strategies has evolved, North American professionals and advocates representing persons with autism have justifiably attempted to eliminate the existence of the most restrictive program prototypes such as large centralized institutional settings. These settings had been the main "therapeutic" arena for autistic youth and adults in Canada and the United States for many years. Dissatisfaction with these settings stemmed from the fact that the environments were often found to be unnatural without any programs to train skills that would be of any value outside the institution. The opponents of institutions observed that clients rarely left the artificial settings largely because the settings themselves promoted a level of dependence that made transition impossible (Wolfensberger, 1972). Goffman (1961) and others have presented a dismal analysis of North American institutional treatment that has been endorsed by American state and national legislatures (e.g., Rehabilitation, Comprehensive Services, and Developmental Disabilities Amendment of 1978 [P. L. 95-602]), in litigious actions taken in the courts (e.g., *Halderman v. Pennhurst,* 1977), and by advocacy societies (e.g., National [United States] Society of Autistic Children, 1980).

Some North American groups have taken these steps further by advocating the abolition of all segregated settings designed exclusively for the treatment of the developmentally disabled (Association of the Severely Handicapped, 1980). These initiatives are intentionally designed to eliminate all forms of residential care; some of which could represent the only feasible option for a large number of autistic individuals. Despite these vigorous and well intentioned efforts, it would appear that we are far from abolishing inpatient or residential treatment for the autistic persons (DeMyer, 1979).

It is true that the historic practice in the United States of placing autistic youth in residential settings is unnecessary especially since many inpatient facilities provide insufficient care and little or no functional training. It is a mistake, however, to conclude that all inpatient care is inappropriate. Unfortunately, some clients, especially the chronic severely disabled, have not been adequately prepared for less restrictive settings. In other cases, no alternatives may exist as in the case of the developmentally disabled client who has no family resources and/or is too severe for the community programs available. Historically, the bulk of what is known about the treatment of autistic youth has been conducted in residential facilities (Luce, 1979). Recently, researchers have begun to study facets of care in restrictive settings that have been so discouraging and in some cases, evidence of long-term, wide-scale change can be accomplished (Christian, 1983; Coughlin, et al., 1984).

In light of 1) the need for a full continuum of services and 2) the promise of recent work demonstrating that transitional residential programming can be very helpful to autistic persons, several authors have recommended that inpatient treatment be included in a continuum of service options for autistic clients. When inpatient facilities are supported by less restrictive options, and the care of the people served in the restrictive components of the agency are geared towards *transition* to less restrictive settings, the advantages of residential care are maximized while the disadvantages are minimized (Luce, 1987).

Table 1. The May Institute continuum of services

Program	Services provided	Location(s)	Clients served
May Institute Residential/Educational Services	Day; Residential	Chatham	43 children; 4-7 yrs old
May Institute Intermediate Care Facilities	Subcontracted day; Residential	Hyannis, Falmouth, Centerville	17 men and women; 22-64 yrs old
May Institute Outreach Group Homes	Residential	West Chatham Hanover*, Sharon*	24 youth; 10-12 yrs old
May Institute Specialized foster homes	Foster placement with specially trained families	Eastern Mass.	3 children; 4-12 yrs old
May Center for vocational training and educational	Vocational and educational	Braintree, Mass.	11 youth; 8-21 yrs old
May Center for early childhood education	Day self-contained and integrated preschool and primary education	Burlington, Mass.	17 children; 3-8 yrs old
May Center for early intervention	In-home parent training and comprehensive preschool education	Eastern Mass.	25 children; 2-8 yrs old

* under construction; eventual client capacity = 24

In his conceptualization of service continua, Bird (1984) noted that many North American mental health professionals have focused primarily on the physical arrangements of the service setting. Specifically, a group home in the community would normally be considered less restrictive than a psychiatric hospital. Unfortunately, such a designation does not consider the programming going on in the setting. Many group homes are less therapeutic and more restrictive than larger settings. Consideration of a service continuum, therefore, must account for many factors beyond "bricks and mortar" (Christian and Hannah, 1983).

To be a functional component of a continuum of services, all forms of care must be *transitional.* The May Institute has established just such a service continuum. Figure 1 shows the service options that are managed by the May Institute available for autistic clients of all ages. It is important to note that while clients often move through several levels of the continuum, at the time each individual client is considered for a move to a less restrictive service option, programs not managed by the May Institute are considered. Most of the clients returned to the community in the last 10 years moved to other programs. The use of programs managed by other groups is possible largely because the staff of the May Institute is very active in the dissemination of techniques it finds effective. This effort has resulted not only in numerous publications (over 100 since 1978) but also in a large number of presentations to professional and lay audiences (over 400 since 1978).

Transitional programming requires that the objectives sought while in the relatively restrictive settings must be based on those skills needed to survive in the less restrictive settings (Luce et al., 1984). Those objectives containing skills that are essentially attained prior to the time of transition are called *transitional priorities.* It is around those priorities that a program must revolve. Unfortunately we have found that most transitional priorities involve training systems that are very difficult to establish. For example, it is common to find that when a child is not able to stay in a community placement, the behaviors that resulted in the failed community placement were not being addressed there.

Ideally, programs should focus on the skill deficits and behavioral excesses that prevent movement to less restrictive settings. Unfortunately, this is not the case in many settings (Anderson et al., 1983). For example, many residential programs are designed to be less intensive therapeutically during the evening, night, and weekend hours. When the true causes of their inpatient placement are derived, Anderson, et al. (1983) found that the actual transitional priorities of a group of residentially placed autistic youth contained behaviors (e.g., independent leisure) that were not addressed in their previous community placements and were further overlooked in residential settings using the typical pattern of staffing. Programs mistakenly devote the bulk of their resources to academic and vocational skills that could more efficiently be addressed in less restrictive settings after discharge from the residential program.

Table 2. Evaluating outcome of transitional service programming

Dependent variables	FY 1978	FY 1988
1. Number of program locations	1	10
2. Number of clients served	37.5	110
3. Age range of clients served (in years)	7-16	3-64
4. Number of clients receiving psychotropic medication	8	1
5. Average level of staff-to-client interaction (Plachek)	40 %	89 %
6. Average (mean) length of stay for children served in Chatham during previous 3 years	4.0	2.9
7. Average (mean) length of stay for clients discharged from Chatham during previous 3 years	7.1	4.0
8. Total number of clients discharged from Chatham during previous nine years	18	86
9. Percentage of clients discharged who returned to natural home or foster home	19 %	55 %
10. Percentage of clients discharged to home or foster home who received no further residential treatment	0 %	90 %

Some of the results of transitional programming at the May Institute are depicted in Table 1. The data were compiled over a 10 year period and were obtained from rating forms and written records which were carefully checked to ensure measurement reliability (Christian, 1983). The number of program options for autistic persons expanded from one to ten and the number of clients served expanded in kind. Data on the therapeutic intensity of the program were compiled using planned activity checks (Doke & Risley, 1972; Dyer et al., 1984) and averaged 89% when measured in 1988. This may account for the decreased dependence on psychotropic medication by 87%.

Of greatest significance perhaps is the decrease in length of stay in our most restrictive, residential or inpatient site for children in Chatham. The number of clients discharged in 10 years after an average treatment period of 4.0 years was 86. Fifty-five percent of those youth discharged returned to their families, a foster family, or an adoptive home in the community. Ninety percent of those youth have successfully remained in their communities.

Task Analyzed Staff Training:
An Effective System of Developing Therapeutic Skills

The May Institute training program is composed of two parts, orientation and skill mastery, that are individually tailored to the needs of the individual. Prior to actual training, *orientation* is conducted. At most of the Institute sites, orientation is accomplished in 3 to 5 days. It is conducted by middle management and administrative staff and focuses on program policy, the nature of the clients being served, as well as the treatment philosophy and methodology. The goal of orientation is *verbal proficiency* regarding the agency and its policies. This phase of training is accomplished through didactic instruction supported by assigned readings, modeling, and role play.

After orientation, skill *mastery* becomes the focus of training. In the development of the agency, it was found that when therapists were appropriately oriented to tasks and sufficiently clear on how to accomplish them, dramatic performance gains were accomplished. For example, Leidholt et al. (1984) and Dyer et al. (1984) demonstrated that the quantity and quality of staff to client interactions could be substantially improved with specific feedback. In both studies, increases in therapeutic activities were attained by informing staff how they could have improved their performance based on random instantaneous time samples or planned activity checks taken in their work environments. In a similar study, Egan et al. (1988) demonstrated that similar checks and feedback improved the records and data maintained on individual clients. Specifically, when employees were told what could be done to their individual casebooks to attain a designated standard, they readily complied and maintained improved performance. While they had previously been given lengthy narrative instructions outlining the standards, case books did not improve until specific corrective instructions were given.

Prompted by the results obtained in the above studies as well as work done elsewhere (Herbert-Jackson et al., 1977; Lattimore et al., 1979), and after three years of research and development at the Institute, we are now capable of training therapists and researchers using *task analyzed checklists* specifically developed for each of the jobs they are required to perform.

Depending on the extent of a therapist's responsibilities, training requires mastery of 7 to 24 checklists. For example, the checklist entitled "Direct Instruction" must be demonstrated by all students and staff in contact with clients, while the checklist on "Giving Feedback" is only administered to those supervisory personnel who have that responsibility.

All therapists in training are given the checklists they are required to master. A supervisor working in the same environment with the same clients observes the trainee engaged in the various checklist tasks (e.g., preparing a meal in the group home) and checks off the essential skills or elements of the task as they are accomplished. If, at the end of the task, all elements of the task were satisfactorily completed, the person is considered trained on that task in that setting. Often one or more elements are not satisfactorily accomplished (e.g., a client is not sufficiently engaged in the meal preparation to the level of their ability). In that case, the trainee is told what could have been done to have met that standard and the checklist is readministered.

Performance evaluation for therapists is also based on task analyzed checklists. Basically, a therapist is rated on the level of feedback needed after training to maintain the level of performance required. As errors occur, supervisors give corrective feedback along a continuum from a verbal reminder to written reprimands. A therapist requiring the latter to maintain performance would be ranked lower than a co-worker who required little or no corrective feedback.

This system of training has been replicated in each of the programs in the Institute's service continuum and currently is being systematically introduced in a large state hospital facility which is affiliated with the Institute (see Christian & Zampini, 1987). The Institute has also been involved in task-analyzing the assessment and development of human service organizations (Christian, 1983; Christian & Romanczyk, 1986).

There are several advantages of such an approach to training behavior therapists. Therapists are more closely supervised, trained and evaluated by working supervisors who have previously mastered the same tasks with the same type of clients. This means that a large number of staff benefit from the experience of training job-related skills as opposed to the more typical and less efficient system of this benefit being limited to a "Director of Training." In addition, unlike most human service settings in the United States, performance is operationalized and there are specific criteria for promotion, bonuses and other reinforcers. Checklists minimize instructor lapses by prompting supervisors to observe and review components of a task that may not always seem essential, and maintenance and quality control are assured with such a system. The desired relationship between staff and supervisor becomes well-established and is continually reinforced using such an approach. Finally, our research has indicated that staff actually prefer on-the-job, pyramidal, task analyzed training to other, more traditional approaches to training (Thibadeau et al., 1982).

As the technology improves (e.g., Luce et al., 1988), additional elements can be changed or added to reflect new developments. In this way, the system is proving to be an effective dissemination mechanism.

Summary

In this condensed discussion about the May Institute, we have attempted to give a brief overview about several program components and a slightly more detailed account of two program systems that we have been found to benefit a large number of autistic clients. For the human service provider interested in more detailed information about these systems, citations have been provided. In the ten years since the May Institute took the rather radical new approach, there have been many changes to the agency. In 1988, the Institute was recognized by the United States Department of Education as one of the nation's *Schools of Excellence*, an honor personally attended by President Ronald Reagan and afforded to only one other special education facility. This and other honors extended by professionals and laymen alike have provided a level of validity that is enjoyed by few.

For the reader or conference participant who is interested in replicating some of our systems in their agency, it should be noted that the result attained in our program locations have been found to be highly generalizable (Campbell & Stanley, 1966) across a variety of settings. Some might be tempted to discount the results achieved at the May Institute as fortuitous and impossible to attain at their research or training facility. It should be noted that many of the programs that have adopted the systems described here were fully operational using systems that were far from adequate. In fact, since the programs that have adopted these practices encompass such a broad range, it is likely that similar replications have are already underway. To date we have found no facility that has not benefitted by the implementation of practices like those described here. With each additional replication, we will not only better serve the clients in our care but gain a better understanding about human service delivery.

ACKNOWLEDGMENTS

The authors gratefully acknowledge the tireless efforts of all the May Institute staff and the many colleagues who have been involved in the replication efforts. In addition, we thank Debra Larsson, Paul Reedy, and Joan Van Keuren for their work in the preparation of this manuscript.

REFERENCES

Anderson, S. R., Avery, D. L., DiPetro, E. K., Edwards, G. L., & Christian, W. P.

(1987). Intensive home-based intervention with autistic children. *Education and Treatment of Children, 10,* 352-366.

Anderson, S. R., Luce, S. C., Newsom, C. D., Gruber, B. K., & Kennedy-Butler, K. (1983, May). Individualized treatment planning for autistic youth. Paper presented at the meeting of the Association for Behavior Analysis, Milwaukee. Association for the Severely Handicapped (1980). TASH adopts resolution calling for abolition of institutions. *Newsletter of the Association for the Severely Handicapped, 6,* 1.

Bird, B. L. (1984). The community-based service continuum. In W. P. Christian, G. T. Hannah & T. J. Glahn (Eds.), *Programming effective human services: Strategies for institutional change and client transition.* New York: Plenum Press.

Campbell, D. T., & Stanley, J. C. (1966). *Experimental and quasi-experimental designs for research.* Chicago: Rand McNally.

Christian, W. P. (1983). A case study in the programming and maintenance of institutional change. *Journal of Organizational Behavior Management, 5,* 99-153.

Christian, W. P., & Hannah, G. T. (1983). *Effective management in human services.* Englewood Cliffs: Prentice-Hall.

Christian, W. P., & Romanczyk, R. G. (1986). Evaluation. In F. J. Fuoco & W. P. Christian (Eds.), *Behavior analysis and therapy in residential programs* (pp. 145-193). New York: Van Nostrand Rheinhold Company.

Christian, W. P., & Zampini, A. J. (1988). *Annual Report: Progress of organizational analysis and development in a state hospital facility.* Unpublished manuscript.

Coleman, M. (Ed.). (1976). *The autistic syndromes.* Amsterdam: North Holland Publishing.

Coughlin, D. D., Maloney, D. M., Baron, R. L., Dahir, J., Daly, D. L., Daly, P. B., Fixsen, D. L., Phillips, E. L., & Thomas, D. L. (1984). Implementing the community-based teaching family model at Boys Town. In W. P. Christian, G. T. Hannah & T. J. Glahn (Eds.), *Programming effective human services: Strategies for institutional change and client transition.* New York: Plenum Press.

DeMyer, M. K. (1979). *Parents and children in autism.* New York: John Wiley and Sons.

Doke, L. A., & Risley, T. R. (1972). The organization of day care environments: Required vs. optional activities. *Journal of Applied Behavior Analysis, 5,* 405-420.

Dyer, K., & Peck, C. A. (1987). Current perspectives on social/communication curricula for students with autism and severe handicaps. *Education and Treatment of Children, 10,* 338-351.

Dyer, K., Schwartz, I. S., & Luce, S. C. (1984). A supervision program for increasing functional activities for severely handicapped students in a residential setting. *Journal of Applied Behavior Analysis, 17,* 249-259.

Egan, P., Luce, S. C., & Hall, R. V. (1988). Use of a concurrent treatment design to analyze the effects of a peer review system in a residential setting. *Behavior Modification, 12,* 35-56. *Halderman v. Pennhurst* 466 F. Supp. 1295 (E.D. Pa., 1977).

Herbert-Jackson, E., O'Brien, M., Porterfield, J., & Risley, T. R. (1977). *The Infant Center: A Complete guide to Organizing and Managing Infant Day Care.* Baltimore, Maryland: University Park Press.

Goffman, E. (1961). *Asylums.* Garden City, N. J: Anchor.

Koegel, R. L., Rincover, A., & Egel, A. (1982). *Educating and understanding autistic children.* San Diego: College-Hill Press, Inc.

Lattimore, J., Jones, M. L., & Calvert, T. L. (1978). *Roadrunner project: Caregiver manual.* Morganton: Western Carolina Center.

Leidholt, P. Lipsker, L. E., Luce, S. C., & Christian, W. P., (1981, May). *A middle management strategy for increasing staff-to-client interaction in a residential treatment setting.* Paper presented at the Annual Convention of the Association for Behavior Analysis, Milwaukee.

Luce, S. C. (1979, December). *Reducing autistic behavior behaviors: A review of the literature.* Paper presented at the annual conference of the Association for the Advancement of Behavior Therapy. San Francisco.

Luce, S. C. (1987). Transitional programming for autistic youth. *Focus on Autistic Behavior, 2,* 1-8.

Luce, S. C., Anderson, S. R., Thibadeau, S. F., & Lipsker, L. E. (1984). Preparing the client for transition to the community. In W. P. Christian, G. T. Hannah, & T. J. Glahn (Eds.), *Programming effective human services: Strategies for institutional change and client transition.* New York: Plenum Press.

Luce, S. C., & Christian, W. P. (Eds.). (1981). *How to work with autistic and severely handicapped youth: A series of eight training manuals.* Austin, TX: Pro-Ed.

Luce, S. C., Dyer, K. D., Taylor, M., & Williams, L. (1988, November). *Improving the therapeutic and supervisory skills of classroom and residential instructors.* Paper presented at the Annual Convention of the Association for the Advancement of Behavior Therapy, New York.

National Society for Autistic Children. (1980). NSAC "Community" policy seeks end to institutionalization. *Advocate, 12,* 1.

Ritvo, E. R., & Freeman, B. J. (1977). National Society for Autistic Children definition of the syndrome of autism. *Journal of Pediatric Psychology, 2,* 146.

Thibadeau, S. F., Butler, K. K., Gruber, B. K., Luce, S. C., Newsom, C. D., Anderson, S. R., & Christian, W. P. (1982, May). *Competency-based orientation and training of human service personnel.* Paper presented at the Annual Convention of the Association for the Advancement of Behavior Therapy, Los Angeles.

Wolfensberger, W. (1972). *The principle of normalization in human services.* Toronto: National Institute on Mental Retardation.

Autism: Specific Problems of Adolescence

CHRISTOPHER GILLBERG and HELEN SCHAUMANN

INTRODUCTION

Taylor (1977), among others, has proposed that in spite of the seemingly excellent compensatory mechanisms of the central nervous system, clinical neuropsychiatric development may be compromised in the long run by brain damage occurring in the fetal or perinatal period. Regression or stagnation in the development of skills could occur years later when, for one or other reason, demands for accelerating development are made. Such demands are made, for instance, around the time of physical puberty. Puberty, of course, also marks the onset of major neurochemical changes, which could affect abnormal brain functions negatively. Other, as yet unidentified factors around the time of puberty could enter into the picture also. For all these reasons, the adolescent period in autism should be of particular interest from both the research and clinical points of view.

Even though it is now almost 20 years since Rutter, in his follow-up of some 60 cases of autism treated in one clinic (Rutter, 1970), commented on the occasional concurrence of autism and deterioration in adolescence, it is not until recently that the matter has attracted interest (Gillberg & Schaumann, 1981; Gillberg, 1984; Gillberg & Steffenburg, 1987). This paper summarizes the changes which occur in adolescence in autism. The empirical evidence in the field is still very limited, but it does provide compelling evidence that adolescence is a critical period of development for a substantial number of young people with autism.

ADOLESCENCE WITHOUT MAJOR COMPLICATIONS

Possibly the majority of children with autism face no more dramatic difficulties during puberty and adolescence than do other children (Brown, 1969; Rutter, 1970; Gillberg & Steffenburg, 1987). However, this majority may not be quite so large as previously believed (Gillberg & Steffenburg, 1987). A number of children with autism actually improve during puberty (Kanner et al., 1972; Rutter & Bartak, 1973; Wing & Wing, 1980). In Kanner's follow-up of 96 children, 11 did rather well as adults and several of these showed marked improvement during the pre-pubertal period and adolescence (Kanner et al., 1972).

ADOLESCENCE WITH MAJOR COMPLICATIONS

Two major and several moderately severe complications often occur in autism during the course of adolescence (Table 1).

TABLE 1. Problems of adolescence in autism.

Complication	Relative frequency	Reference
Epilepsy	20-29 % (males 18 %, females 33 %)	Deykin & MacMahon, 1979, Ohlsson et al., 1988
Deterioration	12-22 % (males 12 % females 50 %)	Rutter, 1970; Gillberg & Steffenburg, 1987
Aggravation of symptoms (often periodic)	35 %	Gillberg & Steffenburg, 1987
Problems associated with sexual maturation/ drive	35 % (males 47 % females 0 %)	Gillberg, 1989
Inertia	?	
Depression/affective illness (particularly in high-functioning individuals)	? (22 (44) %)	Wing, 1981

Epilepsy and deterioration, unfortunately are relatively frequent severe neuropsychiatric complications in pubertal children with autism. Periodic behavioural symptom aggravation, problems associated with sexual maturation/sexual drive, inactivity and depression are also common, but usually represent transient phenomena or at least less severe problems from the point of view of care load.

Some of the increase in problems around the time of puberty in autism is accounted for by sheer physichal growth of the individual with autism. Behaviour problems, self-destructiveness or aggressive outbursts may all remain at a prepubertal level, but the fact that the child is bigger and stronger, can make them more conspicuous and much more difficult to handle.

Epilepsy in Autism

Five - fifteen per cent of all children with autism develop fits in infancy or early childhood (Ohlsson et al., 1988). Infantile spasms are relatively common during this age period (Taft & Cohen, 1971) and can occur before or after the onset of autistic symptomatology.

A quarter to one third of children with autism who have not had fits in early life develop seizures during adolescence or early adult life (Rutter, 1970; Hoeg-Brask, 1970; Deykin & McMahon, 1979; Gillberg & Steffenburg, 1987).

The most common type of seizure disorder appears to be complex-partial (psychomotor) epilepsy. According to a recent population-based study by Ohlsson et al. (1988), 80 per cent of all cases of epilepsy in pre-pubertal children with autism were of the psychomotor variant.

The likelihood of epilepsy is largely inversely related to IQ in that severely mentally retarded children with autism have the highest risk of developing fits (Rutter, 1970). Nevertheless, epilepsy can occur in autism around the time of adolescence even in cases with relatively good intelligence (Gillberg et al., 1987).

Deterioration in Autism

Seven of the 64 cases (12 per cent) of "childhood psychosis" reported by Rutter (1970) deteriorated progressively during adolescence. Some of these simultaneously developed other neurological signs such as seizures and paralysis of the legs.

In the series of "infantile psychosis" reported by Brown (1969), 27 out of 80 cases (34 per cent) for whom adequate information was available, did less well during puberty than during the early school years and 5 (6 per cent) became so disturbed that they required admission to hospital.

Gillberg and Schaumann in 1981 reported that c. one third of all patients with autism deteriorated temporarily or permanently during puberty. They suggested that girls - and especially those with a family history of affective disorder - might be at greater risk than boys of developing pubertal deterioration.

In a more recent publication, Gillberg and Steffenburg (1987) found deterioration in a rather larger proportion of cases. After initial exacerbation of more "common symptoms" associated with autism (such as stereotypies, hyperactivity and self-destructiveness or generally unmalleable behaviour), there sometimes appears a set-back with stagnation/regression of skills - both in the field of daily life activities and language. Altogether c. 25 per cent of all cases with autism deteriorated in the 14 - 20 year-age-period and a majority of these were still in a relatively regressed state 3 years later. Clinical expericence suggests that in a substantial proportion of such cases, positive development can again occur many years later.

There was no clear relationship in this study between onset of deterioration and epilepsy.

ADOLESCENCE WITH OTHER NEUROPSYCHIATRIC COMPLICATIONS

Periodic Aggravation of Behavioural Problems

At the onset of puberty - or a year before or after - there is often a dramatic aggravation of symptoms such as self-destructiveness, restlessness, hyperactivity and aggressiveness. According to the Gothenburg study (Gillberg & Steffenburg, 1987), such aggravation was seen in 50 per cent of the cases. The change in behaviour often prompted some kind of medication. Before puberty less than one in four of children with autism was on medication affecting the nervous system, whereas at age 16 - 23 years, 3 out of 4 were on such treatment (p<.001). A proportion of this increase was due to antiepilectic drugs, but the majority concerned neuroleptics and occasionally lithium.

In some cases, as has already been pointed out, this aggravation is then followed by gradual regression of skills. In others, there is a return to "normal" for at least weeks or months. A new period with exacerbation of symptoms then often occurs. This seems to be the case in particular if there is a family history of affective disorder (Gillberg, 1984). There is now accumulating evidence that autism, while not being specifically geneticallly associated with schizophrenia, may well be correlated with a family history of affective disorder (Tsai et al., 1981; de Long & Dwyer, 1988). It has been our clinical impression that lithium can sometimes be effective controlling pubertal behavioural/"mood" swings in autism.

Problems Associated with Sexual Maturation/Drive

For many individuals with autism puberty is not associated with serious problems in connection with sexual maturation. Many parents of girls with autism worry about what might happen in connection with the onset of menstruation. Often these changes are accepted by the child in a very matter of fact way (Wing, 1980). The growth of sexual drive is usually not accompanied by corresponding growth in the field of social "know-how" which often leads to embarassing behaviour. This seems to be particularly true of moderately mentally retarded adolescent boys with autism (Gillberg, 1984), who may expose themselves, masturbate in public and touch other people's genital regions. Such behaviour can, of course, be very embarassing to those confronted, including parents and siblings. Others may be involved unintentionally in homo- or heterosexual contact (Haracopos, 1988) for the simple reason that they may be lacking in reticence and suspiciousness to such an extent that they may be taken advantage of sexually.

The problems associated with sexual maturation in autism need to be handled with consistency, common-sense and not too much emotion. Simple rules need to be laid down by those caring for adolescents with autism, and these rules will need to be repeated at short intervals (Gillberg, 1983). Medication because of sexual problems is rarely, if ever, indicated. The few female cases in which clothing and underwear are torn and blood may be smeared, might benefit from hormonal suppression of menstruation (Corbett, 1980).

Inactivity/Inertia

In certain individuals with autism the sometimes marked overactivity of early childhood may change to a "state of underactivity" in adolescence. There may be an almost total lack of initiative and yet no clear indications of depressive feeling (Rutter, 1977).

Depression

Feelings of unhappiness or depression are often reported (Wing & Wing, 1980; Rutter, 1982; Newson et al., 1982) and may be particularly likely to present in those cases of autism who are high-functioning or referred to as Asperger syndrome (Wing, 1981; Tantam, 1988). Such individuals may become painfully aware that they are different from other people. Some develop a strong desire for friendship, but may still be totally unable to establish social relationships because they lack the necessary skills. In cases with a family history of affective disorder there is sometimes a typical episode of major depression which might represent a more "primary" rather than "secondary" complication. Occasionally antidepressant medication may be of use (Gillberg, 1984) perhaps in combination with directive supportive psychotherapy in cases with good language skills (Rutter, 1978). Role-playing and videotape feedback followed by systematic training might also be useful when trying to teach these youngsters the requirements of simple social contact and conversation.

Other Psychiatric Problems

In brighter adolescents with autism, now variously described as "high-level", "high-functioning" or "Asperger syndrome" a wide variety of psychiatric complications occur such as negativism, hypoactivity and paranoia-like symptoms (Tantam, 1988). Sometimes such symptoms lead to a suspicion of schizophrenia. I have myself seen quite a number of cases with Asperger syndrome which have been labelled "schizophrenic" or "borderline". Adult psychiatrists need to learn a lot more about high-level autism in order to be able to properly evaluate such cases and avoid, for instance, improper medication. The particular problem of violence developing in young people with Asperger syndrome has been adressed by Baron-Cohen in a case-report (Baron-Cohen, 1988). I have recently examined a number of young persons who have committed violent acts. Asperger syndrome has been common in these cases.

CONCLUSIONS

Adolescence in autism can be a critical period during which epilepsy or deterioration or both may have their onset. A variety of other problems can occur. Girls may be particularly at risk. An association with familial affective disorders is a candidate for future research efforts particularly in those cases in which behavioural/mood swings are prominent. Further investigation into adolescent development in Asperger syndrome is highly warranted.

REFERENCES

Baron-Cohen, S. (1988). An assessment of violence in a young man with Asperger's syndrome. *Journal of Child Psychology and Psychiatry, 29,* 351 - 360.

Brown, W. T. (1969). Adolescent development of children with infantile psychosis. *Seminars in Psychiatry, 1,* 79 - 89.

Corbett, J. (1980). Medical management. In L. Wing (Ed.), *Early Childhood Autism.* Oxford: Pergamon.

De Long. G. R., & Dwyer, J. T. (1988). Correlation of Family History with Specific Autistic Subgroups: Asperger's Syndrome and Bipolar Affective Disorder. *Journal of Autism and Developmental Disorders, 18,* 593 - 600.

Deykin, E. Y., & MacMahon, B. (1979). The incidence of seizures among children with autistic symptoms. *American Journal of Psychiatry, 136,* 1310 - 1312.

Gillberg, C. (1983). Autism in adolescence. Awakening of sexual awareness. *Proceedings of the Second European Autism Conference,* Paris.

Gillberg, C. (1984). Autistic children growing up: problems during puberty and adolescence. *Developmental Medicine and Child Neurology, 26,* 125 - 129.

Gillberg, C., & Schaumann, H. (1981). Infantile autism and puberty. *Journal of Autism and Developmental Disorders, 11,* 365 - 371.

Gillberg, C., & Steffenburg, S. (1987). Outcome and prognostic factors in infantile autism and similar conditions. A population based study of 46 cases followed through puberty. *Journal of Autism and Developmental Disorders, 17,* 273 - 287.

Gillberg, C., Steffenburg, S., & Jakobsson, G. (1987). Neurobiological findings in 20 relatively gifted children with Kanner-type autism or Asperger syndrome. *Developmental Medicine and Child Neurology, 29,* 641 - 649.

Haracopos, D. (1988). *Hvad med mig?* Copenhagen: Andonia Forlag.

Hoeg-Brask, B. (1970). *A Prevalence Investigation of Childhood Psychoses.* Paper given att 16th Scandinavian Congress of Psychiatry.

Kanner, L., Rodriguez, A., & Ashenden, B. (1972). How far can autistic children go in matters of social adaptation? *Journal of Autism and Childhood Schizophrenia, 2,* 9 - 33.

Newson, E., Dawson, M., & Everard, P. (1982). The natural history of able autistic people: the management and functioning in a social context. *Summary of Report to DHSS.*

Ohlsson, I., Steffenburg, S., & Gillberg, C. (1988). Epilepsy in autism and autistic-like conditions. A population-based study. *Archives of Neurology, 45,* 666 - 668.

Rutter, M. (1970). Autistic children. Infancy to adulthood. *Seminars in Psychiatry, 2,* 435 - 450.

Rutter, M. (1978). Developmental issues and prognosis. In M. Rutter & E. Schopler (Eds.), *Autism: a Reappraisal of Concepts and Treatment* (pp 503 - 504). New York: Plenum Press.

Rutter, M. (1982). Personal communication.

Rutter, M., & Bartak, L. (1973). Special education treatment of autistic children: A comparative study. II. Follow-up findings and implications for services. *Journal of Child Psychology and Psychiatry, 14,* 241 - 270.

Taft, L. T., & Cohen H. J. (1971). Hypsarrythmia and childhood autism. A clinical report. *Journal of Autism and Childhood Schizophrenia, 1,* 327 - 336.

Tantam, D. (1988). Asperger's syndrome. *Journal of Child Psychology and Psychiatry, 29,* 245 - 255.

Taylor, D. (1977). Epileptic experience, Schizophrenia and the Temporal lobe. *The McLean Hospital Journal, June,* pp 22 - 39.

Tsai, L., Stewart, M., & August, G. (1981). Implication of a sex difference in the familial transmission of infantile autism. *Journal of Autism and Developmental Disorders, 11,* 165 - 173.

Wing, L. (1980). *Early childhood autism.* Oxford: Pergamon

Wing, L. 1981. Asperger's syndrome: a clinical account. *Psychological Medicine, 11,* 115 - 129.

Wing, J. K., & Wing, L. (1980). Provision of services. In L. Wing (Ed.), *Early Childhood Autism.* Oxford: Pergamon.

Pharmacotherapy of Adolescent Problems

MAGDA CAMPBELL, RICHARD PERRY and RICHARD P. MALONE

INTRODUCTION

Research and clinical trials in psychopharmacology of autism mainly involve young autistic children (for review, see Campbell, 1987). The occasional adolescent or young adult in some studies represents only part of a patient sample with a very wide age range. This is particularly true for most studies of fenfluramine (Ritvo et al., 1986; for review see Campbell, 1987, 1988). It is not clear why these adolescents or young adults were selected to participate in these clinical trials, whether their behavioral symptoms differed from those of young patients. Certainly, it is not known whether autistic adolescents respond in the same way to pharmacotherapy as younger children do. It should be noted that a certain number of autistic persons develop seizure disorder around puberty which deserves careful consideration when prescribing a psychoactive agent (Gualtieri et al., 1987; Tarjan et al., 1957). Side effects of antiseizure drugs are discussed by Gualtieri et al. (1987).

In general, little has been written about autistic individuals in adolescence, with the exception of follow-up studies (for review, see DeMeyer, 1981). Only in recent years have the specific problems and needs of this age group been addressed (Campbell & Schopler, 1989; Cohen & Donnellan, 1987; Marcus & Schopler, 1987; Schopler & Mesibov, 1983; Gillberg & Schaumann, 1981; Wing & Attwood, 1987).

Two types of problems may require psychopharmacologic intervention in this age group of autistic individuals: severe behavioral management and super-imposed psychiatric conditions. A review of the literature suggests that little is known about the latter (Payton, 1987). The behavioral problems requring pharmacotherapy in adolescence typically are aggressiveness, self-mutilation, explosiveness and rage outbursts. No research was conducted to assess critically the efficacy and safety of psychoactive agents in autistic adolescents who display these target symptoms.

The aim of this chapter is first, to present an overview of the pertinent literature as shown in Table 1, and second, to discuss clinical experience concerning pharmacological management of aggressiveness, self-abusiveness, rage outbursts and disruptive behavior in general. Most of the cited literature involves other than autistic patients.

Table 1. Overview of the pertinent literature.

Drug	Design	Daily dose (mg/d)	Diagnosis	Reference	Sample size
Neuroleptics					
Haloperidol and	Double blind placebo controlled	1-9	Autism; Conduct Disorder; MR* Children	Naruse et al., 1982	87
Pimozide	Double blind & placebo controlled	0.75-6.75			
Lithium	Double blind & placebo controlled	-	MR* (adults)	Craft et al., 1987	42
	Double blind & placebo controlled	0.5-0.8** mEq/l	MR*	Tyrer et al., 1984	25
	Open	0.75-1.05 ** mEq/l	MR*	Elliott et al., 1986	2
	Open	>1.0** mEq/l	Autism (children)	Kerbeshian et al., 1972	2
	Open	0.9** mEq/l	MR*	Dostal, 1972	14
Beta-blockers					
Propranolol and	Open	100-300	Autism (Adults)	Ratey et al., 1987	8
Nadolol		120			
Propranolol	Open	40-420	MR* (Adults)	Ratey et al., 1986	19
Nadolol	Open	80	MR* (Adult)	Polakoff et al., 1986	1

Drug	Design	Daily dose (mg/d)	Diagnosis	Reference	Sample size
Propranolol	Open	320-520	Chronic Brain Syndromes (Adolescents, Adults)	Yudofsky et al., 1981	4
Propranolol	Chart review	50-960	Conduct Disorder Explosive Disorder, PDD*** Children, adolescents, adults)	Williams et al., 1982	30

Opioid Antagonists

Drug	Design	Daily dose (mg/d)	Diagnosis	Reference	Sample size
Naloxone	Double blind	0.1, 0.2 0.4	Developmentally Disabled (Adults)	Sandman et al., 1983	2
Naloxone	Double blind	0.1, 0.2 0.4	MR*	Beckwith et al., 1986	2
Naloxone	Open	-	Lesch-Nyhan (Adolescent)	Richardson & Zaleski, 1983	1
Naltrexone	Double blind & placebo controlled	50, 100	MR*	Szymanski, 1987	2
Naltrexone	Open, acute dose range	0.5, 1.0 2.0 mg/kg	Autism (Children)	Campbell et al., 1989	10
Naltrexone	Double blind & placebo controlled	1.0, 1.5 2.0 mg/kg	Autism (Children, Adolescents)	Herman et al., 1986	5
Naltrexone	Double blind & placebo controlled	0.5, 1.0 2.0 mg/kg	MR* (Children, Adolescent)	Herman et al., 1987	3
Naltrexone	Open, acute dose range	1.0, 1.5	Autistic (Adolescents)	Lebouyer et al.,1988	2
Naltrexone	Double blind & ascending dose	12.5-50	MR* (Adolescent)	Bernstein, 1988	1
Naloxone and Naltrexone	Double blind & placebo controlled	0.2, 0.4 50	Autistic (Adolescent)	Barrett et al., 1989	1

*   MR = Mental Retardation
**   Serum Lithium Level
***   PDD = Pervasive Developmental Disorder

OVERVIEW OF THE PERTINENT LITERATURE

Neuroleptics

The neuroleptics are the most studied psychopharmacologic agents in the treatment of autism, and to date have been the most helpful in ameliorating some cardinal behavioral symptoms in this disorder. The high-potency neuroleptics have been found to be preferable to the low-potency neuroleptics, because the latter are often associated with sedation at therapeutic doses (Campbell, Fish, Korein et al., 1972; Fish, 1970).

Chlorpromazine

Though chlorpromazine may be useful in individual adolescents, its effects on decreasing seizure threshold and increasing the frequency of seizures (Tarjan et al., 1957) limit its use in this population.

Haloperidol

In autism, haloperidol has been the most systematically studied of all the psychoactive agents. It has been found to reduce withdrawal and stereotypies (Campbell et al., 1978; Cohen et al., 1980), as well as hyperactivity, abnormal object relations, angry and labile affect (Anderson et al., 1984, 1989). Symptoms of aggressiveness and self-mutilation were not specifically assessed on the Children's Psychiatric Rating Scale, one of the instruments employed. However, temper outbursts decreased significantly $(F(2,68)=3.78)$, p=.03) on haloperidol as rated on the Conners Parent-Teacher Questionnaire in a sample of 45 children (Anderson et al., 1989). Dosages in these studies ranged from 0.25 mg/day to 4.0 mg/day or 0.016 to 0.217 mg/kg/day. However, none of the patients were adolescents in these 4 double blind clinical trials of haloperidol; the subjects' ages ranged from 2.02 to 7.58 years.

Pimozide

Naruse et al., (1982), in a double-blind crossover multicenter trial of pimozide, haloperidol, and placebo, included adolescents. The entire sample consisted of 87 patients, whose ages ranged from 3 to 16 years; it included 34 autistics, and 17 mentally retarded subjects. Pimozide dosages ranged from 1 - 9 mg/day and those of haloperidol from 0.75 - 6.75 mg/day. There was a significant reduction of some forms of aggression ("injury and violence to others", "breaking furniture", p 179) with both drugs over placebo as indicated by several rating scales. However, the effect on self-mutilation did not reach significance.

Studies of neuroleptics in the mentally retarded suggests a role for these drugs in the treatment for irritability, hyperactivity (White & Aman, 1985), aggression and self-mutilation (for review, see Farber, 1987; Lipman, 1986).

The limitations of haloperidol, and neuroleptics in general, are their associations with tardive or withdrawal dyskinesias. Most data on neuroleptic-related dyskinesias are obtained from adults patients (for review; Fann et al., 1980; Campbell et al., 1983; Casey, 1987), mentally retarded children and adolescents (Gualtieri et al., 1984) and prepubertal autistic children (Campbell et al., 1983, 1988a).

Lithium

Lithium was found to have antiaggressive properties in laboratory animals (Weischer, 1969) and in psychiatric patients (for review, see Campbell et al., 1972; Campbell et al., 1984a), including mentally retarded adolescents (Dostal, 1972) and adults (Ziring et al., 1980). The most relevant are perhaps the studies of Dostal and of Campbell et al., 1984b; (for review see Campbell et al., 1984a). The study of Campbell et al. (1984b) involved aggressive children of normal intelligence, diagnosed as conduct disorder.

Dostal (1972) administered lithium to 14 severely retarded boys, ages 11 to 17 years (mean, 14); they were the most aggressive and hyperactive in a group of 60 institutionalized retarded males. The 14 subjects failed to respond to phenothiazine treatment; three suffered from grand mal seizures. They received lithium for 8 months with the aim to maintain a serum lithium level of approximately 0.9 mEq/l. Significant reduction of aggressiveness, anger and psychomotor excitability, restlessness and undisciplined behavior were rated in response to lithium. In addition, a 65 % reduction of incidence of acute outbursts of aggressive behavior were reported by the unit. Side effects were severe polydipsia and polyuria. The author emphasized that the best responders to lithium were those adolescents whose aggressiveness was accompanied by explosive and labile affect. Those patients who did not display explosive and labile affect, and who were hyperactive, who had repetitive and mild sulf-mutilation as well as stereotypic rituals, showed no response to lithium. There is a small literature on the use of lithium in the mentally retarded. Craft et al. (1987) studied the use of lithium in 42 mentally handicapped adults in a double-blind parallel groups design. Lithium was significantly superior to placebo in reducing overall aggression in this 12-week study.

Successful use of lithium in two cases of prepubertal autistic children with aggression has been reported in an open study (Kerbeshian et al., 1987). These children had family histories of affective disorder, and were simultaneously diagnosed as autistic and atypical bipolar disorder.

For measuring lithium levels in saliva, articles by Perry et al. (1984), Shopsin et al. (1969), Vitiello et al. (1988), and Weller et al. (1987) are suggested. For short-term safety of lithium, articles by Campbell et al. (1984a, b), and safety of lithium in general, a paper by Reisberg and Gershon (1979), are recommended.

Megavitamins

It was Linus Pauling (1968) who introduced the concept of orthomolecular treatment in psychiatry (for review, see Hawkins and Pauling, 1973). Megadoses of vitamins, including B6, in the treatment of autism were introduced by Rimland (for detailed review, see Rimland, 1987). Based on the notion that the autistic child "requires more B6 than does a normal child" (Rimland, 1987, p. 402), a total of 191 autistic persons received this treatment: increases in interaction with family members, awareness, and speech, and decreases of temper tantrums and disruptive behaviors were rated. Where megavitamins were supplemented with magnesium, side effects, including enuresis, irritability and sensitivity to sounds have decreased.

A careful analysis of megavitamin therapy and the nutritional interventions was recently presented by Raiten (1987) and Raiten and Massaro (1987).

Gualtieri et al. (1987) argued the therapeutic efficacy of megavitamins and detailed their side effects.

Beta-blockers

The beta-blockers, propranolol, atenolol and nadolol were explored in a variety of patients with target symptoms of aggressiveness, self-mutilation and rage outbursts. The samples usually consisted of patients who failed to respond to pharmacotherapy, particularly to neuroleptic drugs. Most of the studies suffer from methodological flaws and therefore no conclusions can be made: often the sample sizes are small, no controls are employed and the patients continue to receive other psychoactive drugs, while placed on a trial of a beta-blocker. There have been no controlled studies reporting on the effects of beta-blockers in either autistic or retarded populations.

Interest in the beta-blockers as psychoactive agents dates to 1977 when Elliott described the use of propranolol for aggressive behavior in the acutely brain injured, and there were similar other reports in adults (Yudofsky et al., 1981).

Propranolol was reported to be useful in the treatment of children and adolescents with brain dysfunctions who had aggressive outbursts; 2 of the subjects were diagnosed as having pervasive developmental disorder (Williams et al., 1982). The findings are based on a retrospective chart review. Of the 30 subjects, 75 % were found to have decrease of aggressive outbursts. Optimal doses of propranolol ranged from 50 mg/day to 960 mg/day. Sedation occurred as a transient side effect in 6 subjects, and 4 had reversible hypotension. One adolescent with a prior history of depression became depressed while receiving propranolol.

Ratey et al. (1987b) explored beta-blockers in an open trial in 8 autistic adults ranging in age from 25 to 50 years. Six patients were treated with propranolol at doses ranging from 100 mg/day to 360 mg/day, while 2 received nadolol in daily doses of 120 mg/day, on the average for over a year. Aggression and self-injurious behavior were found to be reduced, starting during the first 6 weeks but as late as after 3 months when placed on a beta-blocker. Throughout the trial, the patients remained on neuroleptic medication, except for a 30-year-old man, who received only propranolol (360 mg/day). Subsequently, in six of these subjects decrease of withdrawal and increase of socialization, and in 4 "improved" speech was reported, while receiving propranolol, in doses of 100 to 420 mg/day (Ratey et al., 1987a).

Marked to moderate decrease of self-abusive and aggressive behavior was reported in 16 of 19 profoundly and severely retarded adults whose ages ranged from 22 to 49 years (Ratey et al., 1986). In this open trial, the daily doses of propranolol ranged from 40 mg/day to 240 mg/day (mean, 120) and one person received nadolol, 80 mg/day. Seven patients developed bradycardia or hypotension at doses below 100 mg/day of propranolol; 2 of these subjects were nonresponders (Ratey et al., 1986).

Most of the subjects in the above reports were receiving concurrently with the beta-blocker other psychoactive agents, adding to the difficulty in evaluating their specific effects. Reduction of akathisia (Adler et al., 1985) and increases of neuroleptic levels (Silver et al., 1986) could have contributed to these positive results.

Carbamazepine

Carbamazepine, a tricyclic anti-seizure drug, has a variety of psychoactive, including antiaggressive properties (Post, 1987). Carbamazepine was explored and it is currently in use in affective disorders, in psychotic patients with target symptoms of aggressiveness and excitement, and in episodic dyscontrol syndrome (Post, 1988; for review, see Mattes, 1986; Spencer & Campbell, 1989).

The use of carbamazepine in children with psychiatric disorders has been reviewed elsewhere (Evans, Clay & Gualtieri, 1987; Spencer & Campbell, 1989; Remschmidt, 1976). A recent report involving a sample of treatment - resistant retarded individuals, whose target symptoms included aggression, self-injurious behavior and tantrums, suggests that carbamazepine may be of therapeutic value in this population. Thirty of the 76 patients had a very good response to carbamazepine in this restrospective open trial (Langee, 1989).

To the best of our knowledge, there are no reports on the use of carbamazepine in autism. However, the antiaggressive effects of carbamazepine and its beneficial effects on rage outbursts warrant a critical assessment of this agent in treatment-resistant autistic individuals with these target symptoms.

Naltrexone

The endogenous opioids were implicated in self-injurious behavior; hence the use of opiate antagonists, naloxone and naltrexone in mentally retarded persons with aggressiveness directed against self (for review, see Deutsch, 1986).

In autism, as indicated elsewhere in this book (Campbell, Pharmacotherapy in autism: an overview), the use of naltrexone an oral opiate antagonist, is limited to acute dose-range tolerance trials (Campbell et al., 1989; Herman et al., 1986; Leboyer et al., 1988), with the exception of a single-case study (Walters et al., 1989). Walters et al. (1989) administered naltrexone (1.0 mg/kg/day) over a period of 21 days, to a 14-year-old autistic boy with severe self-injurious behavior. A double-blind and placebo-controlled crossover design was employed. Treatment with naltrexone resulted in complete cessation of self-injurious behavior and increase of social relatedness (Walters et al., 1989). In a well designed experiment, naltrexone administration over a period of 12 days resulted in cessation of self-injurious behavior in a 12-year old autistic girl (Barrett et al., 1989). In an open study 8 of the 10 autistic children had mild to severe aggressiveness, and 5, aggressiveness directed against self. There was only a slight decrease of these symptoms in response to naltrexone (Campbell et al., 1989). It should be noted that this was only a clinical impression, because no specific rating instrument for these maladaptive behaviors was employed. Temper outbursts were reduced at both the

0.5 mg/kg/day and 1.0 mg/kg/day dose of naltrexone, as rated on the Conners Parent-Teacher Questionnaire. The best responder to naltrexone was an extremely aggressive child (Campbell et al., 1989). This was an open acute dose range tolerance trial. In an ongoing double-blind and placebo-controlled trial, aggressiveness against self and others is being measured and the effect of naltrexone on these symptoms is being critically assesssed in autistic children (Campbell, unpublished data).

Herman et al. (1987) administered naltrexone to 3 subjects with self-injurious behavior, two of whom were 17 years of age. One of the adolescents was profoundly retarded, and the other, who had Tourette's syndrome, was of normal intelligence. The greatest reduction of self-injurious behaviors was found at 1.5 mg/kg/day of naltrexone, and in the subject who was most afflicted by this symptom.

Not all reports are in agreement in regard to the efficacy of naltrexone; Szymanski et al. (1987) failed to detect the superiority of naltrexone over placebo in 2 profoundly retarded adults with self-injurious behavior, employing a double-blind crossover design, over a period of 12 to 18 weeks. This too was a placebo-controlled acute dose range tolerance trial, and the ascending doses of naltrexone ranged from 0.5 to 2.0 mg/kg/day. Beckwith et al. (1986) also found no effect of naltrexone on self-injurious behavior.

Naloxone, the other opiod antagonist, is available parenterally, and therefore its clinical utility is limited. There are several case reports of the use of this agent in self-abusive behavior (Sandman et al., 1983) including an adolescent (Richardson & Zaleski, 1983).

Clearly, there has been a paucity of research on the use of opioid antagonists in adolescent autistics, but a few reports involving aggressive retarded persons are encouraging. Furthermore, naltrexone appears to be safe and may help ameliorate some symptoms in autism (Campbell et al., 1989).

The efficacy and safety of naltrexone awaits critical assessment in self-injurious behavior.

CLINICAL EXPERIENCE

Sixteen autistic adolescents were seen for pharmacotherapy consultations, on an outpatient basis. Fourteen children met DSM-III criteria for infantile autism, full syndrome present, and two met criteria for autism, residual state (DSM-III, 1980).

All patients were brought by their parents, some lived at home while others were living in residential schools. The parents were middle or upper-middle class, knowledgeable about autism and its treatment and highly motivated, if not desperate, for help. All of these adolescents had had previous exposure to psychoactive medications. At the time of referral all but four of the adolescents were taking medications prescribed by other physicians, some of whom were psychiatrists.

The adolescents were seen over the past 10 years; only a few psychoactive drugs have been systematically studied in the treatment of autism in this period of time. Moreover, almost all studies have been with preschoool or schoolage samples, haloperidol, fenfluramine, and more recently naltrexone receiving most of the attention. Parents were aware of the studies; three parents requested trials of naltrexone; two requested fenfluramine and one requested haloperidol. Parents of 3 patients consulted at a time their children's dosage of haloperidol was being lowered because of feared side-effects, and the worsening of behavioral symptoms.

The choice of medication was guided by knowledge of the demonstrated effectiveness and safety of medications at the time of each referral. Since this knowledge is forever in flux, a child treated early in the 10-year period was approached differently than one seen later.

The evolving data base can be appreciated by referring to recent review articles of the psychopharmacotherapy of infantile autism (Campbell, 1987). Ten years ago haloperidol was emerging as an effective agent. Over the past 10 years its short-term (Anderson et al., 1984, 1989; Campbell et al., 1978) and long-term (Perry et al., 1989a) effectiveness has been demonstrated. However, in a long-term prospective study the incidence of neuroleptic-related dyskinesias has been shown to be 29.27 % (Campbell et al., 1988a). In all cases the dyskinesias were reversible, bringing hope that low dosage and periodic drug withdrawal can minimize the risk of developing chronic and irreversible dyskinesias.

Fenfluramine received much attention in the early 1980's when initial reports (Ritvo et al., 1983) indicated behavioral and intellectual improvements in the absence of serious side-effects. However, the results of a multicenter trial involving 81 subjects ages 2 to 24 years were more modest (Ritvo et al., 1986), and a few reports failed to show the superiority of fenfluramine over placebo (Campbell et al., 1988b; Ekman et al., 1989; Leventhal, 1985).

Naltrexone is the latest medication to be studied and results are still preliminary (Campbell et al., 1989; Leboyer et al., 1988).

It is of note that to date most patient samples consist of preadolescent children; there is little experience with autistic adolescents and adults.

Patients

The 16 adolescents, 13 males and 3 females, ranged in age from 12 to 19 years.

At the time of referral 12 children were receiving psychoactive medication: 4 received haloperidol, one thioridazine, one chlorpromazine, one clonidine, one triazolam (for sleep) and one received valproic acid. Three children received polypharmacy; one of these, an adolescent, was receiving 6 different psychoactive drugs. The treatment of this adolescent through the years was extremely difficult but his parents were committed to keep him out of an institution.

Target symptoms

The 16 adolescents displayed a variety of symptoms, not necessarily targeted for pharmacotherapy. However, in every case either self-injurious behavior (in 10 children) and/or aggressive behavior (in 8 children) were the target symptoms. The aggressive behaviors included assaultiveness, verbal abusiveness, and frequent and severe tantruming. Symptoms related to deviancies in language, learning and relatedness did not motivate parents to seek consultation. It appears that the parents of these autistic adolescents were resigned to the life-long limitations of their children. The parents' expectations from the consultation were limited to their wish that their children become more manageable at home and at their special school placements, be they residential or community. In some cases medication made it possible for the child to live at home or to be placed in a residential setting.

Results

Reporting the results of the consultations presents some difficulties particularly because no rating instruments were used; the criteria for improvement, as it usually is in private practice, were subjective. The reports of parents, teachers and other involved professionals were sought to determine the effectiveness of drug administration.

The results will be organized around the expericence with haloperidol, fenfluramine, naltrexone and lithium, as shown in Table 2. These were the only medications either continued or introduced by us with the exception of two cases: one in which a child received thioridazine and another, a child who received a brief trial of buspirone.

Table 2. Clinical experience with 16 adolescents.

Drug	Daily doses in mg	Target symptoms	Patient CA* Range in yrs	Therapeutic positive	Response Equvivocal or negative
Haloperidol	1-12	Aggression SIB**	12-19	7	2
Thioridazane	350	Aggression tantrums	15	1	0
Fenfluramine	60	Aggression	12	0	0
Lithium***	900-1800	Aggression verbal outbursts	12-14	1	1
Naltrexone	50-75	SIB	12-18	2	1
Buspirone	15	Aggression verbal outburts	15	0	1

**SIB=Selfmutilating behavior *CA=Chronological age ***Serum Lithium levels 0.5 to 0.7 mEg/L

Haloperidol. Haloperidol was the medication most frequently recommended and used. As was noted above, four children were taking haloperidol at the time of the consultation. In one patient haloperidol was discontinued because of parental disagreement on its use. The patient had a good response, and on lower dosage was much worse. The consultant's recommendation led to raising the dosage with good response. A second child in the group also had a good response to a low dosage but his parents feared dyskinesia. Another physician agreed to discontinue haloperidol and prescribed carbamazepine, nadolol, fenfluramine and chloral hydrate: the response to these drugs was poor. Washout and return to haloperidol yielded a good response. In the third child haloperidol was discontinued leading to severe self-injurious behaviors and abnormal muscle movements which may have been dyskinetic or "tardive-Tourette" (for review, see Perry et al., 1989b). A decision was made to further decrease dosage to help clarify the movement disorder. However, severe agitation and self-abusive behavior ensued; a return to haloperidol was indicated and resulted in a good response. The last patient of this group came to consultation on 12 mg of haloperidol which successfully suppressed self-injurious behavior. The parents wanted to discontinue haloperidol for a trial of fenfluramine. Haloperidol was discontinued resulting in a transient withdrawal dyskinesia; the dyskinetic movements almost ceased within a month. However, the self-injurious behaviors and agitation increased to such a degree that it was decided to reinstate haloperidol with the parents accepting the risk of a chronic dyskinesia. It is likely that without haloperidol this patient who lived at home would have had to be institutionalized, a move dreaded by his parents.

Haloperidol was also successfully used in the case of a girl whose severe self-injurious behaviors responded to chlorpromazine, 150 mg per day. The onset of extrapyramidal side effects, drooling, and, pallor required switch to haloperidol; on 3 mg/day the symptoms were contained without any of the side effects.

For the child who entered consultation on 6 different psychoactive medications, haloperidol was introduced as chlorpromazine, trifluoperazine, and desipramine were discontinued. After 6 months of haloperidol maintenance, severe aggressive, a not compulsive behavior returned and chlorpromazine which in the past had suppressed these symptoms, was substituted for haloperidol. Even at high doses chlorpromazine was ineffective during the exacerbation of self-injurious behavior.

In one case haloperidol was effective but only after trials of fenfluramine (requested by the parent) and of lithium failed to suppress the severe aggressive outbursts. Haloperidol was recommended in another case.

In two cases haloperidol was ineffective. In one, a child entered the consultation on haloperidol with a reported equivocal response. The decision was made to reduce the dosage from 6 to 4 mgs/day. Ten days later the child experienced a seizure. Haloperidol was discontinued, and after one month the child was reported as doing well. Finally an adolescent was started on haloperidol, 2 mg/day, for aggression and perseveration; the drug was effective but akathisia forced a switch to thioridazine which was ineffective. A trial of lithium was successful.

Thioridazine. Thioridazine was used in 2 patients. It was successful in suppressing the tantrums, assaultiveness and insomnia at 350 mg/day in an adolescent girl; side effects were mild extrapyramidal symptoms and weight gain. A trial of thioridazine was unsuccessful in a child who subsequently responded to lithium.

Lithium. Lithium was administered to two adolescents yielding one success and one failure. For another child lithium was recommended to another treating physician. Finally, lithium was just initiated at the writing of this chapter in a high-functioning adolescent whose parents specifically requested its usage to combat the verbally abusive and angry outbursts of their chronically irritable son. Buspirone was tried at first, without any response.

Fenfluramine. Fenfluramine was only tried once, and as noted above, failed in a child who subsequently responded to haloperidol.

Naltrexone. Naltrexone was administered to 3 patients with self-injurious behavior: in two it appeared to have moderate effectiveness, and in the third it failed. An 18 year old, who was a responder to naltrexone, remained on loxitane and lithium because of the pre-existing severity of his self-injurious behaviors.

The patients' ages, target symptoms, daily doses of psychoactive agents, and the patients' clinical response are presented in Table 2.

CONCLUSIONS

It is hoped that the sparcity of data in this area and the severe behavior problems some autistic children develop as they become adolescents, will stimulate research in this field of medicine.

ACKNOWLEDGEMENTS

Part of this work was supported by NIMH grants MH-32212, MH-40177 and 1 T32 MH 18915, and by a grant from the Stallone Fund for Research in Autism. The research was carried out in Bellevue Hospital Center, New York, New York.

REFERENCES

Adler, L., Angrist, B., Peselow, E., Corwin, J., & Rotroen, J. (1985). Efficacy of propranolol in neuroleptic-induced akathisia. *Journal of Clinical Psychopharmacology, 5,* 164 - 166.

American Psychiatric Association. *Diagnostic and Statistical Manual of Mental Disorders, (DSM-III). (3rd ed.)* 1980. Washington DC: Author.

Anderson, J. C., Williams, S., McGee, R., & Silva, P. A. (1987). DSM-III disorders in preadolescent children. *Archives of General Psychiatry, 44,* 69 - 76.

Anderson, L. T., Campbell, M., Adams, P., Small, A. M., Perry, R., & Shell, J. (1989). The effects of haloperidol on discrimination learning and behavioral symptoms in autistic children. *Journal of Autism and Developmental Disorders, 19,* 227 - 239.

Anderson, L. T., Campbell, M., Grega, D. M., Perry, R., Small, A. M., & Green, W. H. (1984). Haloperidol in the treatment of infantile autism: Effects on learning and behavioral symptoms. *American Journal of Psychiatry, 141,* 1195 - 1202.

Barrett, R. P., Feinstein, C., & Hole, W. T. (1989). Effects of naltrexone on self-injury: A double-blind, placebo-controlled analysis. *American Journal of Mental Retardation, 93,* 644 - 651.

Beckwith, B. E., Couk, D. I., & Schumacher, K. (1986). Failure of naloxone to reduce seif-injurious behavior in two developmentally disabled females. *Applied Research in Mental Retardation, 7,* 183 - 188.

Bernstein, G. A., Hughes, J. R., Mitchell, J. E., & Thompson, T. (1987). Effects of Narcotic Antagonists on Self-injurious Behavior: A Single Case Study. *Journal of the American Academy of Child and Adolescent Psychiatry, 26,* 886 - 889.

Campbell, M. (1987). Drug treatment of infantile autism: The past decade. In H. Y. Meltzer (Ed.), *Psychopharmacology: The Third Generation of Progress* (pp 1225 - 1231). New York: Raven Press.

Campbell, M. (1988). Fenfluramine treatment of autism. Annotation. *Journal of Child Psychology and Psychiatry, 29,* 1 - 10.

Campbell, M., & Schopler, E. (Co-chairmen). (1989). Pervasive Developmental Disorders. In T. Byran Karasu (Chairman), *Psychiatric Treatment Manual I (PTM-I), APA Task Force on Treatment of Psychiatric Disorders,* Washington, D C: American Psychiatric Press, Inc.

Campbell, M., Fish, B., Korein, J., Shapiro, T., Collins, P., & Koh, C. (1972). Lithium and chlorpromazine: A controlled crossover study of hyperactive severely disturbed young children. *Journal of Autism and Childhood Schizophrenia, 2,* 234 - 263.

Campbell, M., Anderson, L. T., Meier, M., Cohen, I. L., Small, A. M., Samit, C., & Sachar, E. J. (1978). A comparison of haloperidol, behavior therapy and their interaction in autistic children. *Journal of the American Academy of Child and Adolescent Psychiatry, 17,* 640 - 655.

Campbell, M., Grega, D. M., Green, W. H., & Bennet, W. G. (1983). Neuroleptic-induced dyskinesias in children. *Clinical Neuropharmacology, 6,* 207 - 222.

Campbell, M., Adams, P., Perry, R., Spencer, E. K., & Overall, J. E. (1988a). Tardive and withdrawal dyskinesia in autistic children: A prospective study. *Psychopharmacological Bulletin, 24,* 251 - 255.

Campbell, M., Adams, P., Small, A. M., Curren, E. L., Overall, J. E., Anderson, L. T., Lynch, N., & Perry, R. (1988b). Efficacy and safety of fenfluramine in autistic children. *Journal of the American Academy of Child and Adolescent Psychiatry, 27,* 434 - 439.

Campbell, M., Overall, J. E., Small, A. M., Sokol, M. S., Spencer, E. K., Adams, P., Foltz, R. L., Monti, K. M., Perry, R., Nobler, M., & Roberts, E. (1989). Naltrexone in autistic children: An acute open dose range tolerance trial. *Journal of the American Academy of Child and Adolescent Psychiatry, 28,* 200 - 206.

Campbell, M., Perry, R., & Green, W. H. (1984a). The use of lithium in children and adolescents. *Psychosomatics, 25,* 95 - 106.

Campbell, M., Small, A. M., Green, W. H., Jennings, S. J., Perry, R., Bennett, W. G., & Anderson, L. (1984b). Behavioral efficacy of haloperidol and lithium carbonate. A comparison in hospitalized aggressive children with conduct disorder. *Archives of General Psychiatry, 41,* 650 - 656.

Casey, D. E. (1987). Tardive dyskinesia. In H. Y. Meltzer (Ed.), *Psychopharmacology: The Third Generation of Progress* (pp 1411 - 1419). New York: Raven Press.

Cohen, D. J., & Donellan, A. M. (Eds.) (1987). *Handbook of Autism and Developmental Disorders.* New York: Wiley & Sons.

Cohen, I. L., Campbell, M., Posner, D., Small, A. M., Triebel, D., & Anderson, L. T. (1980). Behavioral effects of haloperidol in young autistic children: An objective analysis using a within-subjects reversal design. *Journal of the American Academy of Child Psychiatry, 19,* 665 - 677.

Craft, M., Ismail, I. A., Krishnamurti, D., Mathews, J., Regan, A., Seth, R. V., & North, P. M. (1987). Lithium in the treatment of aggression in mentally handicapped patients. A double-blind trial. *British Journal of Psychiatry, 150,* 685 - 689.

DeMyer, M. K., Hintgen, J. N., & Jackson, R. K. (1981). Infantile autism reviewed. A decade of research. *Schizophrenia Bulletin, 7,* 388 - 451.

Deutsch, S. I. (1986). Rationale for the Administration of Opiate Antagonists in Treating Infantile Autism. *American Journal of Mental Deficiency, 90,* 631 - 635.

Dostal, T. (1972). Antiaggressive effect of lithium salts in mentally retarded adolescents. In A. L. Annell (Ed.), *Depressive States in Childhood and Adolescence* (pp 491 - 498). Stockholm: Almqvist & Wiksell.

Ekman, G., Miranda-Linne, F., Gillberg, C., Garle, M., & Wetterberg, L. (1989). Fenfluramine treatment of 20 autistic children. *Journal of Autism and Developmental Disorders,* (in press).

Elliott, F. A. (1977). Propranolol for the control of belligerent behavior following acute brain damage. *Annals of Neurology, 1,* 489 - 491.

Elliott, R. L. (1986). Lithium treatment and cognitive changes in two mentally retarded patients. *Journal of Nervous and Mental Disease, 174,* 689 - 692.

Evans, R. W., Clay, T. H., & Gualtieri, C. T. (1987). Carbamazepine in pediatric psychiatry. *Journal of the American Academy of Child and Adolescent Psychiatry, 26,* 2 - 8.

Fann, M. E., Smith, R. C., Davis, J. M., & Domino, E. F. (Eds.) (1980). Tardive Dyskinesia: Research and Treatment. Jamaica, New York: Spectrum Publication, Inc.

Farber, J. M. (1987). Psychopharmacology of self-injurious behavior in the mentally retarded. *Journal of the American Academy of Child and Adolescent Psychiatry, 26,* 296 - 302.

Fish, B. (1970). Psychopharmacologic responses of chronic schizophrenic adults as predictors of responses in young schizophrenic children. *Psychopharmacological Bulletin, 6,* 12 - 15.

Gillberg, C., & Schaumann, H. (1981). Infantile autism and puberty. *Journal of Autism and Developmental Disorders, 11,* 365 - 371.

Gualtieri, T., Evans, R. W., & Patterson, D. R. (1987). The medical treatment of autistic people. In E. Schopler & G. B. Mesibov (Eds.), *Neurobiological Issues in Autism* (pp 373 - 388). New York: Plenum Press.

Gualtieri, C. T., Quade, D., Hicks, R. E., Mayo, J. P., & Schroeder, S. R. (1984). Tardive dyskinesia and other clinical consequences of neuroleptic treatment in children and adolescents. *American Journal of Psychiatry, 141,* 20 - 23.

Hawkins, D. & Pauling, L. (Eds.) (1973). *Orthomolecular Psychiatry.* San Fransisco: W. H. Freeman.

Herman, B. H., Hammock, M. K., Arthur-Smith, A., Egan, J., Chatoor, I., Werner, A., & Zelnik, N. (1987). Naltrexone decreases self-injurious behavior. *Annals of Neurology, 22,* 550 - 552.

Herman, B. H., Hammock, M. K., Arthur-Smith, A., Egan, J., Chatoor, I., Zelnik, N., Appelgate, K., Boeckx, R. L. (1986). Effects of naltrexone in autism: Correlation with plasma opioid concentrations: *American Academy of Child and Adolescent Psychiatry,* Scientific Proceedings for the Annual Meeting, (2), 11 - 12.

Kerbeshian, J., Burd, L., & Fisher, W. (1987). Lithium carbonate in the treatment of two patients with infantile autism and atypical bipolar symptomatology. *Journal of Clinical Psychopharmacology, 7,* 401 - 405.

Langee, H. R. (1989). A retrospective study of mentally retarded patients with behavioral disorders who were treated with carbamazepine. *American Journal of Mental Retardation, 93,* 640 - 643.

Leboyer, M., Bouvard, M. P., & Dugas, M. (1988). Effects of naltrexone on infantile autism. *Lancet,* March 26, p 715.

Leventhal, B. L. (1985). Fenfluramine administration to autistic children: Effects on behavior and biogenic amines. Paper presented at the 25th NCDEU Annual (Anniversary) Meeting, Key Biscayne, Florida, May 1 - 4.

Lipman, R. S. (1986). Overview of research in psychopharmacological treatment of the mentally ill/mentally retarded. *Psychopharmacology Bulletin, 22,* 1046 - 1054.

Marcus, L. M., & Schopler, E. (1987). Working with families: A developmental perspective. In D. J. Cohen & A. M. Donnellan (Eds.), *Handbook of Autism and Pervasive Developmental Disorders* (pp 499 - 512). New York: Wiley & Sons.

Mattes, J. A. (1986). Psychopharmacology of temper outbursts. A review. *Journal of Nervous and Mental Disease, 174,* 464 - 470.

Naruse, H., Nagahata, M., Nakane, Y., Shirahashi, K., Takesada, M., & Yamazaki, K. (1982). A multi-center double-blind trial of pimozide (Orap), haloperidol and placebo in children with behavior disorders, using cross-over design. *Acta Paedopsychiatrica, 48,* 173 - 184.

Pauling, L. (1968). Orthomolecular psychiatry, *Science, 160,* 265 - 271.

Payton, J. B. (1987). Depression in non-retarded autistics. Abstract NR-74A, Scientific Proceedings of the Annual Meeting. Vol. III, *American Academy of Child and Adolescent Psychiatry,* Washington, D. C., October 21 - 25, p 54.

Perry, R., Campbell, M., Grega, D. M., & Anderson, L. (1984). Saliva lithium levels in children: Their use in monitoring serum lithium levels and lithium side effects. *Journal of Clinical Psychopharmacology, 4,* 199 - 202.

Perry, R., Campbell, M., Adams, P., Lynch, N., Spencer, E. K., Curren, E. L., & Overall, J. E. (1989a). Long-term efficacy of haloperidol in autistic children: Continuous vs. discontiuous drug administration. *Journal of the American Academy of Child and Adolescent Psychiatry, 28,* 87 - 92.

Perry, R., Nobler, M. S., & Campbell, M. (1989b). Case Report: Tourette-like symptoms associated with chronic neuroleptic therapy in an autistic child. *Journal of the American Academy of Child and Adolescent Psychiatry, 28,* 93 - 96.

Polakoff, S. A., Sorgi, P. J., & Ratey, J. J. (1986). The Treatment of Impulsive and Aggressive Behavior with Nadolol. *Journal of Clinical Psychopharmacology, 6,* 125 - 126.

Post, R. M. (1987). Mechanisms of action of carbamazepine and related anticonvulsants in affective illness. In H. Y. Meltzer (Ed.), *Psychopharmacology: The Third Generation of Progress* (pp 567 - 576). New York: Raven Press.

Post, R. M. (1988). Time course of clinical effects of carbamazepine: implications of mechanisms of action. *Journal of Clinical Psychiatry, 49,* suppl., 35 - 46.

Raiten, D. J. (1987). Nutrition and developmental disabilities. In E. Schopler & G. B. Mesibov (Eds.), *Neurobiological Issues in Autism* (pp 325 - 338). New York: Plenum Press.

Raiten, D. J., & Massaro, T. F. (1987). Nutrition and developmental disabilities: An examination of the orthomolecular hypothesis. In D. J. Cohen & A. M. Donnellan (Eds.), *Handbook of Autism and Pervasive Developmental Disorders* (pp 566 - 583). New York: Wiley & Sons.

Ratey, J. J., Bemporad, J., Sorgi, P., Bick, P., Polakoff, S., O'Driscoll, G., & Mikkelsen, E. (1987a). Brief report: Open trial effects of beta-blockers on speech and social behaviors in 8 autistic adults. *Journal of Autism and Developmental Disorders, 17,* 439 - 446.

Ratey, J. J., Mikkelsen, E., Sorgi, P., Zuckerman, S., Polakoff, S., Bemporad, J., Bick, P., & Kadish, W. (1987b). Autism: The Treatment of Aggressive Behaviors. *Journal of Clinical Psychopharmacology, 7,* 35 - 41.

Ratey, J. J., Mikkelsen, E., Smith, G. B., Upadhyaya, A., Zuckerman, H. S., Martell, D., Sorgi, P., Polakoff, S., & Bemporad, J. (1986). Beta-blockers in the severely and profoundly mentally retarded. *Journal of Clinical Psychopharmacology, 6,* 103 - 107.

Reisberg, B., & Gershon, S. (1979). Side effects associated with lithium therapy. *Archives of General Psychiatry, 36,* 879 - 887.

Remschmidt, H. (1976). The psychotropic effect of carbamazepine in non-epileptic patients, with particular reference to problems posed by clinical studies in children with behavioral disorders. In W. Birkmayer (Ed.), *Epileptic Seizures - Behaviour - Pain* (pp 253 - 258). Bern: Hans Huber.

Richardson, J. S., & Zaleski, W. A. (1983). Naloxone and self-mutilation. *Biological Psychiatry, 18,* 99 - 101.

Rimland, B. (1987). Megavitamin B6 and magnesium in the treatment of autistic children and adults. In E. Schopler & G. B. Mesibov (Eds.), *Neurological Issues in Autism* (pp 389 - 405). New York: Plenum Press.

Ritvo, E. R., Freeman, B. J., Geller, E., & Yuwiler, A. (1983). Effects of fenfluramine on 14 outpatients with the syndrome of autism. *Journal of the American Academy of Child Psychiatry, 22,* 549 - 558.

Ritvo, E. R., Yuwiler, A., Geller, E., Schroth, P., Yokota, A., Mason-Brothers, A., August, G. J., Klykylo, W., Leventhal, B., Lewis, K., Piggott, L., Realmuto, G., Stubbs, E. G., & Umansky, R. (1986). Fenfluramine treatment of autism: UCLA collaborative study of 81 patients at nine medical centers. *Psychopharmacological Bulletin, 22,* 133 - 140.

Sandman, C. A., Datta, P. C., Barron, J., Koehler, F. K., Williams, C., & Swanson, J. M. (1983). Naloxone attenuates self-abusive behavior in developmentally disabled clients. *Applied Research in Mental Retardation, 4,* 5 - 11.

Schopler, E., & Mesibov, G. B. (Eds.) (1983). *Autism in Adolescence and Adults.* New York: Plenum.

Shopsin, B., Gershon, S., & Pinckney, L. (1969). The secretion of lithium in human mixed saliva: Effects of ingested lithium on electrolyte distribution in saliva and serum. *International Pharmacopsychiatry, 2,* 148 - 169.

Silver, J. M., Yudofsky, S. C., Kogan, M., & Katz, B. L. (1986). Elevation of thioridazine plasma levels by propranolol. *American Journal of Psychiatry, 143,* 1290 - 1292.

Spencer, E. K., & Campbell, M. (1989). Aggressiveness directed against self and others: Psychopharmacologic intervention. In S. L. Harris & J. S. Handleman (Eds.), *Life Threatening Behavior: Aversive vs. Nonaversive Interventions* (in press).

Szymanski, L., Kedesdy, J., Sulkes, S., Cutler, A., & Stevens-Our, P. (1987). Naltrexone in treatment of self injurious behavior: a clinical study. *Research in Developmental Disabilities, 8,* 179 - 190.

Tarjan, G., Lowery, V. E., & Wright, S. W. (1957). The use of chlorpromazine in 278 mentally deficient patients. *American Medical Association Journal of Disturbed Children, 94,* 294 - 300.

Tyrer, S. P., Walsh, A., Edwards, D. E., Berney, T. P., & Stephens, D. A. (1984). Factors associated with a good response to lithium in aggressive mentally handicapped subjects. *Progress in Neuro-Psychopharmacology & Biological Psychiatry, 8,* 751 - 755.

Vitiello, B., Behar, D., Malone, R., Delaney, M. A., Ryan, P. J., & Simpson, G. M. (1988). Pharmacokinetics of lithium carbonate in children. *Journal of Clinical Psychopharmacology, 8,* 355 - 359.

Walters, A. S., Barrett, R. P., Feinstein, C., Mercurio, A., & Hole, W. (1989). The treatment of self-injury and social withdrawal in autism with naltrexone. Paper presented at the Eastern Psychological Association Meeting, Boston, MA, March 1989.

Weischer, M. L. (1969). Über die antiaggressive Wirkung von Lithium. *Psychopharmacologia, 15,* 245 - 254.

Weller, E. B., Weller, R. A., Fristad, M. A., Cantwell, M., & Tucker, S. (1987). Saliva lithium monitoring in prepubertal children. *Journal of the American Academy of Child and Adolescent Psychiatry, 26,* 173 - 175.

White, T. J. R., & Aman, M. G. (1985). Pimozide treatment in disruptive severely retarded patients. *Australian and New Zealand Journal of Psychiatry, 19,* 92 - 94.

Williams, D. T., Mehl, R., Yudofsky, S., Adams, D., & Roseman, B. (1982). The effect of propranolol on uncontrolled rage outbursts in children and adolescents with organic brain dysfunction. *Journal of the American Academy of Child Psychiatry, 21,* 129 - 135.

Wing, L., & Attwood, A. (1987). Syndromes of autism and atypical development. In D. J. Cohen & A. M. Donnellan (Eds.), *Handbook of Autism and Developmental Disorders* (pp 3 - 19). New York: Wiley & Sons.

Yudofsky, S., Williams, D., & Gorman, J. (1981). Propranolol in the treatment of rage and violent behavior in patients with chronic brain syndrome. *American Journal of Psychiatry, 138,* 218 - 230.

Ziring, P. R., & Teitelbaum, L. (1980). *Affiliation with a university department of psychiatry: Impact on the use of psychoactive medication in a large public residential facility for mentally retarded persons.* Paper presented at the conference on use of medications in controlling the behavior of the mentally retarded. September 22 - 24, University of Minnesota, Minneapolis, Minnesota.

Educational Issues in Adolescence

BORGNY RUSTEN

INTRODUCTION

Autism is a casually selected name for a casually selected group. The criteria for its diagnosis have gradually become so extensive that the piece of the jigsaw puzzle for which people were looking originally has become several pieces, indeed almost an entire puzzle, without science having solved the riddle of autism. It is true that research has established that some autistic persons have metabolic disorders or a fragile X-cromosome or damage to or maldevelopment of the cerebellum or other parts of the central nervous system, but just how these defects produce autism remains unknown.

Our son Øystein reached the age of 40 in 1989, so for the last 35 years I have read everything I could find about autism. Formerly such reading-matter was scanty, whereas today the articles are tumbling over each other. In the time of Kanner (1943) and during the next 10 - 20 years the incidence of autism was calculated differently from the present day, the children being so few and so easily recognizable that we could distinguish them ourselves even if we did not know them. One of the biggest changes with regard to the calculation of incidence is that the prerequisite of potentially normal or high intelligence has been dropped. Today it has become accepted that autism may occur at any point on the scale of intelligence.

In teaching autistic young people we need to view the person as a single whole. Methods which take account of the wider conceptions of autism must relate to causative factors and possibilities of development. Constantly diverging diagnoses and alleged causal relations present at great challenge to special teaching methods. As science reveals how the various injuries affect the personality we have to discover new ways. We know that autistic individuals can be influenced and are able to learn, and they are affected by their surroundings, whether we like it or not.

Home and school have a big responsibility in organizing the milieu in which autistic children are placed. I wish researchers would direct attention to this and would cultivate a good working relationship with parents and other professional people who have daily contact with those who suffer from autism.

In order to prepare a plan which fits the individual, one must know the following:

(1)   what financial resources and practical possibilities are available,

(2)   how severe the handicaps of the autistic person are, and

(3)   what manpower one has at one's disposal.

Our most important resources are observation and insight, together with all the information we can acquire from parents and teachers about previous schooling and instruction. In past years all of us who worked with our own and other people's autistic children used the trial-and-error method. But this is to be avoided. We must have definite objectives and intermediate objectives if we are to achieve a satisfactory development. It is the adult who is responsible and must have both himself and the teaching proberly organised.

It is important that the adult should build up a feeling of security in everything he does, as insecurity on that side is easily transferred to the autistic young person.

"I hope he does not notice that I am frightened of him!" says an assistant teacher. This is a vain hope. Human beings and animals alike all notice when you are afraid of them, and it creates apprehension and aggression. Autistic people are the most perceptive of all, and the most prompt to notice who feels secure.

It is also important to consider what the autistic youth learnt in childhood and what habits have been developed. We know too that tasks which such a person can perform under certain conditions cannot be transferred without training to another situation, such as a different room, a different teacher or a different time of day.

WHAT DO WE WANT OUR TEACHING TO ACHIEVE?

* We want to achieve access to the characteristics and potentials of the individual, so as to enhance to the utmost the quality of his adult life.

* We want to try to develop some of the latent capacities, which are so often present.

WHAT PROBLEMS IN AUTISM ARE PARTICULARLY RELEVANT TO THE PROCESS OF TEACHING?

I have heard some educators say that autistic persons forget so much. That has not been my experience - rather I think the opposite applies. We who regard ourselves as normal do not go on remembering everything we learnt at home and at school. Have you not forgotten what the Battle of Stanford Bridge was about and the intricacies of a cow's digestive system? I have. And why? Because they were of no use to me.

In this there lies a challenge to us teachers. We must teach autistic young persons the right things, viz. those which are meaningful and which they can use in adult life. Moreover, it is important that each day should have a good and meaningful content. We must bear in mind that the autistic person we are working with is first and foremost a young human being, and in the second place a victim of autism.

We must beware of expending too much time and effort on unlearning negative behaviour, the really good education method being to teach the autistic person the thing that is correct and constructive. We must reckon with difficulties at the start and not give up. We can put it this way: *When knowledge goes in incivilities go out.*

Autistic young people have puberty problems like other people, with less full control of the body than before and increased difficulties of identification (Gillberg & Schaumann, 1981; Haracopos, 1988). The majority have problems over sexuality. What help can we offer them? In this field there is very little literature: sexuality is, for example, hardly ever mentioned in pedagogical/psychological reports, and the topic is seldom discussed at meetings of treatment. It may well be that attitudes to sexuality in the surroundings are the reason for the reserve with which the topic is treated.

For normal young people the development into adulthood involves difficulties with themselves. Why should this be different for victims of autism? Shall we try to imagine the difficulty of their situation in that phase of life? Perhaps some of them ask themselves or us: *What about me? Will I ever get any relationship with another person? Will I get a wife? Will I get a home and children, like my brothers and sisters? Why do I have all these feelings? What use can I make of them?*

Everybody who works with autistic children ought to recognize the sexual problems they may show in adolescence and try to find individual solutions for them. It is important for the home and school to discuss them openly together and arrive at a common attitude, which must be liberal - "but within limits".

After careful consideration of what subjects most autistic students *can make use of*, and of the way in which the instruction must be carried out, I approve the following:

(1)   training skills of everyday life,

(2)   physical education,

(3)   sign-language or other instruction in communication,

(4)   music and dancing,

(5)   arts and crafts, and

(6)   writing, reading and arithmetic for those functioning on a sufficiently high level to be able to use such skills.

1   Activities of Daily Life

The skills of everyday life are perhaps the area for which it is easiest to construct a simple framework as regards both time and place. Most people get up at about the same time every day; they make themselves ready and dress themselves in the same way; and eat at fixed times, and so on. But observe, that unless we make a plan which everybody agrees to follow, an autistic person's performances will depend on who is with him in the various training situations. Not two adults work alike.

2   Physical education

The most manageable form of physical training are:
-     swimming (or spending time in basin pool)
-     jogging (or going for a walk)
-     ball "games"
-     skiing

Make a cautious start. The person with autism must always be successful. If the proceedings are brought to a happy conclusion, there is good hope that the next time will be successful too. Everyone likes the feeling of being "a success".

A group of students at the Norwegian University of Athletics have written a paper on organized physical activities for autistic persons (Reigstad, 1985). In their study they collected data showing that physical activity helps people with autism at all ages in developing:
-     social abilities,
-     physical abilities, and
-     abilities in relation to one's own personality.

Undesirable deviant behaviour, such as self-stimulation, aggressiveness and self-destruction appear to be considerably reduced by the offer of physical training. Young people are quiet after physical activity, and increased attention and concentration are noted. To achieve mastery through one's own body gives positive experiences and increased self-confidence to many. This in turn will mean improved adaptability, an essential if an autistic person is to live a meaningful life.

3   Communication

All people with autism have communication problems, but all people with communication problems are not autistic.

Difficulties of communication have been present in every handicapped person I have met, though the causes may vary. If there are no obvious organic or psychic inhibitions, then in 90 per cent of the cases our attitudes will put us at a distance. A clever teacher will try to remedy this difficulty be endeavouring to instruct the victim of autism in some method of expressing himself. Communication can be established through several channels, for instance:

body language, gesture and mimicry,

sign-speech,

instruction in talking,

pictures,

writing,

bliss-symbols, and

data programming symbols.

When we are going to give instruction in communication, it is important to decide on which form to choose in the individual case.

If we fail to find a mean of enabling the autistic person to influence his surrounding and express his wishes and needs, the consequence will often be the development of undesirable practices, such as making their own signals, which will not always be understood in their surroundings. This in turn will cause:

withdrawal and self-stimulation

destructiveness (including self-injury) and, last but not least,

aggression.

Excellent methods have been worked out for sign teaching, but it would take too long to go into them here. One of the reasons why it is easier to teach sign than articulation is that most autistic persons apprehend by sight more than by hearing, and it is easier to make signs than to articulate sounds. The teaching of signs is based upon the natural language of the body, and it is never too late to begin.

4   Music and Dancing

I believe autistic people would like to associate with us, but they cannot reach us, because they are not equipped for contact. Can we reach them? One of the means might be music and singing. A discreet humming can often be enough to create quiet in an unquiet mind, and I have seen a young music-therapist catch an autistic individual's attention in such a way that all undesirable behaviour vanished, while the eyes shone and the body relaxed. But it makes a difference what songs we sing or what instrument we play.

When Saul had his dark times of heaviness, David played for him on the harp. Do you suppose it would have had the same effect if he hade beaten a drum?

The National Autism Association of Norway gives summer courses for parents and their autistic children. There is dancing in the evenings. It is astonishing to see the pleasure with which most of the autistic persons take part in that dancing, even though to be near other people can be so burdensome to many of them. Those who can talk benefit most from social gatherings, but I have no doubt that, where there is a capacity for understanding speech, they can profit greatly from being with other people, even if they cannot talk.

5   Arts and crafts

Arts and crafts is a subject of great significance, for like no other they provide a possibility for observation of skills which are relevant to life as an adult. Can I teach somebody to distinguish and remember the names of colours? Has she a sense of shape and the ability to do a jigsaw puzzle? Can he screw a lid off and on etc ?. Can she learn to weave, knit, sew, etc ?

One of our major institutions for the mentally handicapped, where young people with autism live, had a good workshop, of which too little use was made. It was given a new leader who was a craftsman and, as the father of an autistic child, he had had plenty of opportunity to observe the strengths and weaknesses of people with autism. He changed to serial production, which had the advantage that the young autistic workers had to perform the same operations *over and over again, until they had learned their "profession".* After a time he taught them a new part of the production, so that in the end

410

they mastered something like the entire procedure, 70 per cent of the product in some cases, in others up to 95 per cent. The leader is at work every day at 7, and arranges things before the clients arrive at 9.

The young people with autism enjoy being in the canteen, where each of them has his day for preparing coffee, with which pancakes are served. That is their reward. Thus they have found a meaningful place in the adult world, and life is worth living for them.

My contribution is mainly concerned with tasks which parents and teachers can succeed in, and with the importance of dividing the instruction between objectives and intermediate objectives. It says little about methods and roads to success, but one thing is certain: *when you are teaching, you must never let the attention stray for one moment from your pupil.* Else Hansen, the former head of the Sofie School, said it this way: "Remember that, when you are teaching an autistic pupil, it is like taking tea with the Queen" (Hansen, 1970).

For an autistic young person and his helpers the road is a long one, and it means work, work, work!

Winnie the Pooh said once upon a time to his friend Piglet: "What would you do if you had to walk 1 000 miles?" Piglet rubbed his nose and said: "First I would take one step."

REFERENCES

Gillberg, C., & Schaumann, H. (1981). Infantile autism and puberty. *Journal of Autism and Developmental Disorders, 11,* 365 - 371.

Hansen, E. (1970). *Hvorfor stenger de døren?* Copenhagen: Danskernes Forlag.

Haracopos, D. (1988). *Hvad med meg?* Copenhagen: Andonia Forlag.

Kanner, L. (1943). Autistic disturbances of affective contact. *Nervous child, 2,* 217 - 250.

Psychotherapeutical Help in Adolescence

HENRIK PELLING

INTRODUCTION

The attempts to create treatments for autism and schizophrenia on the basis of causality have shown great similarities. This does not, however, mean that autism and schizophrenia have the same causes. Different hereditary patterns and development of symptoms and the fact that the effect of neuroleptic drugs on schizophrenia has no equivalent effect on autism, indicate that there is no such relationship. There is, however, some overlapping of symptoms between autism and childhood schizophrenia; early language abnormalities, lack of social responsiveness, mood lability and abnormalities in sensory, motor and cognitive functioning (Watkin el., 1988). Autism and schizophrenia include many different etiologies of neurological injuries. Continued research into the neuropathophysiological background will eventually give us the explanation of these similarities and differences.

Interpretations of schizophrenia in terms of "the schizophrenogenic mother" and the "double-bind hypothesis" have nor been confirmed, in empirical studies, not been found confirmed. Psychotherapy founded on such theoretical assumptions has not been successful. The impact of family variables on the clinical course of schizophrenia have, however, revealed some important relationships. Patients whose relatives showed a high degree of expressed emotion (EE) at their release from hospital had a considerably higher frequency of relapse than others. Family treatment, aiming at restriction of EE, has proved to be effective. Anderson, Reiss and Hogarty (1986) have in the book "Schizophrenia and the Family" described a model for treatment, including parent education, crisis therapy and family therapy founded on partnership between the parents and the therapist. The promising results of this treatment have been an inspiration to us, not only in the treatment of schizophrenia but also in the family treatment of autism.

ADOLESCENT CHANGES IN AUTISM

In adolescence, new difficulties confront the autistic child. The body and hormonal changes increase the drive pressure as well as the desire for independence, and the manifestations of emotions become more violent. The wish to communicate these new experiences and needs is an additional strain on the limited capability to relate to others and to communicate. Along with body growth, the environment expectations become greater. A nearly grown-up person, even though his retardation is obvious, is thus expected to have acquired some emphathy in terms of other people's feelings and thoughts and to be able to understand the meaning of social signals. The autistic individual is often unable to meet these inner and outer demands, and when his attempts at communication and interaction fail, he is likely to develop behavioural disturbances. Temper tantrums, self-destructiveness and aggressiveness are very difficult to cope with and may lead to a vicious circle in which the autistic person becomes more isolated.

STRAINS ON THE FAMILY

When the autistic child reaches adolescence, the strain on his relatives, parents or siblings, changes in character and like the relatives of schizophrenic patients they may become depressed or develop other psychiatric problems. The lack of contact and the presence of aggressiveness and social isolation are factors present in cases of autism as well as of schizophrenia. The family living with an autistic child has for years been forced to arrange suitable surroundings for the child, to alter the home for safety reasons, to keep constant watch over him and, from time to time, to wrestle with behavioural problems. Conditions do not improve in adolescence. On the contrary, this period often involves an increasing amount of practical problems and situations demanding supervision. Instead of profiting from previous training, the teenager often goes through periods of regression. In addition to true regression, the patient's inability to generalize acquired skills becomes more obvious when he is exposed to more demanding social contacts. Even very young autistic children show attachment behaviour (Shapiro et al.,

1987) thus making the parents feel the need for contact, even if the child's particular handicap makes this contact very rudimentary. The adolescent who shows his preferences to his parents, teachers or nurses, but at the same time tries to have his own way, using his inadequate ability of interaction, is extremely trying to the people around him. Overinvolvement sometimes occurs in an attempt to solve this dilemma, since the autistic adolescent feels most safe with people who are successful in controlling his behavioural symptoms.

A "PSYCHOEDUCATIONAL" MODEL FOR THERAPY

In order to maintain the autistic child's capabilities and skills it is imperative that the persons around him cooperate, without overestimating his ability. The adults must work together in order to create a balance between the elements of training, relaxation and stimulation of communication and interaction.

For obvious reasons, it is more difficult to set limits for the behaviour of the autistic adolescent than for the autistic child. From an early age, the goals of the training must be to implant such rules of behaviour that can also be practised in later life. It may, for instance, be acceptable for very young autistic children to make contact in a bizarre manner, whereas the same behaviour in an adolescent might be frightening. It is therefore important not to encourage *all* attempts to make social contact, but try to direct them into more socially acceptable modes. It is particularly important to make masturbation an accepted outlet for sexuality, but the structure (times and places) should be determined by the grown-ups. Structured education is used from an early age to help the child understand form, colour, concepts, etc. It is, however, important that the education of autistic adolescents does not include too much of these academic activities, but rather concentrates on practical training of social skills. Even leisure time activities must be trained and should be based on the autistic child's personal inclinations to music, simple games and so on.

Many autistic individuals are fond of robust body contact, a need that is difficult to satisfy in a nearly grown-up person. According to our experience, a water setting (bath-tub or swimming pool) offers good opportunities of body contact to the adolescent, while at the same time providing possibilities to improve body image.

Individual therapy sessions are valuable parts of a comprehensive treatment programme, inasmuch as they also focus on emotional expressions. While the patient is performing simple tasks, the therapist may concentrate on all forms of expression, encourage attempts at communication and give such confirmation that the patient is able to comprehend. These sequences are, of course, similar to those in educational sessions, in speech training etc, but sessions void of training elements may increase motivation and improve the means of understanding the autistic child's emotional expressions.

The psychotherapist who develops a keen sensitivity to the patient's signals is an accurate observer of mood changes, often drastic in adolescence, and is thus able to give advice regarding adequate goals for other activities. As the means of communication are unconventional and originating from particular situations, care continuity is particularly important, so that parents, therapists and nursing staff who are familiar with the context in which the message was formulated can help each other understand as well as interpret to others.

Recent research on echolalia and self-injurious behaviour as expressions of a variety of needs and moods (Prizaut & Wetherby, 1987), serve as additional confirmation, from another aspect, of the notion that efforts at interpreting behaviour may be worthwhile. The therapist's display of interest in the autistic person's particular communicative means and his growing ability to give the solicited answers, encourages further interaction. This rapport also facilitates the discrimination between behaviours that should be regarded as means of communication and behavioural symptoms that should be prevented by firm limits.

Unusual care-giving demands on the part of the autistic adolescent often create feelings of inability and guilt in the people around him. Outsiders often add to the feelings of guilt by looking upon the autistic child as either badly brought up or down-right neglected. A vicious circle may thus be activated with the autistic child showing increasingly more behaviour problems and the parents feeling more incompetent and depressed. Both love and forbidden feelings of hatred and rejection may lead to overinvolvement, to the detriment of other family members and many of the parents' personal needs. A desperate wavering may be brought about between hopes for a treatment or a therapist who can really "cure" and a strong belief in one's own unique competence and a derogatory attitude towards other care-givers.

Families under great pressure, caused by serious illness in a child, usually adjust their patterns of behaviour from one given degree of flexibility to a more rigid one. By means of simplifications or by decreasing the number of situations that call for negotiations, the family becomes more concentrated on its most laborous task. Should pressure increase further, there is a risk that the rigid, but at the same time strong, defence collapses into chaos. This model (Lewis, 1986) makes it easier to understand how seemingly dysfunctional patterns become the responses to exceptional situations. The parents, having invented the new rules and modes of acting towards the child, are therefore experts who can work together with therapists on changing them. A psychoeducational model gives the parents an opportunity to do this by endowing them with more knowledge and back-up in crises as well as a partnership with professionals, aiming at solving, step by step, the carefully determined problems. A prolonged such contact may also, if needed, lead to psychotherapeutical help for individual problems when the main problem with the autistic child is under control.

The psychoeducational model is based on the assumed "normality" of the family, a view which has to be reflected in the therapist's attitude. Paradoxically, one also assumes that sometimes the family's competence could be considerably ameliorated by changing its dysfunctional patterns. It is possible that some parents have personality traits specific for a genetic disposition to autism (Wolff et al., 1988). Such personality traits, in the psychotherapeutical sessions, should not be discussed as "environmental" causes or consequences of the child's behaviour problems.

A study of stress in parents of developmentally disabled children has shown a decrease of stress at a high degree of perceived control and spouse support (McKinney & Peterson, 1987). In dealing with these factors, the techniques of traditional family or marriage therapy may be used, although we lack knowledge about the specifics of the stress moderating factors in a family with an autistic child.

The prerequisite for optimal care is a teamwork between different professional categories with expert knowledge of autism. During extended periods of stagnation or regression in the adolescent, supervision is very important in order to maintain professional security and counter-check psychologcial effects.

Different care-givers have to cooperate to clarify the difference between cause and treatment. The causes of a fracture have nothing to do with the plaster of Paris. A stress-vulnerability model helps us to describe correlations between specific stressors and underlying neurological dysfunctions. Treating the stressors with educational and behavioural methods as well as adapted psychotherapies concerning milieu, family and individual is then seen as complementary to pharmacological treatment, sensory integration training, etc.

SUMMARY

The care for disabled children has a long tradition of constructing individual treatment programmes, of encouraging parents to join parents' associations and of using brief periods of planned respite care. In child psychiatry, the therapies used to control behaviour problems and psychoses are becoming more and more specific. In our experience, a psychoeducational model facilitates a cooperation based on experiences accumulated in both these fields. Such a cooperation, regarding organization as well as staff, between child rehabilitation and child psychiatry offers new opportunities to the autistic children and their families.

REFERENCES

Anderson, C. M., Reiss, D. J., & Hogarty, G. E. (1986). *Schizophrenia and the Family. A Practitioner's Guide to Psycho-education and management.* New York: The Guildford Press.

Lewis, J. M. (1986). Family structure and stress. *Family Process, 25,* 235-247.

McKinney, B., & Peterson, R. A. (1987). Predictors of stress in parents of developmentally disabled children. *Journal of Pediatric Psychology, 12,* 133 - 150.

Prizant, B. M., & Wetherby, A. M. (1987). Communicative Intent: A framework for understanding social-communicative behaviour in autism. *Journal of the American Academy of Child and Adolescent Psychiatry, 26,* 472-479.

Shapiro, T., Sherman, M., Calmari, G., & Koch, D. (1987). Attachment in autism and other developmental disorders. *Journal of the American Academy of Child and Adolescent Psychiatry, 26,* 480-484.

Watkins, J. M., Asarnow, R. F., & Tanguay, P. E. (1988). Symptom development in childhood onset schizophrenia. *Journal of Child Psychology and Psychiatry, 29,* 865-878.

Wolff, S., Narayan, S., & Moyes, B. (1988). Personality characteristics of parents of autistic children: A controlled study. *Journal of Child Psychology and Psychiatry, 29,* 143-153.

Autistic Adults

LORNA WING

This chapter is concerned with disorders in the autistic continuum as described in the chapter on diagnosis. The terms "autism" and "autistic" are used for convenience but should be taken to refer to the wider group unless otherwise specified.

There are a small number of studies that have followed autistic children into adolescence and early adult life (DeMyer et al, 1973; Gillberg & Steffenburg, 1987; Kanner, 1973; Lotter, 1974; Rutter, 1970; Wing, 1988). All found that, very approximately, 5 to 10 per cent became independent as adults; another 25 per cent made considerable progress but still needed some supervision, the rest remained severely impaired and required a high level of care. Prognosis was closely related to level of ability in childhood as shown on cognitive and language tests.

There are no epidemiological studies of autism in adults, nor any systematic accounts in the literature of groups of autistic adults followed throughout their life span. Longevity and long term prognosis are therefore unknown. The descriptions in the present chapter are based on information from the above mentioned follow-up studies into early adult life, cross-sectional studies by Shah, Holmes and Wing (1982) and Wing (1988), the clinical experience of the author and colleagues and from accounts provided by parents of autistic adults. A retrospective study by Tantam (1986) of adults with autistic features not diagnosed in childhood but presenting at adult psychiatric clinics has added another dimension to the story. Many aspects of treatment and management of adolescents and adults with autism are dealt with in the book edited by Schopler and Mesibov (1983).

Gillberg (1983, 1984) and Gillberg and Steffenburg (1987) described behavioural and psychiatric problems in autistic and other socially impaired adolescents and young adults.

The manifestations of autism in each of the prognostic groups, their skills, their behaviour, psychiatric complications and the services needed will be described. The groups shade into each other without clear distinction but the arbitrary sub-divisions are useful for purposes of description.

THE GROUP REMAINING SEVERELY IMPAIRED

This is the largest group among all those with the triad of social impairment whose handicaps are recognised in childhood, even if not diagnosed as autistic (Wing and Gould, 1979; Wing, 1988). The majority are aloof in childhood and remain so in adult life, but a minority are passive, or active but odd in social interaction (see the chapter on diagnosis). Epilepsy is particularly common and continues into adulthood (Rutter, 1970). The intelligence level, in most cases, is in the profoundly or severely retarded range. However, a few children who were in the mildly retarded range when young fail to make the expected progress and are severely handicapped as adults (Gillberg & Steffenburg, 1987). There are also a small number of individuals who, although odd in behaviour, make good progress in childhood but undergo a severe regression in skills and behaviour in adolescence and, in adult life, are as severely handicapped as those who have been aloof and severely retarded since early childhood (Wing, unpublished data). The reasons for such a dramatic change are unknown.

Skills

In this group in adult life, all skills are at a low level. Some have simple self care but many need supervision in such tasks or cannot perform them at all. At best, understanding of speech is limited to simple instructions and use of speech to echolalia or a few spontaneous words. Although some were agile in childhood, the adults tend to be odd in posture and gait. The attractive facial appearance so characteristic of many of the children is marred in adult life by the lack of expression and odd grimaces.

During childhood, some of this group enjoy manipulating objects, making marks with pencils or paint and even using simple fitting and assembly toys. In adolescence these simple activities appear to lose their appeal, but are not replaced by more adult interests.

Behaviour

Although some of the group are quiet and amenable in behaviour, many have a range of behaviour problems like those familiar in the children, such as random aggression, destructiveness, aimless pacing or wandering and, most distressing of all, self injury. Unpleasant personal habits, such as smearing excreta, destroying sanitary protection, eating inedible objects picked up from the floor, are more obvious, socially unacceptable and physically harder to cope with in large adults than in small children. Immature manifestations of sexual behaviour, including masturbation in public, can occur and cause much anxiety to parents and care staff (Gillberg, 1984). Stereotypies and resistance to change continue in adult life.

There can be an exacerbation of behaviour problems and deterioration of acquired skills in adolescence that may continue into early adult life. Gillberg and Steffenburg (1987) estimated that about one half of a total population of autistic children developed these problems in adolescence. This was more likely to occur in those who were also mentally retarded. The impression gained from clinical experience in hospitals for adults with mental handicaps is that behavior problems become less marked with increasing age from the thirties onwards. However, some people can continue to be difficult to manage for a surprisingly long time, such as the 70 year old lady seen by the author who was aggressive towards the residents of an old people's home to which she was admitted in error and whose major interest was filling sinks with water and watching it overflow onto the floor while laughing with delight.

Psychiatric Complications

These are difficult, if not impossible, to diagnose in people with minimal or no communication. However, observation of changes in behaviour can indicate possible problems in this area. Increased withdrawal or apathy, loss of appetite, sleep disturbances and the appearance of distress may indicate a depressive illness. Much more common in the severely impaired group are wild swings of mood from manic excitement to intense misery. These may occur in phases of any length. In some, the swings from one extreme to another and back again can occur within a minute or so, without any obvious external cause. Catatonic phenomena can also be seen in young adults. Again, the clinical impression is that these psychiatric problems become less common with advancing age. There is no information available on the occurrence of the dementias of later life in autistic people. Diagnosis of such conditions would present considerable problems.

Services Needed

By the time of adult life, education and training for the severely handicapped group should be directed towards developing basic self care and simple domestic skills, such as helping to lay and clear the table for meals. Progress is likely to be limited and slow. Small successes are most likely in areas associated with experiences enjoyed by the person concerned, such as eating or outings.

Behaviour problems are best dealt with by providing a structured, organised and predictable daily routine with plenty of activities simple enough to be of interest. In the author's experience, the techniques of operant conditioning are of limited or no value, because severely impaired autistic people generally fail to make the necessary lasting connection between their own behaviour and its consequences, however precise the timing. The goals for this group have to be limited, since too much pressure is likely to lead to distress and difficult behavior. Treatment for the affective behaviour disturbances or for catatonic states, if they become severe, is at present unsatisfactory. Medication can be tried, but it is often ineffective and may even exacerbate the problems or produce unacceptable side effects.

The programme of activities should be geared to the level of the members of the group. The daily tasks of self care, that is toilet, washing, teeth cleaning, dressing and grooming and feeding, if the autistic person is encouraged to help, take up a fair amount of time, as do domestic tasks and shopping. Physical activities, such as walking, swimming, horse riding, even dancing and simple forms of physical education with music, are often a source of pleasure. There is also some evidence that physical exertion may lessen stereotypies and reduce the amount of difficult behaviour (Kerr et al, 1982; McGimsey & Favell, 1988; Walters & Walters, 1980). Diversions such as coach rides, picnics and outings to the seaside may also be appreciated. Some may be happy to do jig saw puzzles, finger painting, simple sewing and other sedentary tasks, but many get bored and restless if expected to concentrate on such things.

The skill of the staff who care for people in this group lies in their ability to plan and maintain an environment and programmes that provide appropriate stimulation, minimise behaviour problems and, above all, make life as enjoyable as possible for the autistic adults. It is a task that requires dedication, patience, tolerance, good humour and an empathic understanding of the impairments underlying autism.

Suitable day and residential centres are needed for this group. Some live at home with devoted parents, but most families find it difficult to continue giving the twenty-four hour care that is often required once their autistic child becomes an adult.

In the United Kingdom, most severely handicapped autistic adults are cared for in the services for people with severe mental retardation. Few are admitted to the small number of places in specialised sheltered communities run by the British National Autistic Society. The mixing with sociable mentally retarded people can cause many problems, especially if the autistic individuals have major behaviour problems. Where such placements work reasonably well, there is always a key staff member who is interested in autistic people and understands their needs.

It is still unusual for adults to have been diagnosed as autistic in childhood and the problem is recognised in adult life only if there is a professional person involved who has had relevant experience. There seems little likelihood that all autistic people, however severely handicapped, will ever be provided with a special separate service. But their situation would be much improved if information concerning autistic impairments and the special needs of autistic people were to be imparted to the staff of the mental retardation services during their training, and appropriate help given to autistic people within those services. Other groups among retarded people such as those with hearing or visual impairments or cerebral palsy also have special needs. An ideal service would provide for them all.

In the United Kingdom, it has been suggested that adult psychiatric services should provide treatment for all mentally handicapped people who have psychiatric illnesses. This policy has, up to now, proved inappropriate for most autistic people because of the present lack of knowledge concerning autism in those who work in adult psychiatry. It is impossible to apply in the case of the severely handicapped groups. Services for these adults have themselves to be able to cope with psychiatric complications and the associated disturbance of behaviour.

The Severely Aggressive Sub-Groups

Among severely impaired autistic adults there is a tiny minority who are extremely, even dangerously aggressive, sometimes self injuring as well as attacking others, who have not responded to behaviour management techniques, and who cause problems out of all proportion to their numbers. Those known to the author are adolescents, or adults in their twenties plus one or two in their thirties. It is often difficult to know what precipitates their attacks, which may be directed to their peers or to the staff.

On the whole, they are managed best by staff who are physically strong, calm in temperament and confident of their ability to cope. In the past, such autistic people have been cared for in special wards in institutions, the quality of care varying widely depending on the numbers of staff, their level of skill and experience and the numbers of other residents, small units tending to be better than those catering for large groups. In a few areas in the United Kingdom, individual adults with such problems have been placed as the only resident of small houses or apartments with their own staff, usually two or more carers being present at any time during the day or night. This removes the person away from other handicapped residents, but the degree of success in reducing the aggressive behaviour seems to be variable. The costs are high and the strain on the staff considerable. Careful evaluation of the advantages and disadvantages is needed in order to ascertain how appropriate is this solution for other highly aggressive adults. At the moment there is little certainty concerning the best way of managing such people.

THE GROUP THAT IMPROVE

Approximately one quarter of all autistic children improve significantly as they grow older, although they do not become independent as adults. Most, by the time of adult life, are passive, or active but odd in social interaction, though a few remain aloof except perhaps to parents and siblings. The majority are in the mildly retarded or even normal range of intelligence.

Skills

Understanding and, in most cases, use of language are usually at a level adequate for everyday purposes in adult life, as are self care, domestic and practical skills. Many but not all of this group have made progress in school work and can read, write or calculate. Some even choose to read books related to their particular interests. Most have the characteristic discrepancies in their profiles of skill and some have special islets of ability.

Behaviour

From school age onwards, this group tend to have fewer behaviour problems than those who are severely impaired, though some were equally disturbed in the pre-school years. In a proportion of cases there are difficulties in adolescence but the majority become calmer in adult life.

The major problems in this group, which tend to prevent them becoming more independent, are those arising from the repetitive, stereotyped activities, including rigid adherence to meaningless routines, boringly long winded, repetitive monologues on favourite subjects, peculiar, monotonous vocal intonation, odd facial grimaces and stereotyped movements which occur especially in excitement or distress. These may be overlooked in a child, but stand out in an adult and are potentially alarming to people who are unfamiliar with autism.

The social naivety and immaturity are also potential sources of difficulty outside the home, since inappropriate approaches to other people, especially members of the opposite sex, are not socially acceptable in adults. Manifestations of sexual behaviour require a cool, calm approach on the part of parents or staff and the teaching of rules of appropriate conduct firmly, but without anger or distress (Melone and Lettick, 1983).

Psychiatric Complications

Since this group tends to have more useful language than those who are more severely handicapped, psychiatric complications are easier to diagnose. It is not known what proportions are affected and at what ages, but such conditions can be observed in autistic adults (Gillberg, 1984). Anxiety states and depression are particularly common in clinical work in this field. The present author has seen a very few with manic episodes. Undifferentiated "psychotic" states with bizarre behaviour, rambling speech, strange ideas, perceptual disturbances and catatonic phenomena can occur, often in response to situations that the person concerned finds stressful. Such episodes tend to be short lived, especially if the source of stress can be removed, but occasionally they become chronic. The eventual prognosis is unknown. The present author has not seen any autistic person with typical adult schizophrenia.

Conditions closely resembling obsessional states can occur, usually as an exacerbation of a particular pattern of repetitive behaviour. In some cases, the obsessional thoughts or activities are so dominating that they paralyse all other action. It is sometimes difficult to disentangle what appears to be a combination of the autistic behaviour pattern, depressive lethargy, an obsessional state and catatonia. Treatment of such conditions is particularly difficult.

Services Needed

With the group under discussion, progress in social, domestic, practical and, in some cases, academic skills may continue into early and even middle adult life, so opportunities for learning are needed. Suitable occupation in a sheltered setting, or with an employer who is sympathetic and can provide an appropriate environment, is essential. The right kind of work utilises the skills of the person concerned but also makes allowances for his rigidity, repetitiveness, and the limited, concrete nature of his language and social comprehension.

Appropriate leisure activities are also important. For those living at home this may be the area of life that is most difficult to organise.

Day and residential provision can present problems for this group. Because of their peculiar combinations of skills, handicaps and social impairment they often do not fit into, nor benefit from, placement in centres for non-autistic adults with mental retardation, or those with psychiatric illnesses or physical handicaps. Some do settle in services for these other types of handicaps, usually because of the care and interest of some member of the staff, but others require specialised provision. In the United Kingdom, the National Autistic Society and various local societies have, at the time of writing, set up 17 small sheltered residential communities for autistic adults of all ages, and more are planned. These provide accommodation, occupation and leisure geared to the special needs of the residents.

These developments may appear to be against the trend for integration of handicapped people into the "normal" community. However, every opportunity is taken for the residents to take part in activities available to the local community, including opportunities for employment. This mixing occurs more often and more easily because the residents have a secure environment and an understanding staff to support them, and who can cope with any anxiety or behaviour disturbance that might arise. Such residential centres tend to attract the interest and help of local people who, in turn, enjoy the contact and learn more about autism.

THE GROUP WHO BECOME INDEPENDENT

Those who manage to live and work independently represent only around 5 to 10 per cent of the subjects who have been identified for inclusion in follow-up studies. The precise proportion of all those with developmental social impairment who become independent is currently impossible to estimate, because of an unknown number who have not been included in the published epidemiological studies.

Apart from the inherent likelihood that, in large scale studies, some eligible subjects, especially those with milder handicaps, must escape detection, there are two sources of evidence for doubting the completeness of past studies. First, is the clinical experience of those involved in the field of autism. Such workers are, from time to time, contacted by relatives of adults, who, although living and working independently and never diagnosed as handicapped, have always been odd in behaviour. These relatives make contact because they have read a paper or seen a television programme about autism and have recognised the similarity to the history and behaviour of the person about whom they are concerned. In a few cases, the autistic behaviour was marked in the early years, but rapid progress occurred around 5 to 6 years and continued ever since. The only remaining problem is a subtle lack of empathy. In other cases, many aspects of behaviour in adult life are still a cause for concern. In the present author's experience, numbers of such contacts have been increasing steadily as facts about autism become more widely known. Newson, Dawson and Everard (1982) found many of their subjects for their study of able autistic adults by inserting a description of autistic behaviour in national newspapers.

The second source of evidence is from a study by Tantam (1986). He obtained developmental histories of relatives of adults, some living independently, referred to psychiatric services for various reasons, whom the psychiatrists recognised as odd and eccentric in social interaction and behaviour. Some of these proved to have had the triad of impairments from early childhood, usually in the form described by Asperger (1944) and Wing (1981), although never diagnosed. Those not in this category had become markedly odd and socially withdrawn in adolescence and fitted descriptions of "schizoid personality disorders" (Kretschmer, 1925; Tantam, 1986; Wolff & Chick, 1980). Some of this second group presented similar features and management problems to those with developmental social impairment. The relationship between these groups is of interest for further research.

Types of Social Interaction

Among this group it is possible to find those with aloof, passive, or active but odd social interaction, with the aloof being by far the least frequent. There is also another style of social interaction that is seen in some of the most high functioning autistic adults. They appear polite, aware of other people and able to initiate and give and take in conversational exchanges. Nevertheless, to the careful observer, there is a stilted, even mechanical feel to their social behaviour as if they had learned the rules through intellectual effort rather than by instinct (Shah, 1988). An analogy is that of the speech of someone conversing in a foreign language they have learnt well, but through study as an adult rather than by long exposure to it as a young child.

Skills

Those who become independent are in the normal range of intelligence, at least in most areas of function. The most successful are those with special skills and interests that are useful for employment, and a strong desire to live as normal a life as possible. Temple Grandin, who utilized her visuo-spatial skills and interest in cattle handling systems to set up her own business, is one of the most remarkable examples of a successful autistic adult (Grandin and Scariano, 1986).

Behaviour

Independence in adult life is possible only for those who have never had or have outgrown the aggression, destructiveness and other major behaviour problems common in autistic children. Nevertheless, the subtle social and language impairments and the rigidity and repetitiveness of behaviour have their effects. The daily life of high functioning autistic adults tends to follow a set routine, disruptions to which can produce considerable anxiety and occasionally inappropriate, angry or confused responses. For example, one man who travelled to work by public transport was so cross when his usual bus was late that he hit the driver. In all other circumstances he was gentle and mild mannered.

Some who live by themselves become increasingly eccentric as the years go by. They may fill their rooms with an accumulation of junk, dress in a bizarre fashion and behave oddly in public. They may be known to the neighbourhood and regarded with pity or derision, but they usually refuse offers of help and resent interference.

In marked contrast to the obviously eccentric sub-group are those who are in regular employment and appear to lead a normal, conventional life, but whose behaviour pattern, especially at home, is a worry and a burden to their relatives. They are among those, mentioned earlier, who have never been diagnosed as autistic or handicapped and do not seek help for themselves, but whose relatives learn about autism by chance, recognise the connection, and then seek advice. In some cases the people concerned, mostly men, are married and have children. The behaviour that concerns the relatives, particularly the wives, is the egocentricity, the lack of empathy and emotional responsiveness, the inability to give emotional support to the family, the insistence on following routines that may be taken to absurd limits, and the childish rages if their daily pattern is upset in any way. Those who are married tend to be good financial providers but to be dependent on their wives to manage all the details of everyday life. The hardest thing for these wives is the knowledge that, if they ended the marriage, their husbands would not be able to cope without them.

Although some apparently independent autistic adults are difficult and strange in behaviour, this should not obscure the fact that others do gradually learn enough of the rules of social life to cope without being an impossible burden to others, and make their contribution to society through their special skills and through the open innocence of their interactions with everyone they meet, regardless of age, sex or social class.

Psychiatric Complications

The autistic adults with enough self awareness to wish to be "normal" are also aware that they differ from others. Odd behaviour, gait and posture attract attention and the occasional stare or rude comment. Some autistic people become hypersensitive and interpret any glance or remark as critical, even to a degree that could be described as paranoid. A few have been in trouble with the law because of aggressive responses to real or fancied insults.

Affective disorders are fairly common, especially in response to partial insight into the developmental abnormalities, or a desire for a friend or a partner of the opposite sex and repeated failure to find anyone to fill these roles.

As with the other autistic groups, unclassified "psychotic" states can occur in response to stress, with the features as previously described. Again, typical adult schizophrenia appears to be very rare and has never been seen by the present author.

Obsessional and catatonic states can also, rarely, occur.

It is very uncommon for this group to commit crimes in pursuit of their circumscribed interests, since those who become independent have to have a basis of social rules that they follow.

Psychiatric illnesses can interrupt the working career of high functioning autistic people at any stage. When seen by adult psychiatrists unfamiliar with autism, diagnosis is a problem, especially if no developmental history is available or requested.

Services Needed

By definition, the autistic adults who become independent do not need the day and residential services required by the other groups. One of the most important sources of help for the high functioning people is a concerned, supportive and understanding family. Even those who graduate to living alone still tend to need the tactful supervision, prompting to maintain proper self care, and all round emotional support provided by the mother or other relative. If there is no one in the family available to act in this capacity, some other person to take on the role of counsellor is needed, but not easy to find.

Success in employment is most likely if the work is appropriate to the person's skills and the employer is understanding, ensures that the autistic person is accepted by workmates, and values the positive qualities of the person concerned.

As for all autistic people, leisure can be a problem even if employment goes well. Many autistic people need guidance to find activities they do enjoy, such as joining clubs for the pursuit of their special interests. Groups of earnest train spotters, bird watchers, stamp collectors or chess players have provided life-lines for some autistic people who would otherwise have lived solitary lives.

The need for workers in adult psychiatry to recognise and understand autism in the presence of complicating psychiatric illness is of particular importance for the independent adults. They are the most likely to be referred to such services if they become ill, and are vulnerable to the prescription of inappropriate treatment and management.

THE FAMILIES OF AUTISTIC ADULTS

Problems occur at all stages in the lives of autistic people up to and throughout adult life. The types of difficulties and the needs change at different phases of the life cycle so parents and families have to adapt to a series of new challenges. The stress of caring never goes away (DeMyer and Goldberg, 1983; Bristol and Schopler, 1983). Even if the autistic person is in a residence away from home, the involved parents still retain an anxious concern for his or her welfare, because of the life-long vulnerability that is an inherent part of autism.

Parents and families need continuing advice and support from experienced and concerned professional workers. In the U.K., some families with autistic children receive such help, but it is rare to find this continued when the child becomes an adult. Because few of the older autistic adults have been diagnosed, their families are very unlikely to have had access to any source of information or counselling.

Whatever the age of the autistic person, parents gain comfort and support from meeting others with similar problems and some experience satisfaction from working together to set up services for autistic people. It is therefore important to tell parents of the existence of relevant voluntary associations so that they can choose to join if they wish.

CONCLUSION

Information concerning autistic adults is gradually increasing, but there are still large gaps in our knowledge. Studies of the epidemiology, changes in middle and later life, sex differences in outcome, physical and psychiatric complications and longevity are all needed. Such information is necessary for the development of services needed to care for those who remain dependent all their lives and to support and encourage those who have the ability and determination to become independent.

REFERENCES

Asperger, H. (1944). Die autistischen Psychopathen im Kindesalter. *Archiv für Psychiatrie und Nervenkrankheiten, 117,* 76-136.

DeMyer, M. K., Barton, S., DeMyer, W. E., Norton, J. A., Allen, J., & Steele, R. (1973). Prognosis in autism: a follow-up study. *Journal of Autism and Childhood Schizophrenia, 3,* 199-246.

Gillberg, C. (1983). Psychotic behaviour in children and young adults in a mental handicap hostel. *Acta Psychiatrica Scandinavica, 68,* 351-358.

Gillberg, C. (1984). Autistic children growing up: problems during puberty and adolescence. *Developmental Medicine and Child Neurology, 26,* 125-129.

Gillberg, C., & Steffenburg, S. (1987). Outcome and prognostic factors in infantile autism and similar conditions: a population based study of 46 cases followed through puberty. *Journal of Autism and Developmental Disorders, 17,* 273-287.

Grandin, T., & Scariano, M. M. (1986). *Emergence - Labelled Autistic.* Tunbridge Wells: Costello.

Kerr, L., Koegel, R. L., Dyer, K., Blew, P. A., & Fenton, L. R. (1982). The effects of physical exercise on self-stimulation and appropriate responding in autistic children. *Journal of Autism and Childhood Schizophrenia, 12,* 399-420.

Kanner, L. (1973). *Childhood Psychosis: Initial Studies and New Insights.* New York: Winston/Wiley.

Kretschmer, E. (1925). *Physique and Character.* London: Kegan Paul, Trench & Trubner.

Lotter, V. (1974). Factors related to outcome in autistic children. *Journal of Autism and Childhood Schizophrenia, 4,* 263-277.

Melone, M. B., & Lettick, A. L. (1983). Sex education at Benhaven. In E. Schopler & G. M. Mesibov (Eds.), *Autism in Adolescents and Adults.* New York: Plenum.

McGimsey, J. F., & Favell, J. E. (1988). The effects of increased physical exercise on disruptive behaviour in retarded persons. *Journal of Autism and Developmental Disorders, 18,* 167-180.

Newson, E., Dawson, M., & Everard, P. (1982). *The Natural History of Able Autistic People: Management and Functioning in a Social Context.* London: Report to the Department of Health and Social Security.

Rutter, M. (1970). Autistic children: infancy to adulthood. *Seminars in Psychiatry, 2,* 435-450.

Schopler, E., & Mesibov, G. (Eds.) (1983). *Autism in Adolescents and Adults.* New York: Plenum.

Shah, A. (1988). *Visuo-Spatial Islets of Abilities and Intellectual Functioning in Autism.* London: PhD Thesis (unpublished).

Shah, A., Holmes, N., & Wing, L. (1982). Prevalence of autism and related conditions in adults in a mental handicap hospital. *Applied Research in Mental Retardation, 3,* 303-317.

Tantam, D. (1986). *Eccentricity and Autism,* London: PhD Thesis (unpublished).

Watters, R. G., & Watters, W. E. (1980). Decreasing self-stimulatory behaviour with physical exercise in a group of autistic boys. *Journal of Autism and Developmental Disorders, 10,* 379-388.

Wing, L. (1988). The continuum of autistic characteristics. In E. Schopler & G. Mesibov (Eds.), *Diagnosis and Assessment in Autism.* New York: Plenum.

Wing, L., & Gould, J. (1979). Severe impairments of social interaction and associated abnormalities in children: epidemiology and classification. *Journal of Autism and Childhood Schizophrenia, 9,* 11-29.

Wolff, S., & Chick, J. (1980). Schizoid personality in childhood: a controlled follow-up study. *Psychological Medicine, 10,* 85-100.

Addendum: Is the Primary Lesion in Autism Related to the Locus Coeruleus?

ANNICA B. DAHLSTRÖM

In the autistic child a diversity of symptoms can be present, but some major common traits are obvious. One major sign of autism in childhood is the lack of a normal interest in people, things and events. Some children with autism even avoid actively to become at all involved with people or other aspects of the environment. They may dislike input from the surroundings, be it the loving touch of a parent, direct eye contact or other stimuli of any of their 5 senses.

Having worked in the field of neurobiology for more than 25 years, and having had the opportunity to participate in the first discovery and description of the major monoaminergic pathways in the CNS (Fuxe & Dahlström, 1964, 1965), what has struck me when listening to descriptions of the clinical findings in autism was "The locus coeruleus". This utterly important, although small, nucleus has been demonstrated to be the key center to deal with impulse input from our 5 senses, and to mediate information of such input of a variety of cortical regions in such a way as to initiate an optimal response of the organism to what is happening in the surroundings (cf. rev by Svensson, 1987).

Therefore I have been surprised that so little reference has been made to noradrenaline (NA), or to any of the major metabolites of NA, e. g. 3-methoxy-4-hydroxy-phenylethyleneglycol (MHPG) in the neuro-chemical studies of autism, be it on CNS tissue proper or on cerebrospinal fluid (CSF) chemistry. The other monoamines, dopamine (DA) and 5-hydroxytryptamine (5-HT) on the other hand have been discussed frequently.

The reasons why I would like to put forward the locus coeruleus (LC) as a key structure which may be impaired in the autistic syndromes are severalfold, and professor Gillberg has asked me to discuss these here.

1) The LC is a paired, small and rather compact nucleus, located in the floor of the 4th ventricle, rather close to the midline, under the cerebellar pedunculi. About 2 000 nerve cells in the rat LC are responsible for the absolute majority of noradrenergic nerve terminals in the forebrain, the hypothalamus, the hippocampus and all regions of the cerebral cortex as well as NA-ergic terminals in the spinal cord grey matter. In man the number is around 10 000. These nerve cells thus display an unusually wide-spread innervation pattern (cf. Loughlin et al., 1982; Aston-Jones et al., 1986). In fact it has been shown with the retrograde tracing technique that a single LC nerve cell can innervate at least 5 different, widely separated, areas like the cerebral cortex, hippocampus, hypothalamus, cerebellum and spinal cord (Loughlin et al., 1980; 1982). Other cells innervate "only" the spinal cord and hypothalamus. Groups of LC neurons have a topographical orientation within the LC (Mason & Fibiger, 1979; Loughlin et al., 1986). These investigations have been made mainly in the rat, but studies in the monkey indicate that in principle the same organization of the LC is found also in higher mammals (Foote et al., 1980; Felten & Sladek, 1982; Morrison et al., 1982).

Comment: Many authors now seem pessimistic as regards finding a special lesion which could explain all the diverse symptoms expressed by the patients with autism. Considering the projection pattern of the LC and of various areas with the LC, the LC could well be the locus which is lesioned, or malfunctioning, in one way or the other (there are a large number of possible mechanisms) in the child with autism.

The muscular dystonia found in many autistic children could also be related to the LC functions, since LC neurons innervate not only the motor cortex, but also the motoneurons in the spinal cord (Nygren & Olsson, 1977). Thus the anatomical basis for modulation of muscle tone by LC neurons is present.

2) In the adult animal the LC is of vital importance for dealing optimally with both enteroceptive and exteroceptive sensory input, for maintaining alertness during the day, and for allowing the animal to adjust himself properly to the environment i. e. for vigilance (cf. rev. by Svensson, 1987). Mild sensory stimulation evokes a typical electrical pattern in LC neurons, recorded with various neurophysiological recording techniques (Aston-Jones & Bloom, 1981; Aghajanian, 1978; Foote et al., 1980; Elam et al., 1986a, b). Merely touching an animal causes a burst of activities in LC neurons, which are then conveyed to the various brain areas innervated by the LC. Even arousal caused by e. g. smoking and nicotine passes via the LC from peripheral sensory input. It

has recently been demonstrated that, contrary to belief, nicotine arousal does not operate via stimulation of nicotinic acetylcholine receptors in cortical areas, but depends upon capsaicin-sensitive sensory neurons (Hajos, 1987). The LC is constantly active, more or less, except in one situation, and that is, during sleep. REM sleep is the only state in which LC neurons are actively suppressed to absolute silence. The mind is then purposely shut off from the environment.

Comment: One might conceptualize the LC as the key sensory mediator in the CNS. Could damage to LC (the whole nucleus or to subdivisions in it) explain the total inability of autistic patients to deal properly with the surrounding? Autistic children frequently have sleep disturbances. It is not known which phase of sleep is disturbed, however.

3) The LC is of particular importance during fetal life, as has been demonstrated in the rat. The NAergic fibres from the LC grow out very early during the prenatal development, and constitute the dominating neuronal elements in some layers of the developing cortex during a period when the cortex is still very immature (Schlumpf et al., 1980). For this reason it has been suggested that the noradrenergic nerve terminals in this region are "pioneer structures", which are involved in the development and maturation of the cerebral cortex. Support for this view has come from results of experiments in which the noradrenergic terminals in the cortex had been selectively lesioned by neurotoxins early in development. This led to altered morphology of the cortex, where pyramidal cells showed abberrant development of apical and/or basal dendritic trees (Felten et al., 1982). It is known that alcohol and opiates administered to the fetal brain, suppress the LC neurons. The mental retardation seen in some children of mothers with addictive problems could be related to the LC lesions (cf. Jonsson, 1985).

Comment: Children with autism are often diagnosed relatively early in life. The mother often notices that her child differs in behaviour to that of other children already during the first few days of life. Thus, the abnormality is likely to be present at birth and to be due to abnormal prenatal development of areas of the brain.

However, in a few cases autism has been reported to occur suddenly after a traumatic event in the child's life. For instance, one previously normal child was said to become autistic suddenly at age 2 years after having been accidentally severly burnt by boiling water. Keeping in mind the LC as the relay nucleus of sensory input might one not speculate that a sudden explosive shower of painful sensory stimuli could cause harm to the LC neurons exposed to such intensive stimulation? It has been shown that cutaneous noxious stimuli, especially of thermal character, strongly activate both central and peripheral NA systems (Elam et al., 1986a). If peripheral sensory neurons are eliminated by pretreatment with capsaicin this responsiveness of LC neurons to cutaneous thermal stimuli is markedly reduced (Hajos et al., 1986).

4) Many reward systems of the CNS operate via noradrenergic nerve terminals from the LC (cf. Engel, 1989). Intracranial self stimulation behaviour is elicited if electrodes are inserted in the locus coeruleus region (Crow et al., 1972) Also the voluntary ingestion of alcohol (Amit et al., 1977; Brown et al., 1977) or opiates (Brown et al., 1978) is suppressed if dopamine-ß-hydroxylase is inhibited and thereby NA synthesis blocked. Thus, if LC is damaged or operating abnormally, the ability of the individual to experience pleasure is decreased or missing.

Comment: In many autistic children, it appears that it is hard to elicit pleasure. Caresses, nursing, talking etc. can appear to cause unpleasentness, contrary to what is seen in normal children.

5) The LC is located in the floor of the 4th ventricle, under the cerebellum. In many cases computer tomography studies of children with autism have revealed slightly enlarged 4th ventricles and somewhat thinner pons regions. This is the area where the LC is located, and this may support the hypothesis that LC is involved. The total number of nerve cells here has been counted in a few postmortem studies of individuals with autism (Mary Coleman, personal communication) and found not to differ from normal cases. However, even if the number of nerve cells in normal, the dendritic tree of those cells may be abnormal, or organized in abberant patterns. Also, the axon ramifications of these cells may be inadequate, or may not have reached their target cells in the cortex properly. A very detailed morphological study of various parts of the brain stem and of cortical areas is warranted in autism to explore these possibilities. Golgi-like stains, demonstrating dendritic ramifications of individual neurons are particularly important.

6) "The fragile X-syndrome" includes traits of autism. Here medical intervention with amphetamine-like drugs has been beneficial in some cases (Randi Hagerman, personal commucination). Amphetamine exerts its action mainly by releasing newly synthesised transmitter from noradrenergic (and dopaminergic) nerve terminals. One might speculate that in this syndrome the LC could be functioning subnormally and that the nerve terminals in the untreated fragile X-patient release insufficient amounts of transmitter. By administering amphethamine more NA is released from the nerve endings, and this could provide an explanation for a possible therapeutic effect of this drug. Amphetamine has been tried in other patients with autism too, but usually without much success. The reason for this could be that in the severely autistic child there are no, or an insufficient number of, noradrenergic nerve endings from which the drug can release NA.

Suggestions for Future Research

1) When postmortem material is available, take particular care to investigate the LC neurons, count number of cell bodies and map the dendritic fields of these somata.

Study the distribution and chemical content of nerve terminals in many different cortical areas by immunocytochemical and biochemical techniques with the following questions in mind: Is the density and distribution of dopamine-beta-hydroxylase (DBH)-positive terminals normal in the various laminae of the cortex? Do the terminals contain normal contents of the NA-synthesising enzymes (tyrosine hydroxylase, dopa-decarboxylase, and DHB)? Has the area a normal content of NA.

Using radiolabelled receptor ligands for studying the presence of adrenergic receptors, the number and density of 1, a2, and ß-receptors post- and presynaptically warrant investigation.

2) In living patients the CSF should be investigated not only for DA and 5-HT and their metabolites, but in particular NA and NA-metabolites should be studied.

Computerized tomography investigations should focus on the LC-region. Perhaps MRI-studies could provide more detail of the region of the floor of the 4th ventricle. PET-scans will be possible to perform with new labels for the noradrenergic system.

3) Neurophysiology studies: Evoked potentials, stimulating peripheral sensory fields and recording from various cortical areas might yield information on LC-functions.

4) The sleep pattern of autistic children should be studied in detail. Such studies could give further important information of the pattern of REM sleep and give information on possible involvement of the LC.

Finally, I would like to point out that the above has been written in a hurry, by someone who, despite being rather familiar with basic neurobiological phenomena, lacks clinical experience of the autistic child. I apologize if sometimes the statements made above sound blunt; space and time simply have not allowed more detailed discussion. However, I have tried to collect a number of useful references, and refer the reader to these for a more in-depth discussion on the role of the LC in the experimental animal, and possibly also in the human mind.

REFERENCES

Amit, Z., Brown, Z. W., Levitan, D. E., & Ögren, S. O. (1977). Noradrenergic mediation of the positive properties of ethanol: I. Suppression of ethanol consumption in laboratory rats following dopamine-beta-hydroxylase inhibition. *Archives internationale de Pharmacodynamie et de Thérapie, 230,* 65 - 75.

Aston-Jones, G. (1985). Behaviour functions of the locus coeruleus derived form cellular attributes. *Physiological Psychology, 13,* 118 - 126.

Aston-Jones, G., Enni, M., Pieribone, V. A., Nickell, W. T., & Shipley, M. T. (1986). The brain nucleus coeruleus: Restricted afferent control of a broad efferent network. *Science, 234,* 734 - 737.

Brown, Z. W., Amit, Z., Levitan, D. E., Ögren, S. O., & Sutherland, E. A. (1977). Noradrenergic mediation of the positive reinforcing properties of ethanol: II. Extinctions of ethanol-drinking behavior in laboratory rats by inhibition of dopamine-beta-hydroxylase. Implications for treatment procedures in human alcoholics. *Archives internationale de Pharmacodynamie et de Thérapie, 230,* 76 - 82.

Brown, Z. E., Amit, Z., Sinoyr, D., Rockman, G. E., & Ögren, S. O. (1978). Suppression of voluntary ingestion of morphine by inhibition of dopamine-beta-hydroxylase. *Archives internationale de Pharmacodynamie et de Thérapie, 232,* 102 - 110.

Crow, T. J., Spear, P. J., & Arbuthnott, G. W. (1972). Intracranial self-stimulation with electrodes in the region of locus coeruleus. *Brain Research, 26,* 275 - 287.

Elam, M., Svensson, T. H., & Thorén, P. (1986a). Locus coeruleus neurons and sympathetic nerves: activation by cutaneous sensory afferents. *Brain Research, 358,* 77 - 84.

Elam, M., Svensson, T. H., & Thorén, P. (1986b). Locus coeruleus neurons and symphathetic nerves: activation by visceral afferents. *Brain Research, 375,* 117 - 125.

Engel, J. (1989). Personal communication.

Felten, D. L., Hallman, H., & Jonsson, G. (1982). Evidence for a neurotrophic role of noradrenaline neurons for the postnatal development of rat cerebral cortex. *Journal of Neurocytology, 11,* 119 - 135.

Felten, D. L., & Sladek, J. R. (1983). Monoamine distribution in primate brain. V. Monominergic nuclei: Anatomy Pathways, and local organization. *Brain Research Bulletin, 11,* 171 - 284.

Foote, S. L., Aston-Jones, G., & Bloom, F. E. (1980). *Impulse activity of locus coeruleus neurons in awake rats and monkeys is a function of sensory stimulation and arousal.* Proceedings of the National Academy of Sciences of the United States of America, 77, 3033 - 3037.

Foote, S. L., & Bloom, F. E. (1979). Activity of locus coeruleus in the unanesthezised squirrel monkey. In E. Usdin, I. J. Kopin & J. Barchas (Eds.), *Catecholamines: basic and clinical frontiers, vol 1. Proceedings of the 4th Int Catecholamine Symposium* (pp 625 - 628). New York: Pergamon.

Foote, S. L., & Bloom, F. E., & Aston-Jones, G. (1983). Nucleus locus coeruleus: new evidence of anatomical and physiological specificity. *Physiological Review, 63,* 844 - 914.

Foote, S. L., Freedman, R., & Oliver, A. P. (1975). Effects of putative neurotransmitters on neuronal activity in monkey auditory cortex. *Brain Research, 86*, 229 - 242.

Fuxe, K., Dahlström, A. (1964). Evidence for the existence of monoamine containing neurons in the central nervous system. I. Demonstration of the monoamins in the cellbodies of nervcells in the brain stem. *Acta Physiologica Scandinavica, 62, suppl, 232.*

Fuxe, K., Dahlström, A. (1965). Evidence for the existence of monoamine containing neurons in the central nervous system. II. Experimentally induced changes in the intraneuronal aminolevels. *Acta Physiologica Scandinavica, 64, suppl 247.*

Hajos, M. (1987). *Capsaicin and brain monoaminergic mechanisms: Neuropharmacological and thermoregulatory aspects.* University of Göteborg, Thesis.

Jonsson, G. (1985). Hjärnan - en "dator" med plastiska egenskaper. (The brain - a "computer" with plasticity). *Läkartidningen 82,* 3178 - 3180 (Summary in English).

Kitahama, K. L., Denoroy, N., Goldstein, M., Jouvet, M., & Pearson, J. (1988). Immunohistochemistry of tyrosine hydroxylase and phenylethanolamine-N-methyltransferase in the human brain stem: description of adrenergic perikarya and characterization of longitudinal catecholaminergic pathways. *Neuroscience, 25,* 97 - 111.

Loughlin, S. E., Foote, S. L., & Fallon, J. H. (1982). Locus coeruleus projections to cortex: topography, morphology and collateralization. *Brain Research Bulletin, 9,* 287 - 294.

Loughlin, S. E., Foote, S. L., & Grzanna, R. (1986). Efferent projections of nucleus locus coeruleus: Morphologic subpopulations have different efferent targets. *Neuroscience: 18,* 307 - 319.

Molliver, M. E., Grzanna, R., Lidov, H. G. W., Morrison, J. H., & Olschowka, J. A. (1982). In *Cytochemical methods in Neuroanatomy* (pp 255 - 277). New York: Alan R Liss Inc.

Morrison, J. H., Foote, S. L., O'Connor, D., & Bloom, F. (1982). Laminar, tangenital and regional organization of noradrenergic innervation of the monkey cortex: Dopamine-ß-hydroxylase immunohistochemistry. *Brain Research Bulletin, 9,* 309 - 319.

Nygren, L. G., & Olsson, L. (1977). A new major projection from locus coeruleus: The main source of noradrenergic nerve terminals in the ventral and dorsal columns of the spinal cord. *Brain Research, 132,* 85 - 93.

Ponzio, F., Hallman, H., & Jonsson, G. (1981). Noradrenaline and dopamine interaction in rat brain during development. *Medical Biology, 59,* 161 - 169.

Svensson, T. H. (1987). Peripheral, autonomic regulation of locus coeruleus noradrenergic neurons in brain: putative implications for psychiatry and psychopharmacology (Review). *Psychopharmacology, 92,* 1 - 7.

Autism: Diagnosis and Treatment. The State of the Art, May 1989

LENA ANDERSSON, MICHAEL BOHMAN, MAGDA CAMPBELL, MARY COLEMAN, UTA FRITH, CHRISTOPHER GILLBERG, RANDI HAGERMAN, DEMETRIOUS HARACOPOS, PATRICIA HOWLIN, MARGARET LANSING, GILBERT LELORD, IVAR LOVAAS, HENRIK PELLING, AUDRIUS PLIOPLYS, BORGNY RUSTEN, ERIC SCHOPLER, SHEILA SPENSLEY, SUZANNE STEFFENBURG, LUKE TSAI, LYNN WATERHOUSE, and LORNA WING.

Autism (infantile autism, childhood autism, autistic syndrome, autistic disorder) which almost always has its onset before 36 months of age is a behaviourally defined syndrome of neurological impairments associated with multiple medical conditions. Pathophysiology and behavioural dynamics in this spectrum of disorders are not yet fully understood. The spectrum is developmental and is manifested early in childhood by impairments in social relatedness, communication and imagination. These impairments vary in degree and also in form over time. They constitute severe biological handicapping conditions in the child which can lead to deleterious secondary effects on the family and other close persons. The behaviour pattern seen in autism may or may not be associated with other disabilities/disorders, such as mental retardation, epilepsy, dysphasia, and hearing and visual deficits. Social deficits vary from severe to mild. If the child has severe social deficits, diagnosis is more likely to be made in the first few years of life. In cases with milder social deficits, diagnosis may be postponed for many years. Cognitive deficits too vary from profound mental retardation to normal and - in exceptional cases - high IQ. "High - level" autism and so called Asperger syndrome now appear to be clearly overlapping clinical entities.

The clinical picture may change appreciably with age and regular reassessments should be made to ensure that the child continues to receive the most appropriate kind of intervention. Many children become more communicative and are able to relate to others, albeit in a limited fashion. However, long-term problems nearly always persist in the areas of communication, social adjustment and work.

There is no known cure for autism. A small proportion do well in adult life seemingly regardless of intervention. Habilitation and treatment have to be tailored to the needs of the individual child depending on his/her underlying medical condition, language development, IQ, family conditions and personality. A correct early diagnosis and medical work-up is essential in all cases. Possible underlying causes range from PKU and rubella embryopathy to tuberous sclerosis and the fragile X syndrome. Information to the family and treatment strategies for the child have to take such diagnoses - and additional handicaps, such as epilepsy - into account. The family should be involved in the habilitation of the child from the start.

Any treatment plan must include educational and behavioural approaches. Some children are given medication because of extreme behaviour problems. There can be no "30 minutes a day exclusively" treatment for children with autism. A multidisciplinary integration of approaches in which parents and siblings are actively involved is called for in most cases. A high degree of structure, a calm environment and continuity as regards time, place and persons are all essential elements in the habilitation programme.

Multidisciplinary teams specializing in autism must be available for diagnosis and follow-up. A long-term perspective (usually lifelong) must be taken from the start. A variety of "integrated" and "separated" services must be provided for people with autism in the preschool age period, during the school years, in adolescence, and throughout adult life.

Göteborg, Sweden

May 10, 1989

Contributors

LENA ANDERSSON, RFPB, Stockholm, Sweden

CATHERINE BARTHELEMY, Centre Hospitalier Regionale et Universaire de Tours, Hôpital Bretonneau, Tours Cedex, France

INGA LILL BOHMAN, Department of Child and Adolescent Psychiatry, University of Umeå, Umeå, Sweden

MICHAEL BOHMAN, Department of Child and Adolescent Psychiatry, University of Umeå, Umeå, Sweden

KATHERINE CALOURI, Department of Psychology, University of California, Los Angeles, California, U S A

MAGDA CAMPBELL, Department of Psychiatry, NYU Medical Center, New York, New York, U S A

WALTER P. CHRISTIAN, The May Institute Inc., Chatham, Massachusetts, U S A

MARY COLEMAN, 450 East Heather Lane, Lake Forest, Illinois, U S A

ANNICA B. DAHLSTRÖM, Department of Histology, University of Göteborg, Göteborg, Sweden

DEBORAH FEIN, Trenton State College, Child Behavior Study, Trenton, New Jersey, U S A

UTA FRITH, MRC Cognitive Development Unit, London, England

CHRISTOPHER GILLBERG, Department of Child and Adolescent Psychiatry, University of Göteborg, Göteborg, Sweden

RANDI J. HAGERMAN, The Child Development Unit, The Childrens Hospital, Denver, Colorado, U S A

LAURENCE HAMEURY, Centre Hospitalier Regionale et Universaire de Tours, Hôpital Bretonneau, Tours Cedex, France

DEMETRIOUS HARACOPOS, Sofieskolen, Copenhagen, Denmark

PATRICIA HOWLIN, The Maudsley Hospital, Institute of Psychiatry, Children's Department, London, England

JACQUELINE JADA, Department of Psychology, University of California, Los Angeles, California, U S A

MARGARET D. LANSING, University of North Carolina at Chapel Hill, Chapel Hill, North Carolina, U S A

GILBERT LELORD, Centre Hospitalier Regionale et Universaire de Tours, Hôpital Bretonneau, Tours Cedex, France

IVAR LOVAAS, Department of Psychology, University of California, Los Angeles, California, U S A

STEPHEN C. LUCE, The May Institute Inc., Chatham, Massachusetts, U S A

RICHARD P. MALONE, Department of Psychiatry, NYU Medical Center, New York, New York, U S A

HENRIK PELLING, Department of Child and Adolescent Psychiatry, Akademiska Hospital, Uppsala, Sweden

RICHARD PERRY, Department of Psychiatry, NYU Medical Center, New York, New York, U S A

AUDRIUS V. PLIOPLYS, Division of Neurology, The Hospital for Sick Children and Surrey Place Center 2, Surrey Place, Toronto, Ontario, Canada

BORGNY RUSTEN, Ramstadsåsvägen 13, Hovik, Norway

HELEN SCHAUMANN, Department of Child and Adolescent Psychiatry, University of Göteborg, Göteborg, Sweden

ERIC SCHOPLER, Division TEACCH, 310 Medical School Wing E, University of North Carolina at Chapel Hill, Chapel Hill, North Carolina, U S A

EVA SJÖHOLM - LIF, Department of Child and Adolescent Psychiatry, University of Umeå, Umeå, Sweden

SHEILA SPENSLEY, 96 Laurel Way, Totteridge, London, England

SUZANNE STEFFENBURG, Department of Child and Adolescent Psychiatry, University of Göteborg, Göteborg, Sweden

LUKE Y. TSAI, Division of Child and Adolescent Psychiatry Service, University of Michigan, Ann Arbor, Michigan, U S A

LYNN WATERHOUSE, Trenton State College, Child Behavior Study, Hillwood Lakes, Trenton, New Jersey, U S A

LORNA WING, MRC Social Psychiatry Unit, Institute of Psychiatry, De Crespigny Park, Denmark Hill, London, England

PAMELA YATES, The Maudsley Hospital, Children's Department, Institute of Psychiatry, Denmark Hill, London, England

Index